D1823424

Internet of Things

Technology, Communications and Computing

Series Editors

Giancarlo Fortino, Rende (CS), Italy
Antonio Liotta, Edinburgh, UK

The series Internet of Things - Technologies, Communications and Computing publishes new developments and advances in the various areas of the different facets of the Internet of Things. The intent is to cover technology (smart devices, wireless sensors, systems), communications (networks and protocols) and computing (theory, middleware and applications) of the Internet of Things, as embedded in the fields of engineering, computer science, life sciences, as well as the methodologies behind them. The series contains monographs, lecture notes and edited volumes in the Internet of Things research and development area, spanning the areas of wireless sensor networks, autonomic networking, network protocol, agent-based computing, artificial intelligence, self organizing systems, multi-sensor data fusion, smart objects, and hybrid intelligent systems.

Internet of Things is covered by Scopus.

More information about this series at http://www.springer.com/series/11636

Chinmay Chakraborty • Uttam Ghosh
Vinayakumar Ravi • Yogesh Shelke
Editors

Efficient Data Handling for Massive Internet of Medical Things

Healthcare Data Analytics

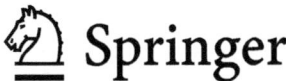
Springer

Editors
Chinmay Chakraborty
Electronics and Communication
Birla Institute of Technology, Mesra
Deoghar, Jharkhand, India

Vinayakumar Ravi
Division of Biomedical Informatics
Cincinnati Children's Hospital
Medical Center
Cincinnati, OH, USA

Uttam Ghosh
Vanderbilt University
Nashville, TN, USA

Yogesh Shelke
Aranca Technology Research & Advisory
Mumbai, Maharashtra, India

ISSN 2199-1073 ISSN 2199-1081 (electronic)
Internet of Things
ISBN 978-3-030-66635-4 ISBN 978-3-030-66633-0 (eBook)
https://doi.org/10.1007/978-3-030-66633-0

This Springer imprint is published by the registered company Springer Nature Switzerland AG
The registered company address is: Gewerbestrasse 11, 6330 Cham, Switzerland

Contents

Introduction

Background

This book would focus on recent advances and different research areas in multimodal data fusion under the healthcare informatics and would also seek out theoretical, methodological, well-established, and validated empirical work dealing with these different topics. It aims at bringing together the latest industrial and academic progress, research, and development efforts within the rapidly maturing health informatics ecosystem. It also highlights various technologies and concerns regarding energy-aware and secure sensors and how they can reduce energy consumption. It also discusses the life cycle of sensor devices and protocols with the help of energy-aware design, production, and utilization, as well as Internet of Things (IoT) technologies such as tags, sensors, sensing networks, and internet technologies. In a nutshell, this book will give a comprehensive overview of the state-of-the-art theories and techniques for massive data handling and access in medical data and Smart health in IoT, and provide useful guidelines for the design of the massive Internet of Medical Things (IoMT).

In the past decades, the number of deployments for sensor networks grew drastically. The health monitoring and diagnosis for the target structure of interest are achieved through the interpretation of collected data. The rapid advances in sensor technologies and data acquisition tools have led to the new era of Big Data, where massive heterogeneous data are collected by different sensors. The enhancing accessibility of the data resources gives new scopes for health monitoring, while the data aggregated from multiple sensors to make strong decisions remains a challenging problem. Challenges for data fusion in health monitoring will be the focus through these quality chapters. Fusion is a multi-domain developing field; it is mainly categorized as contextual information, observational data, and learned knowledge. Data fusion systems provide dynamically changing situations by integrating sensors outcome, knowledge bases, databases, user mission, and contextual information. Sensor technologies become more demandable in healthcare for development, testing, and trials, intending to be a part of both hospitals and homes.

This book will also offer valuable perceptions to researchers and engineers on how to design sensor systems and how to improve patient's information delivery care remotely. The end-to-end clinical data connectivity involves the development of many technologies that should enable reliable and location-agnostic communication between a patient and a healthcare provider. However, the main challenge in sensors is how to manage concerning critical applications, where several connected devices generate a large amount of medical data. This large volume of data, often called big data, cannot readily be processed by traditional data processing algorithms and applications. By intelligently investigating and collecting large amounts of healthcare data (i.e., big data), the sensor can enhance the decision-making process and early disease diagnosis. Hence, there is a need for scalable machine learning and intelligent algorithms that lead to more interoperable solutions and that can make effective decisions in emerging sensor technologies. Nevertheless, their rapid and widespread deployment, along with their participation in the provisioning of potentially critical healthcare services raises numerous issues related to the data acquisition and data analysis of the performed operations and provides services.

Recent developments in sensor technology, wearable computing, the Internet of Things, and wireless communication have given rise to research in ubiquitous healthcare and remote monitoring of human health and activities. Health monitoring systems involve processing and analysis of data retrieved from smartphones, smartwatches, smart bracelets, and various sensors and wearable devices. Such systems enable continuous monitoring of patients' psychological and health conditions by sensing and transmitting measurements such as heart rate, electrocardiogram, body temperature, respiratory rate, chest sounds, or blood pressure. Pervasive healthcare, as a relevant application domain in this context, aims at revolutionizing the delivery of medical services through a medical assistive environment and facilitates the independent living of patients. The optimization algorithms can be applied because of acquiring the sensor data from multiple sources for fast and accurate health monitoring.

In this book, we discuss

- Data collection, fusion, ownership, and privacy issues.
- Models, concepts, technologies, and solutions for data-driven or evidence-based healthcare data processing and analytics.
- Effective display (AR/VR, data visualization, and mixed reality).
- Recent trends of emerging technologies and robust systems.
- Examples of case studies and practical solutions.

This book aims at addressing these topics across multiple abstraction levels, ranging from architectural models, the provisioning of services, protocols, and interfaces to specific implementation approaches. Furthermore, additional focus will be given to areas related to the role of data mining and machine learning in modeling and deploying secure and trustworthy sensor networks IoMT systems.

Book Organisation

The book is structured well using an efficient healthcare data analytics perspective. This book consists of 15 excellent chapters in the field of the Internet of Medical Things technology, and a brief summary of each is presented here.

An Overview of the Internet of Medical Things and Its Modern Perspective

This chapter aims to provide an updated overview of the Internet of Medical Things (IoMT), addressing its evolution and branch of application potential, showing and approaching its success relationship, with a concise bibliographic background, synthesizing the potential of technology. IoMT allows more refined monitoring of the patient in real time and it is possible to issue alerts and inform health professionals more easily, even before the situation becomes more critical for the patient. One of the greatest advantages of IoMT among many others is access, by health professionals, concerning data consistent with the patient's reality, as the lack of information about the patient is a common and serious problem.

Big Medical Data Analytics Under Internet of Things

This chapter is aimed to provide researchers a review of recent advances in Internet of Things (IoT)-based medical Big Data analytics. It presents the sources of Big Data in health care, its tools and platforms, and its significance in health care. It also discusses the challenges of BDA and recent advances in IoT-based Dig Data. Big Data is the massive amount of data sets of structured and unstructured data that are complex. The massive data analytics of the health care system are crucial owing to the large amount of data observed in the health care sector such as medical imaging data, clinical notes, and patient data collected from the large number of patients using various sensors, including heartbeat rate sensors. So, extraction of valuable data and discarding useless information is a significant process.

Big Medical Data Analytics Using Sensor Technology

This chapter discusses the top-level view of many wearable gadgets of various sorts which have been established in clinical and domestic atmospheres as being useful in the standard of health improvement of adults. The current advancement in microchip technology devices and microelectronics techniques permit the improvement of low-value gadgets which can be extensively utilized by human beings as tracking equipment for well-being or precautionary resolutions. Sensors are utilized in electronics, clinical, and non-clinical systems and convert diverse types of important symptoms into electric indications. Sensors may be used for life-helping transplants, protective events, long-time period tracking of disabled or unwell persons.

Smart Healthcare Technologies for Massive Internet of Medical Things

Machine learning and deep learning allow auto-diagnosis of disease and detect the disease at an earlier stage in a systematic way from the acquired dataset from the patient. A smart health care system is required to handle the large volume of data produced by the Massive Internet of Medical Things. Smart healthcare systems use information and communication technology of IoT, data analytic, machine learning, deep learning, augmented reality, and cloud technologies to realize efficient, personalized, convenient health care systems. Augmented Reality (AR) helps surgeons to diagnose the disease accurately, perform surgery precisely with the help of quick real-time data of the patient. mHealth system utilizes mobile applications to easily reach the community of patients to provide health care services.

Sensor Informatics of IoT, AR/VR, and MR in Healthcare Applications

In this chapter, the essential informatics of various sensors used in distinct applications based on emerging technology such as IoT, AR/VR, and Mixed Reality (MR) in healthcare applications are conferred. With the day-to-day advancements in manufacturing and optimization technology, sensors are becoming a powerful supporting device in every field which gives ease in the collection of data. The collection of information is done with the help of sensors like MEMS sensors, position tracking sensors, etc., for the respective network technology from the real world at various locations in a distributed physical environment. Apart from the advancement in technologies, there is a trade-off between data collection and data handling. Big Data analytics itself is an extreme part of these emerging technologies since all these advancements are based on data.

Body Sensor Networks as Emerging Trends of Technology in Health Care System: Challenges and Future

This chapter aims to present a comprehensive overview of Big Data, digitization of health records, improved patient care, electronic medical records, and telemedicine. It describes key challenges of technology in public health as technological progress does not guarantee equitable health outcomes. The authors focus on the future of developed technologies in the healthcare sector due to lower costs, increase efficiency, and, most importantly, improve quality of care, which will help the readers to effectively use the information for their research endeavors.

Smart Sensor Technologies for the Healthcare System

The chapter begins with a summary of IoT smart sensors. It elaborates on the walk-on part of IoT in healthcare, several sensors, and smart gadgets used in healthcare, fitness, and well-being care units. Expeditious growth in semiconductor, computing, and transmission technologies have contributed to the innovative production of sensors otherwise known as "smart" sensors, which have the potential for far-flung wireless communication, information exchange between themselves, and computerized data processing. The emergence of microsensors amalgamated with intelligent sensor framework technology permits a forefront production of sensor framework escorted by remarkably inflated proficiencies, and very little size, weight, and energy usage.

Cloud and IoMT-Based Big Data Analytics System During COVID-19 Pandemic

This chapter presents the COVID-19 biomedical data analytics using cloud-based IoMT. The data gathered from diverse wearable sensors like body temperature, glucose, heartbeat, and ECG sensors were conveyed via IoMT gadgets to the integrated cloud with the data analytics layer. The cloud database HadoopMapReduce methods can be used to process the vast amounts of data collected during COVID-19 monitoring and surveillance in parallel. For speedy tracking, evaluation, decision-making, and improved care approvals from doctors via IoMT devices to the advanced cloud and data analytics layer, data are gathered from diverse wearable sensors.

Remote Human Health and Activities Monitoring Using Wearable Sensor-Based Systems: A Review

Work in this chapter critically appraises recent research in wearable systems by assessing the functionality and performance of sensor devices. The objective is integrating the inputs from different sensors and to study the shortcomings of the integration. The potential improvement of wearable sensor systems will modernize future healthcare systems. This chapter focuses on the current research on wearable sensors for various diseases like diabetes, heart diseases, and Alzheimer's. Data collected from sensors can be viewed by patients, and it is also stored in the cloud and retrieved at the hospitals for continuous assessment of patient's health by the doctors.

A Healthcare Resource Management Optimization Framework for ECG Biomedical Sensors

In this chapter, three levels of processing are provided: edge, fog, and cloud. In this multi-agent systems play the main role to connect all processing levels. A deployment scenario of a smart home has been explained and the expected result is shown. A Healthcare Resource Management Optimization framework is proposed to mitigate the issue. Fog computing as an intermediate layer has been implemented to overcome the limitation of cloud computing. The main duty of fog computing in this work is to process healthcare-critical tasks by fog nodes through the implementation of multi-agent systems.

Diabetes Detection and Sensor-Based Continuous Glucose Monitoring: A Deep Learning Approach

In this chapter, all the different deep learning algorithms used for noninvasive computer-aided diabetes diagnosis, making use of HRV input, are briefly discussed. Hybrid deep learning network and the deployment of very large-sized input datasets for training these networks can further better the efficacy of abnormality detection. The process of continuous glucose monitoring and the development of sensors and analysis of the collected data from sensors are hot topics of the research presented. Continuous glucose monitoring sensors are portable devices that allow measurement of blood glucose concentration in real-time almost continuously for several days.

"Sensing the Mind": An Exploratory Study About Sensors Used in E-Health and M-Health Applications for Diagnosis of Mental Health Condition

This chapter is divided into three main sections: Firstly, a basic understanding of depression and its types are given, then a literature survey to identify the gap between current scenario and the future roadmap. The third segment discusses different sensor devices used in this area. This chapter has performed an exploratory study over several research papers working in this area and the basic trends have been identified. This chapter covers the aspect of different sensors and IoT devices that are being used for the detection of mental health problems from words, expressions, and body language.

Role of Sensors, Devices, and Technology for the Detection of the COVID-19 Virus

This chapter presents a review of the key biological properties of SARS-CoV2 utilized to evolve facile, sensitive, and robust detection techniques for COVID-19. The scope of the review includes the existing diagnostic techniques with their details from classical biological techniques like RT–PCR to most recent techniques involving novel biosensors, electronics tools, artificial intelligence, machine learning, and IoT. The review elaborates on key methods that can be employed in the future for better managing the COVID-19 outbreak, thereby guarding against future pandemics.

Implementation of Internet of Medical Things (IoMT): Clinical and Policy Implications

This chapter explores the impact of IoMT on the key stakeholders, patients, physicians, providers, payors, government, and regulators, and touches on some of the best practices from across the world. Recent advances in computing, data storage, and sensors match up to the rate of increase in medical research, venture capital, and private equity investments in healthcare.

Applicability of Blockchain Technology in Healthcare Industry: Applications, Challenges, and Solutions

The chapter highlights the need and applicability of blockchain technology in healthcare applications. It outlines several unresolved challenges that can pave way for future research directions in this field. The authors explore the applicability of blockchain technology in the healthcare sector and present various applications, advantages, challenges, and future research strategies of blockchain technology in the healthcare industry.

Big Medical Data Analytic Using Sensor Technology

This chapter offers a top-level view of many wearable gadgets of various sorts which have been established in clinical and domestic atmospheres as being useful in the standard of health improvement of adults. Remote healthcare is primarily constructed on epidemic sensors and device and present-day conversation and records technology gives green answers that lets in human beings to stay of their comfortable domestic environment, is by hook or by crook protected. Healthcare groups like coverage agencies want real-time, reliable, and correct diagnostic outcomes supplied by way of sensor structures that may be observed remotely, whether or not the affected person is in a clinic, hospital, or at home.

Mesra, Jharkhand, India   Chinmay Chakraborty

Chapter 1
An Overview of the Internet of Medical Things and Its Modern Perspective

Reinaldo Padilha França, Ana Carolina Borges Monteiro, Rangel Arthur, and Yuzo Iano

1.1 Introduction

It is undeniable that one of the best technological developments that are seen in a new era is found in the area of health. New forms of treatment, medication control, patient monitoring, equipment, and much more are just some of the applications available with the medical Internet of Things, which promises to make work in hospitals and clinics much more dynamic and efficient [1, 2].

The assimilation of the Internet of Things by the health sector in all content converges toward a single certainty: the fact that the connection between different devices and the Internet only tends to contribute to the advancement of the medical segment [2–4].

Representing the connection between the physical world and the constant transmission of virtual data, the Internet of Things (IoT) allows all objects to be connected through the internet [5–7]. When it comes to medical devices, technology is commonly called the Internet of Medical Things (IoMT) [1–7].

The health area has always been a niche where the most advanced technological developments were sought, precisely because it has a focus on human well-being. In this sense, an immense evolution in the equipment is available in the medical area, since different technological aspects started to be implemented, such as connectivity technology, in these environments [2–9].

The medical Internet of Things has already been transforming the way patients are kept safe and healthy, considering the great increase in the demand for low-cost

R. P. França (✉) · A. C. B. Monteiro · R. Arthur · Y. Iano
School of Electrical and Computer Engineering (FEEC),
University of Campinas – UNICAMP, Campinas, SP, Brazil
e-mail: padilha@decom.fee.unicamp.br; monteiro@decom.fee.unicamp.br;
rangel@ft.unicamp.br; yuzo@decom.fee.unicamp.br

© The Author(s), under exclusive license to Springer Nature Switzerland AG 2021
C. Chakraborty et al. (eds.), *Efficient Data Handling for Massive Internet of Medical Things*, Internet of Things,
https://doi.org/10.1007/978-3-030-66633-0_1

solutions for hospitals and clinics, and IoMT has precisely met this demand with a technology that still optimizes the service, which makes the job of doctors much easier [2–9].

The various connectivity and traceability technologies being implemented in the Internet of medical things opened new doors to invest in this medium differently, aiming at the effectiveness of new technologies for the treatment of illnesses, management, and observation of patients at long distance and a lot more [2–9].

Monitoring, for example, is one of the most positive aspects of the Internet of Medical Things. With this technology, it is possible to notify and inform professionals more easily and even directly activate service providers with the capacity to identify the problem, before the situation becomes much more critical, thus preventing the loss of life with this technology [4–11].

Much more than a data connection, the Internet of Medical Things is the perfect integration between indispensable information from the patient's reality and the availability of data for consultation with doctors. Through this technology, medicine can benefit from greater agility in the verification of hospital conditions and even the early preparation for possible failures of both patients and medical equipment [4–11].

This chapter is motivated to provide a scientific major contribution related to the discussion and overview of the Internet of Things (IoT) toward the Medical and Health area, addressing their key points and their importance, which are a complex and heterogeneous concept but which involves the technology's potential of the Internet of Medical Things (IoMT).

Therefore, this chapter aims to provide an updated overview of the Internet of Medical Things, addressing its evolution and branch of application potential, showing and approaching its success relationship, with a concise bibliographic background, and synthesizing the potential of technology.

1.2   Methodology

This research study was developed based on the analysis of scientific papers and scientific journal sources referring to the Internet of Things toward the Medical and Health area, aiming to gather pertinent information regarding thematic concerning evolution and fundamental concepts of technology.

The differential of this paper is that it deals with an approach to the studied theme through current examples of the applicability of the concept of IoMT, which focuses on the role of IoMT in modern perspectives. Thus, it is also possible to boost more academic research through the background provided through this study.

1.3 Internet of Medical Things Concept

The IoT (Internet of Things) concept describes the universe of objects connected to the internet and their assignments and seeks to develop devices connected to the internet and with communication power, since through the web, it could be accessed by other smart devices, not just for sending messages but also for receiving [6–11].

The potential of the Internet of Things has as its main characteristic the exchange of information, in line with the characteristic that it is formed by components connected to the internet, which interconnected to an ecosystem, aiming to improve the management of a given system of which the device is part and also increase its performance through external data [6–13].

The digital transformation was one of the main responsible for bringing IoT, along with new technologies, such as Big Data, AI (Artificial Intelligence), Cloud Computing, and derivatives (Fog and Edge), among other technologies, into the most diverse types of companies, organizations, and institutions. In this application bias, the Internet of Medical Things (IoMT) emerges, as an aspect of IoT within the health field [10–16].

In medicine, wearables and connected medical equipment are a clear example of the use of IoT to capture data and optimize the routine of professionals and patients. These wearable devices connect the various actors that form the health triangle that has patient, doctor, and healthcare environments (clinics, hospitals, laboratories, medical equipment, and medication companies, health plans, and preventive medicine, among others) [8–16].

Through these solutions, it is possible to monitor and generate data on the status of patients, whether in the office, in the hospital, or even at home. Technology allows decision-making by the attending physician, and it is not intended to replace medical care. On the contrary, it helps the patient to follow medical recommendations, helping to prevent diseases and treating health problems in the best way, or even in the way of treating health problems, chronic or not, through the collected data, more accurate diagnoses, and treatments with better, more assertive results [8–16].

1.3.1 Internet of Medical Things (IoMT)

Representing the connection between the physical world and the constant transmission of virtual data, the IoT allows all objects to be connected to each other over the internet. In that sense, applied this technological concept for medical devices, the technology is called the Internet of Medical Things (IoMT) [14–18].

IoMT is the IOT technology that can be treated as the evolution of the original concept, focused exclusively on the health sector. With the objective of providing personalized service, considering the technologies used to achieve these goals, they can take various forms, such as mobile devices equipped with smart applications, medical equipment for home use, service applications, and emergency care kits, among others to provide data-driven treatment through the use of devices adapted to patients [14–18].

When it comes to health and application of IoT, with a new specification, the IoMT concept is more closely linked to healthcare environments and the maximization of care together with an improvement of results for the patient. Precisely, because it has a focus on human well-being, the health area is a niche where the most advanced technological developments and the evolution of equipment available in the medical area are sought. This relates to new forms of treatment, patient monitoring, medication and equipment control, and applications available with IoMT, making work in hospitals and clinics more dynamic and efficient. Just as, it is worth highlighting the impulse that the health area had through the different technological aspects related to connectivity technology [14–20].

The fact that the connection between different devices and the Internet only tends to contribute to the advancement of the medical segment is exemplified in the common application of IoMT in the form of bracelets and watches, a form of wearables, which monitor a series of characteristics, such as heartbeat, movement, and number of steps, among other aspects [14–20].

IoMT technology makes items such as cardiac pacemakers and ingestible sensors and pills the size of vitamin supplements that replace invasive procedures, capable of monitoring vital signs and even detecting types of cancer early and capturing and transmitting images of the gastrointestinal tract intelligent and passive and the colon, for example. Along with them, there are hundreds of technologies that, like nanosensors that are ingested and go into the bloodstream, where they send information about the cardiovascular system or use RFID (Radio Frequency IDentification) tags, which allow monitoring and management of medical assets and equipment through radio frequency within a given environment, which is through the crossing of data, are revolutionizing the interaction between patients and medical institutions [15–22].

IoMT goes far beyond a data connection, responsible for the perfect integration between essential information from the patient's reality, which through this technology, medicine can benefit from greater digital agility in the verification of hospital charts, and even considering the availability of data for consultation with doctors, allowing early preparation by the doctor through a general clinical view of the patient through these data [14–22].

1.3.2   IoMT Applications

IoMT is used in the transport and storage of vaccines, since one of the causes associated with the problem of the vaccine not reaching its destination is the lack of safe transport and storage systems for these inputs, since they need refrigeration to be preserved [23–25]. In this context, IoMT can work through sensors found in the portable refrigerator itself, creating effective systems that keep vaccines protected, connected with an IoT platform capable of monitoring in real time the status and quantity of these inputs. Therefore, IoMT technology helps inputs to reach regions where conditions are more precarious, with the guarantee that people can be vaccinated without prejudice, as in countries on the African continent [20–28].

IoMT is used in the monitoring of medicines related to waste in health linked to the wrong dispensing of medicines or even poor packaging, which in this respect, enables the control of temperature and humidity of medicines in healthcare environments, clinics, or even hospital pharmacies. Smart beds are used, which perform the reading of several vital indicators of the patient, informing a central system about their condition, and checking the medication at the bedside before being administered to the patient. Installing IoMT making hospital beds "smart" assists nurses and other professionals in accommodating and securing patients at risk of falling out of their beds, as long as it is possible for them to inform professionals about the best position to accommodate the patient, collaborating to make them comfortable and recover quickly, evaluating daily monitoring, and making it possible to detect any problem in the dosage of medicines instantly, which means more hope for patients. Or even, the smart bed technology can send messages to health professionals, if they have not been properly repositioned after feeding or cleaning a particular patient [21–29].

IoMT is also used in activity trackers in the treatment of cancer, for example, in order to collect lifestyle data from patients who are treating multiple myeloma, a type of cancer that attacks plasma cells or even other types and classes of disease, allowing healthcare professionals to have the ability to diagnose patients more quickly, since the collaboration of technology through cloud computing services and IoMT gadgets makes the medical routine safer and more effective, allowing the creation of personalized treatments and more adapted to the unique profile of each patient [21–31].

IoMT is also used to monitor the evolution of Parkinson's symptoms, which is a neurological, chronic, and progressive disease. However, by combining sensors and mobile devices and monitoring information such as the level of appetite or fatigue, doctors have the ability to analyze each reaction in a unique and personalized way, which, through machine learning, provides information on symptoms in real time for clinical professionals. Thus, making decisions about the course of treatment is easier and more accurate [21–32].

Still evaluating the use of IoMT in monitoring the evolution of symptoms of depression, in patients with depression, through wearable devices, such as smartwatches, equipped with applications and other systems that can monitor symptoms and behaviors of people diagnosed with this disease at medium to moderate level. Collecting data, assessments of the patient's mood and even assessing their cognition, among others, while these IoMT devices performing routine tasks based on questionnaires for the patient and collecting other corresponding data, and then this information is sent and analyzed by doctors and other specialists. Based on the information recorded, health professionals opt for more assertive treatments that improve the quality of life of those who suffer from the disease [2, 8, 17, 20–32].

Or even the use of IoMT to monitor the response of patients to Alzheimer's treatment, monitoring the real-time progress of treatment in each patient suffering from this condition, since this disease causes the patient to gradually lose their motor functions due to damage to the central nervous system, causing stiffness and tremors, among other severe consequences. Although there is still no cure, treatment is done with drugs, which aim to control symptoms and enable patients to have a better quality of life. Through the integration of sensors with smartphones, using a tracking bracelet, it is possible to track hand tremors from the user, better identifying the progress of the disease, and the impact it has on the person's routine. This results in a gain in quality of life, since that person will have more security in your routine and other situations in which the disease may affect your daily life [21–34].

IoMT can still be used in the possibility of remote operation of these types of equipment (remote control), reducing the need for personnel in loco or even the monitoring of prediction in the maintenance of medical equipment. The information collected by these medical types of equipment makes it possible to anticipate breakages and increase the availability of the installed product [21–34].

IoMT combined with AI (Artificial Intelligence) makes it possible to identify, in advance, through the data collected and analyzed by AI that return insights with the results, in relation to patients at risk or in the circumstances of developing a generalized infection (sepsis). It is found that hospital infections are still responsible for part of hospitalizations, since inpatients generally acquire some infection during their hospital stay. Thus, through systems with IoMT, they monitor in real time the hygiene of the professionals that circulate in the environments. The technology records by alcohol gel totems, for example, equipped with sensors, which identity who is or is not with clean hands, linking the identification to that information on the employees' own badge [12, 20–35].

IoMT contributes to a vital function in hospitals, related to hygiene in hospital environments, used by means of sensor systems, and monitors that control hygiene practices in these environments, preventing possible contamination and even the death of patients from infection (sepsis), in addition to reporting real-time compliance data to the correct standards [21–35].

IoMT also contributes to the detection of breast cancer with wearables, which detect patterns and identify temperature variations in the breast region, using sensors, since the patient wears the device as if she were wearing a bra, which collects and transmits body information to a medical professional's smartphone, for example, verifying the data in real time even from a distance. The purpose of this type of IoMT can be seen as a good alternative for patients who need to examine the region on a monthly basis. Thus, it is possible to identify the clinical picture as soon as possible, noninvasively, and at a good cost [17, 20–29, 36].

IoMT can also be used as smart contact lenses that measure the glucose levels of patients with diabetes through their tears, evaluating that this type of contact lens connected to the internet stores the data collected on a mobile device. Or even this type of IoMT can be used to control and assist in the treatment of other diseases that require continuous control. Still those IoMT acting as intelligent CGM (Continuous Glucose Monitor) are evaluated, since CGM allows diabetes (a chronic disease that needs daily monitoring) to be evaluated through instant and accurate data. Currently, there are several ways to apply (wearables) this type of functionality to equipment that monitors the glucose levels of diabetics, allowing them to record patterns and point out abnormalities, which can be useful for these people, their doctors, and caregivers [20–29, 34–38].

IoMT can also be used in digital exam records considering those digital devices for diagnostic exams (X-ray, ultrasound, computed tomography, magnetic resonance, and electrocardiogram, among others), capable of generating and storing data digitally, eliminating the use of paper. This has a green impact, since this possibility preserves the environment, reduces the need for physical space for files, and ensures the conservation of documents, i.e., digital files, without any additional care, such as handling radiographic films, which can be easily damaged. Still reflecting on the aspect that information, in a digital state, allows greater simplicity in sharing, which can be done via e-mail or messaging applications, or even specific healthcare systems, between medical teams [14–21, 30–38].

IoMT can also be used as a smart cardiac pacemaker with an IoT device, i.e., implanted (connected) in the patient, which facilitates patient monitoring, thus representing that these types of devices collect, store, and send information in real time about the cardiovascular system to a cardiologist who has the conditions to be able to monitor the health conditions of the patient from a distance, intervening when necessary, being able to make decisions to improve their quality of life [14–21, 24–30, 39].

1.3.3 The Benefits and Advantages of IoMT

IoMT allows more refined monitoring of the patient in real time, since this is one of the most critical advantages of the Internet of Medical Things related to having the vital data of the patient in the bedsides in a centralized and updated way at every moment (real time) brings an enormous reduction potential of costs with adverse events [17–20, 30–39].

With this technology, it is possible to issue alerts and inform health professionals more easily, even before the situation becomes more critical for the patient. It is possible to directly call service providers with the ability to identify the problem, thus preventing the loss of lives with IoMT technology [17–21, 30–39].

Reflecting on the millions of devices connected through IoMT to medical systems over the network, performing data collection and information, and data transmission, assessing that this is in constant use of monitoring parts of patient bodies, accelerating and assisting medical decisions. In the same sense as giving patients a better chance of getting out of health risk situations without the slightest sequel [14–21, 30–39].

IoMT allows a more detailed and refined self-care of the patient, evaluating that the wearable and implantable medical devices makes it possible to place the patient in the center of his own care, clinically assessing the evolution of his health status, still reflecting that in some cases, the person himself (or elderly companion) can intervene at home since he has already been instructed by the doctor, and even going to any health institution is not necessary, and so the patient can anticipate scheduling elective appointments instead of going through an emergency [14–21, 30–39].

IoMT also allows benefits through ingestible sensors (microdevices) that, when swallowed, allow doctors to monitor the level of medication at a distance, or even via Bluetooth technology, making it possible for the health professional, elderly companion, or even the patient himself to carry out monitoring smartphone, related to the treatment of diseases [14–23, 30–39].

The purpose of IoMT technology is to have the largest number of data about the patient before and during treatment, which makes it possible to assess the best way to conduct the therapeutic process. Representing that from this and new information, it is possible, for example, to significantly reduce adverse reactions to certain types of treatments. In the same sense, controlling more assertively each of the symptoms that afflict patients comes to limit the lifestyle of these people in some way [40, 41].

One of the greatest advantages of IoMT is access, by health professionals, with respect to data consistent with the patient's reality. Since the lack of information about the patient is a common and serious problem, reflecting on a patient, depending on his/her social level, too little is directed to medical assistance and, therefore, does not allow the collection of a lot of data about him, which hinders more assertive care, based on his history, i.e., data past [14–21, 37–41].

It is consistent to point out that data are transformed into actions through technology, specifically dealing in the field of health, IoMT, since the data collected allow a better understanding of the patient's health, which from the combination of sensors, mobile devices, and machine learning, possibly transform it into objects that assist in health care in the daily life of this patient, making health professionals follow and receive data and information in real time about each patient, or even from a wearable that groups the patients 'health data and sends them facilitating the doctors' work, allowing a more effective medical assistance [12, 14–21, 37–44].

Another advantage of IoMT is related to the remote access of patients by doctors and health professionals, which represents the release of medical care centers such as hospitals and clinics, allowing patients to be monitored employing remote access, which prevents them from having to be kept in the clinic or hospital environment, and depending on the situation they may come to catch sepsis or other types of contamination, for example [12, 14–21, 37–44].

In the same sense, the advantage of IoMT corresponds to the personalized care of this patient, through the volume of consistent data collected through the use of devices implanted in the patient, or through the use of wearables, it guarantees an analysis and a personalized service for each case and each patient [12, 14–21, 37–44].

The other advantage of IoMT can be found in disease prevention, through real-time access to data on the health of a specific patient, relating sleep quality and heart rate from a wearable, and it helps in making decisions for a lifetime healthier. Ensuring greater comfort and tranquility of this patient, through monitoring by the doctor or health professional, resulting in continuing with all his activities normally, and if any problem arises, this patient can get in direct contact with this professional [2, 8, 14–21, 45].

Another great advantage of IoMT is closely linked to patient satisfaction and engagement, through the most detailed and assertive data through the IoMT, such as the discovery of habits, health problems, and other information that help in a later treatment or even to avoid the appearance of some complication, which provides an optimized type of medical care, benefiting both the journey of this patient in a healthy environment and the work and operation of health services, which promotes awareness of this patient so that he follows all medical recommendations, since he is satisfied with the compromise of the system as a whole. Similarly, a user is satisfied with a certain application, i.e., the transparency of the technology for this user is optimal [37–45].

The advantage of IoMT related to the constant feedback related to the monitoring facilitated by the devices allows a constant response about the patient's reactions in relation to the applied treatment [37–45].

In the same sense, the advantage of IoMT is to obtain advanced management of medical care for patients using smart accessories, sending real-time alerts to patients and/or health professionals, such as blood glucose and temperature monitoring, cardiac performance, among other signals. This optimizes the workflow of healthcare environments, checking in real-time the patient's behavior and clinical status according to the treatment administered, deciding between continuing or changing a particular medical approach, ensuring more comfortable care for the patient [37–45].

1.3.4 IoMT Challenges

Even in full growth, the use of IoMT is still initial, evaluating the existence of a few devices connected in healthcare environments, monitoring patients [33, 40–45].

Still reflecting that in these health environments (hospitals, clinics, and clinics), containing access to the Internet through a wired connection (RJ-45 among others) or wi-fi. This represents one of the main challenges, including the insertion of connectivity means in these health environments, allowing devices to communicate (collect and send data), resulting in an increase in the number of intelligent medical equipment. Considering that IoMT applications generally require moderate bandwidth, in this sense, it is necessary to determine the dimensioning of the WAN links, due to the data volumes and interactions that the IoMT causes in the digital structure, this requires a restructuring of networks and data transfer systems information [33, 37, 43–47].

Another challenging point is the complexity of the IoMT, still mentioning its importance is on information security, representing the volume of generation, collection, and transmission of confidential data about patients in the face of the imminent threat of cybercriminals and increasing the number of attacks in search of this information [33, 37, 43–49].

Still considering that the IoMT market is in full growth and the reason is the improvement that this technology can bring to the health sector, an estimate reveals how much is expected of this technology regarding its implantation and adoption by most health professionals around the world, through greater control of patient conditions, ensuring more comfort to them. Reflecting on this estimate that comes from one of the main reasons for the advancement of IoMT is the increase in chronic diseases and the aging of the world population, which consequently will require more care and better care for these patients. This represents a challenge for health systems with an interest in adding IoMT and all its corresponding digital structure [33, 37, 43–49].

The use of Big Data technology for IoMT can be considered one of the most complex challenges, since it requires a digital structure on data storage, filtering, and analysis so that it can offer a clearer view, from a strategic point of view, for the information collected [1, 3, 11, 15, 33, 37, 43–49].

Still reflecting on Digital Security in IoMT, devices must be protected by effective technological measures that can be avoiding infection by ransomware, causing the device to be blocked, turning off a health monitoring system, or entering a private health system patient manipulating the data, and can only be used freely again after permission from criminals, for example, still assessing the occurrence of denial of service attacks of the type DoS (Disk Operating System) or DDoS (Distributed Denial of Service), leading to the disruption of the provision of health services [33, 37, 43–49].

The issue of Privacy in IoMT in the face of the huge amount of data collected and stored is a challenge, since these data must be properly encrypted so that there is no risk of theft, sale, or even misuse against patients [33, 37, 43–49].

The factor of Storage in IoMT linked to the premise of "to get more and more data available," it is worth noting that these data are personal to patients and health environments. Representing that the infrastructure to store all these data must be built with effective security standards, in the same sense, data centers must meet the need for storage through the growing and continuous volume of data [33, 37, 43–49].

The challenge of maintaining IoMT Information Confidentiality in relation to the connected IoMT devices generating and collecting data and information must be promptly established, through policies aimed at the concern with the privacy and confidentiality of patient information [33, 37, 43–50].

As well as the challenge of maintaining the Integrity and Availability of IoMT Information, by capturing signals from IoMT sensors, avoiding the collection and transmission of wrong information, which can occur through poor configuration and calibration of sensors and medical equipment [17, 20, 23, 26, 30, 33, 37, 43–50].

The challenge of unavailability and lack of integrity in the signal collected from these IoMT sensors are concerned for health managers, since this factor impacts the unavailability of databases and servers, resulting in the unavailability of health systems. In this sense, there is a need for an Event Treatment Policy that ensures compliance with what is and will be and when it will be done, thus guaranteeing the correct operation of all actors in a healthcare system, whether human or machine [33, 37, 43–51].

Thus, the impact caused by IoMT must have two central focuses, related to the data generated and collected (volume), understanding that Big Data can be a useful tool for the result of information increasingly collected in the most diverse mobile devices' medical reality, and the visibility of that data, combined with the need for easy and clear access to that data, ensuring a security aspect, in an attempt to prevent problems from arising in the rapid recovery of the system, in case there is a problem [1, 3, 11, 15, 33, 37, 43–51].

1.4 Health Informatics Concepts

The collection of data about patients and their illnesses is used to assess the progress of their personal health conditions and provides data analysis that is vital for the functioning of IoMT systems that allow safe decision-making of doctors regarding treatment and health professionals [48–54].

In this sense, e-Health is the use of information and communication technologies in health, such as IoMT to perform treatment of patients, research, monitoring diseases, and monitoring the health of the patient. The development of wearable technology, static devices, and applications connected to IoMT in addition to creating a connected ecosystem has provided the creation of potentially integrated solutions and has helped to collect and process vital data for health informatics [37–42, 48–55].

Health informatics is evaluated as an interdisciplinary field that studies and investigates the effective use of data, information, and knowledge for scientific research and develops computer systems to support medical activities with respect to the analysis and digital processing of bioelectric signals, digital image processing medical, patient monitoring systems, diagnosis and decision support, and intelligent computer-aided instruction systems. Further development is through the study of design and adaptation of innovations based on Information Technology (IT) in the management of medical data, planning, and provision of patient-oriented health services, such as problem-solving and medical decision-making, with a focus on improving human health [37–42, 48–55].

In this sense, data analysis through Big Data in health care is a technology that when implanted tends to allow better management of patient data, showing that this technology has brought even more precision to the decision-making in the health area, regarding the use of Big Data to aid in the diagnosis and treatment of patients, managing to develop treatments in the short-, medium-, and long-term, and analyzing the current state of the patient and trends for the future [1, 3, 11, 15, 37–42, 48–55].

Considering that medical computerization and the arrival of IoT and later IoMT, in view of this, the health scenario has undergone transformations with real impact for patients and doctors. Pondering its applicability from the integration of health management systems to diagnostic imaging devices, both for the diagnosis of diseases and for the treatment of diseases [14–19, 37–42, 48–55].

Big data in medicine represent large conglomerates of information, through large volumes of data, which are compiled into databases and/or software, with the aim of creating trends and improving knowledge about the management and health status of patients. It is still worth noting the difference between Big Data and other ways of obtaining information, related to volume, speed, variety, variability, and complexity. This makes management processes more efficient, enabling the generation of insights, reducing costs, saving time, developing more assertive treatments, as well as making decisions more intelligent [1, 3, 11, 15, 37–42, 48–55].

In this sense, wearable devices, like other IoMT devices that propose to monitor blood pressure and heart rate, among other data, are used to collect data about the patient's symptoms and conditions, processed by Big medical Data analytics (Big Data Analytics in health care). Even using this information, appropriate AI algorithms can measure results equivalent to that of human professionals, being able to perform a complete analysis, identifying the probable diagnosis [2, 8, 14–21, 37, 45, 55].

The application of Health Informatics can be found in the Electronic Patient Record (PEP), Clinical decision support, Monitoring of chronic patients, Electronic Health Record (RES), Patient flow management, Digital processing of signals and images (PACs), Telemedicine, Collection, storage (data warehousing), Data analysis related to biostatistics through Business Intelligence (BI), Administrative, financial and logistics management through IoMT, statistical analysis of medical data, and Interoperability [37, 42, 53–59].

Still considering the fact that machines are not able to offer patients the same empathy as a doctor, despite technological advances in AI software, or even that it is still not possible to fully rely on deep learning and machine learning, indicating that despite all the technological support applied, it is necessary to analyze and decide by health experts [2, 8, 14–21, 37, 42, 59].

The promotion of the transformation of healthcare systems focused on data collected as laboratory results, medical diagnoses, and hospitalization records, among other categories, through the tools of Informatics in Health, provides a complete health history, supported by advanced artificial intelligence and learning of machine, which focuses on individual patients to suggest changes in their care, through the incorporation of decision support techniques and focus on patient safety [2, 8, 14–21, 37, 42, 48–54, 59].

Health Analytics is the concept defined as a set of methodologies used in order to analyze large volumes of data through Big Data technology in the health sector, contributing to the clinical care of the patient and the management of health resources. The concept is also applied to health management, and one of the main contributions is in reducing waste and improving the quality of the services offered, in addition to sustainable productivity in patient's health care [1, 3, 11, 15, 37–42, 48–52, 59].

The set of systems and tools that are part of BI comes from IT to take tailor-made solutions regarding the transformation of data, which are apparently disconnected, in essential information that guides the decision-making of health professionals with a consolidated basis. Applied in the medical field, the implementation of BI and Health Analytics in health institutions enables the search and interpretation of information collected and stored in the system, aimed at supporting decisions within the patient's life cycle and stay at the health institution [1, 3, 11, 15, 37–42, 48–55, 59].

Health management software is used for the control and management of patient data, with the objective of providing greater security in the care and provision of medical services, assessing that the most diverse IoMT devices collect data that are aimed at the management and improvement in the offer of health services and not at sharing sensitive data with third parties and without authorization [1, 3, 11, 15, 37–42, 48–59].

Medical Informatics is then a field of activity where Health Informatics transforms health through the analysis, design, implementation, and evaluation of information and communication systems, assessing the information and knowledge needs of health professionals and patients. By improving the individual results of each patient, they increase patient safety in the care process, improving the synthesis of large health databases collected and enhancing the management of medical services and medical research, in the same sense as strengthening the doctor-patient relationship, and even characterizing, evaluating, and refining clinical processes performed by technology, developing, implementing, and perfecting clinical decision support systems, in order to promote safe, efficient, effective, timely, patient-centered, and impartial customized patient care. Still evaluating that through Medical Informatics together with information technologies, it is possible to develop analysis, implementations, and evaluations of IoMT technologies that improve the individual health results of patients [37–42, 48–52, 57–61].

1.4.1 Benefits of Big Data in Health

The health area is quite complex and is closely related to people's lives, which requires a constant search to improve efficiency and quality, in general by scientific evidence, in terms of both diagnoses and the treatment of patients. Through Big Data, better results are promoted for health professionals, patients, and health institutions, since it is possible to generate better documentation, data analysis, and statistical and mathematical methods to obtain relevant data for the health area [59–65].

Big Data can help significantly with the customized treatment of patients, and its use is efficient for this area, since it is possible to obtain a large volume of information from patients, through IoMT devices [59–65].

Through Big Data, it is possible to reduce costs in clinics, through management based on data, collected by IoMT equipment and devices, managing to better analyze the entire structure of the health institution and enabling a more focused action of activities in clinics and hospitals, with no waste or loss of quality of service, without affecting the care offered to patients [59–65].

The data collected through the IoMT allow for a more adequate planning of actions, such as adequate maintenance of equipment, cost reduction, and improvement in emergency operations, allowing data to be analyzed in an easier way. Through the relationship between IoMT and Big Data related to the possibility that a large volume of data is collected in detail, this ensures that all this data is stored (Big Data) allowing the combination of this data with other technologies (AI), making correlations and analysis [59–65].

With Big Data, it is possible to perform a better cross-checking of data in relation to medical procedures, enabling personalization of medicine, bringing more inputs and data so that the health professional can identify which types of treatments are best for a particular type of patient, and reflecting on the existence of initiatives that seek to identify the DNA data of people with the premise of developing precision medicine. Still considering the objective of generating knowledge about the genetic variations found in the population, which allows the development of personalized treatments [59–69].

In this sense, the adoption of data and the application of Big medical Data analytics technology enable a greater sharing of information and more effectiveness in health as a whole. In addition to providing insights into the type of treatment that may be more effective for a particular type of patient, there is also a reduction in the risk of errors in treatments, indications of medications, or even in cases of hospitalizations [59–69].

1.5 Discussion

It is a fact that advances through the democratization of the internet generate a greater number of system interactions supporting the application of IoT in medicine, the well-known IoMT. With this growing adhesion in relation to connected devices, whether in hospitals, homes, clinics, laboratories, companies, or healthcare establishments, IoMT has become a major trend for the medicine of the future.

IoMT is the technology intended to enable advanced services through the interconnection between things (physical and virtual), based on information and communication technologies (ICT), applied to the medical field, emphasizing that this technological use can contribute to the advancement of several medical applications that guarantee greater access and efficiency in the provision of health services to patients.

As mentioned in previous sections, through IoMT technologies and the improvement and evolution of ingestible sensors, which would release medications directly in the region to be treated and monitor their results, they have a therapeutic approach.

In the same sense that the IoMT provides reinforcement in the personalization of medical treatments, considering several technologies of connectivity and traceability, generating an analysis of diverse patient data, as well as expanding the innovation in the medical monitoring of the patient. It also aims at the effectiveness of new technologies for the treatment of diseases, management, and medical observation of patients at long distance, becoming more effective with the collection of body information in real-time. In this way, it provides more accurate diagnoses, as the patient profile is created with long-term records. Thus, these patients gain a better quality of life, with fewer diseases, through better medical monitoring.

The application of IoMT in the health environment contributes to facing the challenge related to the increase in health spending, mainly due to the aging of the population, which is a worldwide trend, and the consequent decrease in the economically active people. In this sense, investments in health are necessary, which can contribute both to improving the quality of life of people and to increasing the efficiency of health units, through the use of powerful technologies such as IoMT.

Digital health through IoMT, although in the early stages of development, will revolutionize the healthcare industry due to the advancement of wireless technology, the advancement of smartphones, Cloud technology, and sensors that have enabled the miniaturization of medical equipment and their ability to make diagnostic, treatment, and prevention costs decrease.

In the same derived bias as with the advances with IoMT, it was possible to mix nanotechnology, biomedicine, and bioengineering, with the potential to use their technologies together, in order to carry out exams with speeds and facilities through connected gadgets that send diversified information to internal systems of hospitals, clinics, and derivatives, allowing the creation of digital medical records and making the workflow more dynamic, flexible, and modern. Through a digital medical history, it can be updated automatically, informing all the conditions that the patient has had and is running at the time of the medical request, allowing the best management of patients and accelerating care in different medical environments.

IoMT reached the main challenges in the health area, since the connectivity and traceability of IoMT fit in the most diverse places, with respect to the treatment of chronic diseases. It is possible to better monitor by means of technology, health promotion and prevention, and improving management efficiency.

Through wearable devices and components connected to the internet, which interconnected generate an ecosystem, they formed a health triangle relating patient, doctor, and healthcare environments (hospitals, clinics, laboratories, health insurance, and preventive medicine institutions, or even equipment industries doctors and medicines).

1.5.1 IoMT in Hospitals

Many devices have the ability to be connected to the Wi-Fi network or other types of networks in a hospital, clinic, or laboratory, generating large amounts of data, having their activities and health conditions monitored, and allowing the tracking of information.

Still pondering that the stress levels of health professionals, can be monitored, allowing to reduce factors such as pressure and work overload, which increases security for making important medical decisions in the treatment of patients.

Regarding the patient, it can reduce the number of hospitalizations and keep the patient well cared for at home since IoMT devices identify that in some cases. They are quite simple problems, representing that technology makes their interaction with the doctor much more powerful and useful, in addition to giving more control and quality of life to the patient and preventing people from being tied to waiting in hospitals or outpatient clinics.

The greatest impact of IoMT is on the side of health services, including hospitals and clinics, with regard to improving patient management, which can streamline the care process, as long as data such as blood type, health history, and patient age, collected in the emergency room, serve to guide as to possible diagnoses and treatments.

In the same sense, the IoMT also has a positive impact on the management of the structure of a hospital, allowing the tracking of drugs and other products, which can be relocated to avoid waste, or even equipment with high technology can be analyzed daily, so that activities' preventive maintenance is carried out in the correct period, which avoids repairs and constant replacement of these devices.

1.5.2   IoMT and Telemedicine

This relationship was born from the joint use of information and communication technologies, by using telemedicine as a provider of remote exam interpretation services, which can be considered as a modality of application of IoMT. The possibilities of IoMT multiply and make medicine an essential instrument with greater control of the conditions of patients, guaranteeing more comfort to users, in order to achieve the quality of life that every human being wants and deserves.

Considering remote patient monitoring platforms, telemedicine should encourage changes in behavior and change the health landscape in the coming years, indicating that the disruptive power of IoMT increases the quality of life of patients, improving the management and medical monitoring of chronic diseases. Thus, the use of IoMT technology allows the creation of new treatments that are more accurate and with a greater wealth of information, which optimize the care of patients with serious illnesses or facilitate the identification of risk patterns.

Aligned with the goal of health care to maintain efficient monitoring of patients, health institutions, clinics, and hospitals are based on reality with information obtained in real time, ranging from the blood pressure of patients to the number of steps a person takes. Through Big Data technologies, AI, and machine learning systems, patterns are more easily identified, and new solutions to diverse health problems can be identified more easily.

Reflecting on the sharing of data collected by digital devices IoMT during diagnostic tests, via a telemedicine platform, with health professionals at a distance, these data are sent to the patient's records, and are available for interpretation and analysis by health specialists, enabling the issuance of distance reports with quality and efficiency. Still considering the characteristics of sending data to an application on patients' smartphones as well as sending to doctors, since this also allows monitoring by them.

This reality can be achieved as long as health institutions, clinics, and hospitals use digital equipment in their diagnostic tests, and from there, collect information and transmit it through connected devices, taking advantage of the potential of IoMT. What sequences, these data are shared and accessed by qualified specialists for interpretation of the exams. By supporting the information available in the patient's digital medical record, it has the properties to better evaluate the exams and produce the report at a distance, supporting the choice of the best treatment through adverse events.

1.5.3 Sensor Data Analytics

The processing of data collected by the IoT, i.e., intelligent IoMT sensors, changes the way healthcare institutions view patients. Through the volume of random information and unstructured data, and with the infinity of usage data made available by sensors and chips embedded in medical devices, there is also a need to make the most of them, transforming them into information, through tool analytics.

Considering that a lot of unstructured data becomes important for medical analysis, these data can be crucial to better capture trends in prognosis and make predictive analysis. It is possible, therefore, that many analytical tools oriented to Analytics can also be used to generate solutions related to IoMt data analysis. This can also be used as functions present in cloud-based services, allowing high-volume data processing with greater flexibility and less cost than doing it internally, with its own infrastructure.

Mining data from different sources such as IoMT sensors and supported by algorithms, health professionals can count on powerful analytical tools to identify pathologies, receive recommendations for defining the most appropriate treatments, and even accelerate the development of new drugs based on group tests monitored individuals, also correlated with Artificial Intelligence to analyze health data received from connected IoMT devices and sensors, allowing the creation of a platform that integrates medical equipment for the extraction and analysis of information collected through medical records, imaging tests, and wearables [70] and providing a revolution of IoT in precision medicine, supported by the association of Artificial Intelligence with robotics and even technology in cloud computing, ensuring a greater quality of life for patients.

Analytics solutions using data collected by IoMT sensors offer the ability to add a variety of data from hundreds of different sources in real time. This means increasing commitment to the patient, providing more effective and personalized interactions with the patient, which ends up achieving a longer relationship with the patient. Therefore, these solutions provide complete patient profiles, which allows for more personalized experiences. Thus, Analytics helps healthcare organizations take advantage of their data and use it to lead them to smarter businesses, more efficient operations, higher profits, and more satisfied patients.

1.6 Trends

In the area of Health, IoMT devices can collect and monitor the vital signs of patients and send them to a cloud, using mobile technology, which concentrates the data, and these can be accessed through software that shows indications of evolution and analyzes machine learning, which assists in doctors' decision-making [71–76].

The monitoring of information through smart watches and IoMT wearables reaches more and more levels of greater detail in relation to patients. Since it is important to monitor whether your patient is recovering adequately with a given treatment, evaluating this becomes ever closer to the doctor, retaining patients to the doctor's office, clinics, or health institutions [77–82].

Other applications of IoMT technology aim at safer surgeries through the identification of each of the instruments used in the operating room, which through traceability helps in the management of prostheses and special materials, devices, and materials with high added value. This impacts the identification of the exact location of each medical instrument, and prevents, for example, cases of forgetfulness within the patient [82–84].

Through Big Data technologies and AI that analyze the volumes of data collected from connected IoMT devices, they are able to correlate them with information from the medical literature, thereby generating insights and making it possible, for example, to identify regions where there is a higher incidence of certain pathology or infectious disease [84–86].

Artificial intelligence (AI) will make it possible to understand the scenario even better, model, and predict medical demand, through an ideal cut and according to the type of activity or behavior of patients. From the information generated continuously, based on data obtained (IoMT), in the hospital management system modules, medical professionals will be able to make even more assertive decisions regarding diagnostic processes, identification of predispositions to diseases, and even treatment prescriptions, even using the information collected by hospital equipment for AI learning [24, 87].

1.7 Conclusions

IoT is a technology that advances more and more in daily routine tasks and needs, in addition to being applied in industry and several commercial sectors, creating a more sophisticated interaction between objects and people.

Applied in the area of health, IoMT, the benefits are numerous, ranging from improving communication between patient and doctor and speeding up the diagnosis for the treatment of chronic diseases, thereby allowing the doctor to have the patient's health history to assess digitally and access to a patient's history at anytime, anywhere there is a connection; improving the quality of medical service; and even cost reduction and patient awareness about the technological role in managing one's own health.

IoMT's applications range from the use of intelligent patient monitoring sensors, the use of applications to record heartbeat, a number of steps, calories consumed, to the integration of medical devices, such as performing CT scans, among other exams using digital record.

Still considering the use of IoMT as a way to transform the way health care is through mobile applications with characteristics of the connection to various devices to obtain and the ability to report data on the patient's body in search of medical insights. These innovations can make people's lives more uncomplicated, using visual identification algorithms and natural language capable of describing the state of a person and reading texts and answers to questions, capable of identifying emotions. This type of technology can be used with the help in the treatment and monitoring of diseases of psychological and neurological profile.

One of the benefits through the application of IoMT is the integration with telemedicine, linked to the strategic use of information generated by this type of technology, enabling the analysis of exams and the issuance of medical reports at a distance, representing a cost reduction with the hiring of specialists, and adding agility to the results of exams.

IoMT is able to increase patient satisfaction in relation to treatment, through the use of sensors, wearable, and specific medical devices to improve their medical services, by increasing the level of healthcare customization. In this sense, it improves engagement with health specialists, with the ability to humanize the relationship between medical professionals and their patients.

Other benefits of IoT are the reduction of human errors through the use of machine learning and AI applications, cost reduction in health institutions; improvement in exam results, improvement in clinic management, and optimization of the work pace through new models of health management, where doctors and healthcare companies can better monitor the state of the patient's body in search of healthier routines, improved communication between all healthcare system agents, and even increased productivity, even showing the exponential growth and even the interest in the development of new technologies and solutions related to IoMT and offering patients new ways of prevention, treatment, and health care.

References

1. D.V. Dimitrov, Medical internet of things and big data in healthcare. Healthc. Inform. Res. **22**(3), 156–163 (2016)
2. M. Haghi, K. Thurow, R. Stoll, Wearable devices in medical internet of things: Scientific research and commercially available devices. Healthc. Inform. Res. **23**(1), 4 15 (2017)
3. V. Jagadeeswari et al., A study on medical internet of things and big data in personalized healthcare system. Health Inform. Sci. Syst. **6**(1), 14 (2018)
4. F. Hu, D. Xie, S. Shen, On the application of the internet of things in the field of medical and health care, in *2013 IEEE International Conference on Green Computing and Communications and IEEE Internet of Things and IEEE Cyber, Physical and Social Computing*, (IEEE, 2013)

5. G. Fortino, P. Trunfio (eds.), *Internet of Things Based on Smart Objects: Technology, Middleware and Applications* (Springer Science & Business Media, 2014)
6. C. Savaglio et al., Agent-based Internet of Things: State-of-the-art and research challenges. Futur. Gener. Comput. Syst. **102**, 1038–1053 (2020)
7. G. Fortino et al., Agent-oriented cooperative smart objects: From IoT system design to implementation. IEEE Trans. Syst. Man Cybern. Syst. **48**(11), 1939–1956 (2017)
8. S.M.R. Islam et al., The internet of things for health care: A comprehensive survey. IEEE Access **3**, 678–708 (2015)
9. N. Bui, M. Zorzi, Health care applications: A solution based on the internet of things, in *Proceedings of the 4th International Symposium on Applied Sciences in Biomedical and Communication Technologies*, (2011)
10. I. Chiuchisan, H.-N. Costin, O. Geman, Adopting the internet of things technologies in health care systems, in *2014 International Conference and Exposition on Electrical and Power Engineering (EPE)*, (IEEE, 2014)
11. D. Metcalf et al., Wearables and the internet of things for health: Wearable, interconnected devices promise more efficient and comprehensive health care. IEEE Pulse **7**(5), 35–39 (2016)
12. M. Usak et al., Health care service delivery based on the Internet of Things: A systematic and comprehensive study. Int. J. Commun. Syst. **33**(2), e4179 (2020)
13. A.C.B. Monteiro et al., Methodology of high accuracy, sensitivity and specificity in the counts of erythrocytes and leukocytes in blood smear images, in *Brazilian Technology Symposium*, (Springer, Cham, 2018)
14. A.C.B. Monteiro et al., A comparative study between methodologies based on the Hough transform and watershed transform on the blood cell count, in *Brazilian Technology Symposium*, (Springer, Cham, 2018)
15. B. Sanjukta, C. Chinmay, Machine learning for biomedical and health informatics. Ch. 4, 353–373, in *CRC: Big Data, IoT, and Machine Learning Tools and Applications*, (2020., ISBN 9780429322990). https://doi.org/10.1201/9780429322990
16. M. Ge, H. Bangui, B. Buhnova, Big data for Internet of Things: A survey. Futur. Gener. Comput. Syst. **87**, 601–614 (2018)
17. A. Ghosh, D. Chakraborty, A. Law, Artificial intelligence in Internet of Things. CAAI Trans. Intellig. Technol. **3**(4), 208–218 (2018)
18. P.J. Escamilla-Ambrosio et al., Distributing computing in the internet of things: Cloud, fog and edge computing overview, in *NEO 2016*, (Springer, Cham, 2018), pp. 87–115
19. A. Gatouillat et al., Internet of medical things: A review of recent contributions dealing with cyber-physical systems in medicine. IEEE Internet Things J. **5**(5), 3810–3822 (2018)
20. F. Al-Turjman, H. Zahmatkesh, L. Mostarda, Quantifying uncertainty in Internet of medical things and big-data services using intelligence and deep learning. IEEE Access **7**, 115749–115759 (2019)
21. F. Alsubaei, A. Abuhussein, S. Shiva, Ontology-based security recommendation for the internet of medical things. IEEE Access **7**, 48948–48960 (2019)
22. F. Qureshi, S. Krishnan, Wearable hardware design for the internet of medical things (IoMT). Sensors **18**(11), 3812 (2018)
23. S.R. Khan et al., IoMT-based computational approach for detecting brain tumor. Futur. Gener. Comput. Syst. **109**, 360–367 (2020)
24. R. Chatterjee et al., A novel machine learning-based feature selection for motor imagery EEG signal classification in Internet of medical things environment. Futur. Gener. Comput. Syst. **98**, 419–434 (2019)
25. W.N. Ismail et al., CNN-based health model for regular health factors analysis in internet-of-medical things environment. IEEE Access **8**, 52541–52549 (2020)
26. S. Anand, A. Sharma, Internet of medical things: Services, applications and technologies. J. Comput. Theor. Nanosci. **16**(9), 3995–3998 (2019)
27. F. Al-Turjman, M.H. Nawaz, U.D. Ulusar, Intelligence in the Internet of medical things era: A systematic review of current and future trends. Comput. Commun. **150**, 644–660 (2020)

28. R. Basatneh, B. Najafi, D.G. Armstrong, Health sensors, smart home devices, and the internet of medical things: An opportunity for dramatic improvement in care for the lower extremity complications of diabetes. J. Diabetes Sci. Technol. **12**(3), 577–586 (2018)
29. M. Irfan, N. Ahmad, Internet of medical things: Architectural model, motivational factors and impediments, in *2018 15th Learning and Technology Conference (L&T)*, (IEEE, 2018)
30. S. Vishnu, S.R.J. Ramson, R. Jegan, Internet of medical things (IoMT)-an overview, in *2020 5th International Conference on Devices, Circuits, and Systems (ICDCS)*, (IEEE, 2020)
31. J. Flore, Ingestible sensors, data, and pharmaceuticals: Subjectivity in the era of digital mental health. New Media Soc. (2020). https://doi.org/10.1177/1461444820931024
32. K. Zhang, Internet of Things technology in animal vaccine cold chain management. Revista Cientifica-Facultad de Ciencias Veterinarias **29**(2) (2019)
33. Buitendach, Henning, Immanuel N. Jiya, and Rupert Gouws. "Solar-Powered Peltier Cooling Storage for Vaccines in Rural Areas." (2019)
34. J.N.S. Rubí, P.R. de Lira Gondim, Interoperable Internet of Medical Things platform for e-Health applications. Int. J. Distrib. Sens. Netw. **16**(1), 1550147719889591 (2020)
35. M. Elhoseny et al., Effective features to classify ovarian cancer data in internet of medical things. Comput. Netw. **159**, 147–156 (2019)
36. P. Borovska, D. Ivanova, I. Draganov, Internet of medical imaging things and analytics in support of precision medicine for the case study of thyroid cancer early diagnostics. Serdica J. Comput. **12**(1–2) (2018)
37. B. Klímová, K. Kuča, Internet of things in the assessment, diagnostics and treatment of Parkinson's disease. Heal. Technol. **9**(2), 87–91 (2019)
38. U. Khan et al., Internet of Medical Things–based decision system for automated classification of Alzheimer's using three-dimensional views of magnetic resonance imaging scans. Int. J. Distrib. Sens. Netw. **15**(3), 1550147719831186 (2019)
39. S.S. Aljehani et al., iCare: Applying IoT technology for monitoring Alzheimer's patients, in *2018 1st International Conference on Computer Applications & Information Security (ICCAIS)*, (IEEE, 2018)
40. L. Yang et al., Monitoring and control of medical air disinfection parameters of nosocomial infection system based on internet of things. J. Med. Syst. **43**(5), 126 (2019)
41. G. Manogaran, N. Chilamkurti, C.-H. Hsu, Emerging trends, issues, and challenges in Internet of Medical Things and wireless networks. Pers. Ubiquit. Comput. **22**(5–6), 879–882 (2018)
42. M. Kim et al., An electrochromic alarm system for smart contact lenses. Sensors Actuators B Chem. **322**, 128601 (2020)
43. O. Geman, I. Chiuchisan, M. Hagan, Body sensor networks and Internet of Things for management and screening of patients with diabetic neuropathy, in *2018 International Conference and Exposition on Electrical and Power Engineering (EPE)*, (IEEE, 2018)
44. F. Alsubaei et al., IoMT-SAF: Internet of medical things security assessment framework. Internet of Things **8**, 100123 (2019)
45. A. E. Hassanien, N. Dey, S. Borra (eds.), *Medical Big Data and Internet of Medical Things: Advances, Challenges, and Applications* (CRC Press, 2018)
46. R.K. Mahendran, P. Velusamy, A secure fuzzy extractor based biometric key authentication scheme for body sensor network in Internet of Medical Things. Comput. Commun. **153**, 545–552 (2020)
47. F. Lamonaca et al., An overview on Internet of medical things in blood pressure monitoring, in *2019 IEEE International Symposium on Medical Measurements and Applications (MeMeA)*, (IEEE, 2019)
48. J. Wang et al., An efficient and privacy-preserving outsourced support vector machine training for internet of medical things. IEEE Internet Things J. **8**, 458–473 (2020)
49. Z. Guan et al., Achieving data utility-privacy tradeoff in Internet of medical things: A machine learning approach. Futur. Gener. Comput. Syst. **98**, 60–68 (2019)
50. Y.-Z. Hsieh, Internet of things pillow detecting sleeping quality, in *2018 1st International Cognitive Cities Conference (IC3)*, (IEEE, 2018)

51. R. Ivanov et al., Open ice-lite: Towards a connectivity platform for the internet of medical things, in *2018 IEEE 21st International Symposium on Real-Time Distributed Computing (ISORC)*, (IEEE, 2018)
52. S.P. Raja, T. Dhiliphan Rajkumar, V.P. Raj, Internet of things: Challenges, issues and applications. J. Circuits Syst. Comput. **27**(12), 1830007 (2018)
53. G. Hatzivasilis et al., Review of security and privacy for the Internet of Medical Things (IoMT), in *2019 15th International Conference on Distributed Computing in Sensor Systems (DCOSS)*, (IEEE, 2019)
54. Y. Sun, F.P.-W. Lo, B. Lo, Security and privacy for the internet of medical things enabled healthcare systems: A survey. IEEE Access **7**, 183339–183355 (2019)
55. F. Alsubaei, A. Abuhussein, S. Shiva, Security and privacy in the internet of medical things: Taxonomy and risk assessment, in *2017 IEEE 42nd Conference on Local Computer Networks Workshops (LCN Workshops)*, (IEEE, 2017)
56. W. Sun et al., Security and privacy in the medical internet of things: A review. Secur. Commun. Netw. **2018**, 5978636 (2018)
57. E. Coiera, *Guide to Health Informatics* (CRC Press, 2015)
58. E. J. S. Hovenga, M. R. Kidd, S. Garde (eds.), *Health Informatics: An Overview*, vol 151 (Ios Press, 2010)
59. J. A. Magnuson, B. E. Dixon (eds.), *Public Health Informatics and Information Systems* (Springer Nature, 2020)
60. K.F. Hollis, L.F. Soualmia, B. Séroussi, Artificial intelligence in health informatics: Hype or reality? Yearb. Med. Inform. **28**(1), 3 (2019)
61. K. do Carmo Neves et al., Benefits and disadvantages of implementing the electronic patient record for the health service. Res. Soc. Develop. **9**(7), 735974630 (2020)
62. L.H. Schinasi et al., Using electronic health record data for environmental and place-based population health research: A systematic review. Ann. Epidemiol. **28**(7), 493–502 (2018)
63. A.F. Qasim, R. Aspin, F. Meziane, Integration of digital watermarking technique into medical imaging systems, in *2019 10th International Conference on Dependable Systems, Services, and Technologies (DESSERT)*, (IEEE, 2019)
64. T.A. Emon et al., Telemedicine and IoMT: Its importance regarding healthcare in Bangladesh. Int. J. Sci. Eng. Res. **9**(2), 5 (2018)
65. Y.-M. Kim, D. Delen, Medical informatics research trend analysis: A text mining approach. Health Informatics J. **24**(4), 432–452 (2018)
66. P. Kokol, K. Saranto, H.B. Vošner, eHealth and health informatics competences. Kybernetes **47** (2018). https://doi.org/10.1108/k-09-2017-0338
67. M. Elhoseny et al., A hybrid model of internet of things and cloud computing to manage big data in health services applications. Futur. Gener. Comput. Syst. **86**, 1383–1394 (2018)
68. M. Zheng et al., An emerging wearable world: New gadgetry produces a rising tide of changes and challenges. IEEE Syst. Man Cybern. Mag. **4**(4), 6–14 (2018)
69. G.E. Simon, Big data from health records in mental health care: Hardly clairvoyant but already useful. JAMA Psychiat. **76**(4), 349–350 (2019)
70. R. Gravina et al., Multi-sensor fusion in body sensor networks: State-of-the-art and research challenges. Inform. Fusion **35**, 68–80 (2017)
71. G. Fortino et al., Enabling effective programming and flexible management of efficient body sensor network applications. IEEE Trans. Hum. Mach. Syst. **43**(1), 115–133 (2012)
72. G. Fortino et al., Platform-independent development of collaborative wireless body sensor network applications: SPINE2, in *2009 IEEE International Conference on Systems, Man, and Cybernetics*, (IEEE, 2009)
73. G. Fortino et al., SPINE2: Developing BSN applications on heterogeneous sensor nodes, in *2009 IEEE International Symposium on Industrial Embedded Systems*, (IEEE, 2009)
74. S. Iyengar et al., A framework for creating healthcare monitoring applications using wireless body sensor networks, in *Proceedings of the ICST 3rd International Conference on Body Area Networks*, (2008)

75. V. Xafis et al., An ethics framework for big data in health and research. Asian Bioeth. Rev. **11**(3), 227–254 (2019)
76. E. Vayena, A. Blasimme, Health research with big data: Time for systemic oversight. J. Law Med. Ethics **46**(1), 119–129 (2018)
77. G. Manogaran et al., A new architecture of Internet of Things and big data ecosystem for secured smart healthcare monitoring and alerting system. Futur. Gener. Comput. Syst. **82**, 375–387 (2018)
78. S. Smys, J.S. Raj, Internet of things and big data analytics for health care with cloud computing. J. Inf. Technol. **1**(01), 9–18 (2019)
79. G. Aceto, V. Persico, A. Pescapé, Industry 4.0 and health: Internet of things, big data, and cloud computing for healthcare 4.0. J. Ind. Inf. Integr. **18**, 100129 (2020)
80. S. Tahir et al., An energy-efficient fog-to-cloud Internet of Medical Things architecture. Int. J. Distrib. Sens. Netw. **15**(5), 1550147719851977 (2019)
81. B. Sivathanu, Adoption of internet of things (IoT) based wearables for healthcare of older adults – a behavioural reasoning theory (BRT) approach. J. Enabling Technol. (2018)
82. M. Bargh, Digital health software and sensors: Internet of things-based healthcare services, wearable medical devices, and real-time data analytics. Am. J. Med. Res. **6**(2), 61–66 (2019)
83. J. Cecil et al., An IoMT based cyber training framework for orthopedic surgery using Next Generation Internet technologies. Inform. Med. Unlocked **12**, 128–137 (2018)
84. Y. Ushimaru et al., Innovation in surgery/operating room driven by Internet of Things on medical devices. Surg. Endosc. **33**(10), 3469–3477 (2019)
85. D.-N. Le et al. (eds.), *Emerging Technologies for Health and Medicine: Virtual Reality, Augmented Reality, Artificial Intelligence, Internet of Things, Robotics, Industry 4.0* (Wiley, 2018)
86. H. Nagano, Big data, information and communication technology, artificial intelligence, Internet of things: How important are they for gastroenterological surgery? Ann. Gastroenterol. Surg. **2**(3), 166 (2018)
87. Z. Liu et al., Deep reinforcement learning with its application for lung cancer detection in medical Internet of Things. Futur. Gener. Comput. Syst. **97**, 1–9 (2019)

Chapter 2
Big Medical Data Analytics Under Internet of Things

Arij Naser Abougreen

2.1 Introduction

Nowadays, the concept of Big Data is a very popular concept [1]. Data is generated with huge volume and very high speed and it is increased exponentially [2, 3]. Big data is not a novel concept. However, researches change the way of defining it continuously [4]. Recently, Big Data is defined by fifteen characteristics while in the past it was identified by three characteristics which are volume, variety and velocity [5–7]. Big Data in healthcare is an active research topic [7]. The size of Big Data in Healthcare was about 150 Exabytes in 2011, and it is increased by a rate between 1.2 and 2.4 Exabytes annually [8]. Big Data are complex data that cannot be managed and analyzed using conventional software and hardware [9]. Researchers from all over the world have difficulty in handling multidimensional healthcare data [10]. So, improved algorithms and approaches are required to obtain the best outcomes. Researchers have been developing novel techniques and algorithms to handle Big Data [2]. BDA plays a significant role in extracting the valuable information from huge volume of data [11, 12]. Healthcare is a data-rich sector [5]. Patient's health monitoring is useful for detecting various types of diseases [13]. It is predicted that the number of medical staff in 2030 will be forty-three million and this number will be much lower than what the world needs. So, alternatives are needed [14]. One of the most useful technologies that can help healthcare industry is IoT [13]. Machines which communicate with themselves and share data between each other are known as IoT [15]. These devices are linked and an IP address is assigned to each device [16]. To get IoT data, usually sensors are deployed to aggregate data and these data are transmitted to the centralized server. IoT permits generating huge amount of

A. N. Abougreen (✉)
Electrical and Electronic Engineering Department, University of Tripoli, Tripoli, Libya
e-mail: a.abougreen@uot.edu.ly

© The Author(s), under exclusive license to Springer Nature Switzerland AG 2021
C. Chakraborty et al. (eds.), *Efficient Data Handling for Massive Internet of Medical Things*, Internet of Things,
https://doi.org/10.1007/978-3-030-66633-0_2

data [17]. IoT is one of the internet applications which can improve our life and it includes machine to machine learning (M2M) [15, 17]. Extracting the useful data from IoT data is not an easy task. So, BDA tools are needed to analyze real-time data of IoT. Combining BDA with IoT makes IoT more valuable [15]. Big Data can be employed in healthcare field to analyze and manage a large amount of health data [18]. Privacy and security are the main challenges in IoT and BDA [10, 15, 19, 20]. The purpose of this chapter is to summarize Big Data characteristics, Big Data sources, BDA-related work, challenges of BDA in healthcare, BDA platforms and tools, Integrating BDA with IoT challenges, and recent advances in IoT-based Big Data.

This chapter is aimed to provide researchers a review on recent advances in IoT-based medical Big Data analytics.

The major contributions of this chapter are as follows:

- It reviews Big Data platforms and Tools.
- It reviews the work that has been done on BDA in healthcare. It also highlights the significance of Big Data in healthcare.
- It discusses the challenges of BDA in healthcare.
- It reviews different types of sensors in healthcare monitoring system and discusses the challenges that sensors face.
- It discusses the challenges of Integrating IoT with BDA.
- It reviews the recent advances in IoT-based Big Data.
- It will empower researchers to further work on BDA under IoT.

This chapter is organized as follows: in Sect. 2.2 Big Data definition is presented. Section 2.4 presents the healthcare Big Data sources. Section 2.5 reviews Big Data platforms and tools. In Sect. 2.6 BDA-related work is presented. Section 2.7 discusses the significance of Big Data in healthcare. The challenges of BDA are discussed in Sect. 2.8. Sections 2.9, 2.10, 2.11, 2.12, and 2.13 discuss IoT, sensors, sensor challenges, integrating IoT with BDA challenges and recent advances of IoT-based Big Data respectively. Figure 2.1 depicts the structure of the chapter.

2.2 Big Data Definition

The first property of Big Data that comes minds is size. However, there are other characteristics [21]. Big Data means huge data which involves structured, unstructured, and semi-structured data [11]. Most authors define Big Data by the three characteristics which are volume, velocity, and variety and they also known as three V's [11]. Volume is the large amount of data which are produced continuously from several sources. Velocity is the data which are produced rapidly and need to be processed in a rapid way for extracting useful information [9, 11]. Variety is the Big Data which are produced from different sources and in many formats. However, some authors and scientists have added more characteristics to give a better definition [11]. IBM has introduced the fourth V, which is veracity. Veracity indicates that

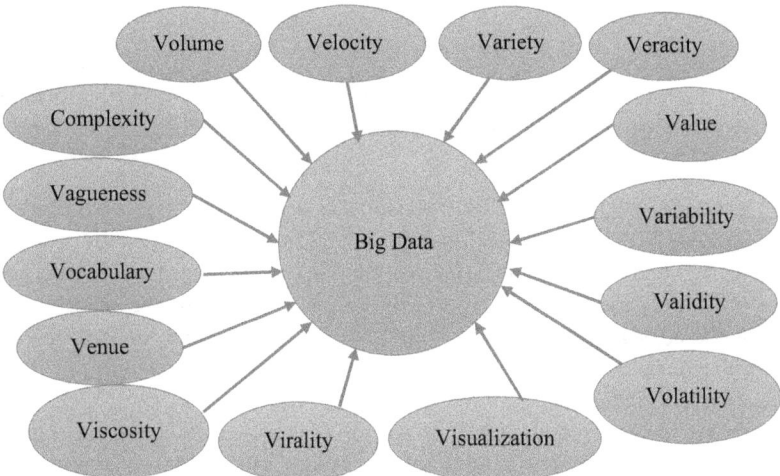

Fig. 2.1 Big Data characteristics

there are some unreliable sources of data [21]. It also refers to data quality and the degree of certainty [9]. Other authors have defined Big Data by six characteristics which are denoted as six Vs. These authors have added value and variability to the characteristics. Value refers to the useful outcomes of the analysis [9]. Variability relates to the data flow rate variance [21]. The authors in [6] describe Big Data by fifteen characteristics (Fourteen Vs and a C). Thus, Validity, Volatility, Visualization, Virality, Viscosity, Venue, Vocabulary, Vagueness, and Complexity have been added to the characteristics [6]. Complexity refers to the difficulty of organizing and analyzing Big Data due to evolving data relationships [11]. Figure 2.1 exhibits the Big Data characteristics.

2.3   Big Data Sources

There are essential sources of Big Data which are social data, machine data, and transactional data. Social data generates from likes, tweets, comments, and video updates. Machine data generates from industrial equipment such as sensors. These kinds of data are growing exponentially as IoT grows continuously. Transactional data generates from the daily transactions such as payment orders and storage records [22].

2.4   Healthcare Big Data Sources

1. *Physiological Data*

These data are enormous as far as volume and speed are concerned:

(a) *Volume*

An assortment of signals is gathered from different sources to monitor patient attributes involving blood pressure, blood glucose, and heart rate.

(b) *Velocity*

Data are collected rapidly. In healthcare sector, data is generated at high speeds [23]. The increased growth in data resulting from continuous monitoring needs to be processed in real time in order to assist making the appropriate decision. Effective approaches are needed to analyze and process the gathered signals to give useable data to the healthcare experts and other related partners [24].

2. *Electronic Medical Records/Electronic Health Records*

Electronic medical record (EMR) is a digital record which contains the medical activity information of the patient and it is usually used to make a treatment decision [1]. Electronic health records (EHRs) are the most important source for Big Data which are the digitized healthcare data from a patient [24, 25]. The EHR are gathered from and exchanged by clinics, and insurance agencies. EHR view, store, and gather all details of the patient's health like vital signs, immunizations, results from the test of radiology or laboratory, past clinical history, pathology reports, allergies, active medical problems, and medications [25–27]. EHR contain both structured and unstructured data [1, 25]. The difference between EHR and EMR is that EHR contains the whole patient records from birth to death in one place. So, EHR contains the patient's record from several doctors [1, 25].

3. *Medical Images*

These images produce a massive amount of data which can help experts for distinguishing or recognizing disease. Medical images are unstructured data which involve X-ray and CT scans. They play a significant role in diagnosis. Due to the complexity, dimensionality, and noise of the gathered images, effective image processing approaches are needed to offer appropriate data for patient care [24, 28]. One of the systems that can be employed for storing medical imaging are Picture Archival &Communication Systems (PACS) [25].

4. *Clinical Notes*

Clinical notes contain claims, recommendations, and decisions and they are one of the biggest unstructured wellsprings of healthcare Big Data. Due to the diversity in format, dependability, completeness, and exactness of the clinical notes, it is difficult to assure that the healthcare provider has the right information. Effective data mining and natural language processing techniques are needed to extract useful data [24].

5. *Behavioral Data*

The sources of this data are social network data and sensors data [25, 28]. Sensors collect data from patients. Diseases and their related symptoms are tracked continuously for providing best cure [28].

6. *Genomic Data*

   This data addresses aspects of DNA in structural and serial order of different functions of genes. There is a need for a particular program that can store and process this data. A repository named genomic database includes human genomes and association rules related to genomes. This repository identifies the identical symptoms that affect health and its related infections [28].

2.5 Big Data Platforms and Tools

1. *Advanced Data Visualization (ADV)*

   It is helpful for handling with various data types and it can be used easily. Moreover, it assists analysts to explore data. It achieves perfect results and it is employed for extraction of medical hidden patterns in healthcare data [25, 28].

2. *Presto*

   Presto is a distributed SQL Query engine which is employed to analyze a large amount of clinical data. Using Presto, data analysis can be performed rapidly [25, 28].

3. *Hive*

   Hive was at first evolved by Facebook; however, it is currently utilized and developed by different organizations such as Netflix and Amazon [24]. It is employed to handle with large-scale data records. Compared to Presto, Hive is slower. However, it is an effective tool which can perform all Excel sheet missions efficiently. It is commonly used to store and retrieve medical records [25, 28]. Data stored in Hive can be accessed by Presto [25]. Hive is utilized for Big Data analysis, summarization, and queries [3].

4. *Vertica*

   It is similar to Presto and is used to process a massive volume of clinical data which can be used later for data analytics. Also, it is affordable and its architecture has the advantage of simplicity. In addition, it has other advantages such as operational costs and accelerating healthcare reports and documentation which assist in analyzing health patterns of patients [25, 28].

5. *Key Performance Indicators (KPI)*

   They use electronic healthcare records to determine practices of people. Patients who are more susceptible to clinic environment may be exposed to KPI tool to improve outcomes [28].

6. *Online Analytics Processing (OLAP)*

   In OLAP, data is ordered in multidimensional patterns and statistical computation can be performed rapidly. It increases data safety restrictions and improve quality control. Also, it tracks healthcare records and assists in disease diagnosis [25, 28].

7. *Online Transaction Processing (OLTP)*
   It is used to process registration of patients. It is also employed for analyzing different operations of patients [28].

8. *Apache Hadoop*
   It was utilized for the first time by Yahoo and Facebook. It is an open source data processing framework which can store and process A massive volume of data on a cluster of hardware [29]. This framework is based on Java [30]. Hadoop consists of many components and the most significant ones are Hadoop Distributed File System and the MapReduce programming model. HDF is employed for storing data, while MapReduce is utilized for processing these data [29]. There are many benefits of Hadoop such as high scalability and flexibility, cost-effectiveness, and reliability to manage and process a large volume of structured and unstructured data [31].

9. *The Hadoop Distributed File System (HDFS)*
   HDFS improves the performance of clinical data analytics due to the partition process of massive data sets into small ones. These small data samples are distributed across whole system. It assists in diagnosis [25, 28].

10. *Casandra File System (CFS)*
    It is very similar to HDFS and it is employed to deal with analytical processes and tolerates errors [28].

11. *Map Reduce System*
    This system handles with a large amount of data. It segments the chore into subchores and gathers its yield. It efficiently incorporates different operational computations into the system. It monitors each server where the chore is being performed. It can perform parallel errands effectively [28]. It is cost-effective [3].

12. *HBase*
    It is a column-oriented management database. It runs on the top of HDFS. It is suitable to process the real-time data [32]. It is used to gather and analyze billions of rows in a short time [3].

13. *Cloud Computing*
    Cloud computing has a great impact in healthcare field. It makes healthcare more valuable via reducing costs, increasing the productivity and data analysis. It also offers excellent security [25].

14. *1010data*
    1010data contains of a columnar database and it is commonly used to handle with semi-structured data like such as IoT data. It can visualize, report, and integrate data. It is an advanced analytic tool. It can provide optimization and statistical analysis services. In addition, it supports large-scale infrastructure. The drawback of this tool is the inefficiency of extraction and transformation of data [29].

15. *Cloudera Data Hub*
    It is a Hadoop-based platform which is used for process and analyze the massive IoT data. To obtain more reliable service and excellent performance and data access control, the Cloudera Data Hub integrates Cloudera Manager, Navigator, and its backup and recovery components [29].

16. *Infobright*

It is employed to solve data management and analytic issues. About fifty tera-bytes of data can be analyzed via this tool. It is appropriate for IoT data. This tool is commonly employed with Hadoop [29].

17. *Hortonworks*

It builds a massive IoT data analytics and management framework based on Hadoop. The Hortonworks Data Platform (HDP) possess a free open source software distribution and concentrates on the enhancement of Hive. However, with its HDP plugin, it doesn't have the ability to decrease the number hosts per node group in the produced cluster [29].

18. *HP-HAVEn*

The Hadoop Autonomy Vertica Enterprise (HAVEn) security was presented by HP. It is a novel large IoT data platform architecture for a large number of HP systems which is employed with any number of applications. HP offers refer-ence equipment setups for the major distributors of the Hadoop software. Autonomy's IDOL software offers search and exploration services for unstruc-tured data [29].

19. *MongoDB*

It can be employed as a file system. It can manage data which change fre-quently. Also, it can be utilized for unstructured or semi-structured [24].

20. *Apache Spark*

It is an open source framework which is utilized to process a large amount of data. It outperforms Hadoop MapReduce in speed and simplicity. It supports real-time processing machine learning algorithms [3, 7, 33].

21. *Apache Mahout*

Apache mahout is a highly scalable and it supports machine learning techniques for smart data analysis applications [33].

2.6 Big Data Analytics–Related Work

A large volume of data is generated continuously. So, advanced data analysis is needed for better understanding and extracting the valuable information. There are many challenges of BDA such as the complexity of data which is a heterogenous data. BDA is an active research field. There are various analytical techniques involv-ing data mining, visualization, statistical analysis, and machine learning [11, 34]. Data mining can help in diagnosis of diseases and providing efficient treatments [35].

BDA has the capability for handling a huge amount of data efficiently. Healthcare field produces a massive amount of data. These data could be structured or unstruc-tured which makes processing them a challenging task. In [36], EMR which has been generated from many medical devices and apps was induced into MongoDB via Hadoop framework. So, better understanding for data was achieved and decision can be taken quickly [36].

Heterogenous data are generated in healthcare sector. Without BDA data are use-less [37]. In [37], a survey on BDA in healthcare is presented. It was found that Hadoop can performs BDA effectively. Thus, urgent cases can be predicted.

BDA can support doctors' decision [38]. In [38], authors present a review on BDA in healthcare. BDA platforms, algorithms, and challenges have been presented.

In [39], Big Data framework for healthcare systems was proposed. These sys-tems can provide services based on the analysis of vital signs such as ECG. Algorithms for extracting feature values from raw data were added to Hadoop platform due to the inability of Hadoop to handle unstructured bio-signals.

In [40], authors present a review on utilization of BDA in heart attack prediction. Also, privacy concerns and challenges of BDA were discussed. It was found that BDA can be utilized to predict and prevent heart attack effectively.

In [41], the authors present a system for gathering EHR using Hadoop frame-work. These EHRs is stored in Hbase which is the database employed by Hadoop ecosystem. MapReduce functions are employed to split the data into parts. Each subpart is mapped to a specific node in the cluster for processing purpose. Medical data can be updated and statistics can be viewed.

Healthcare sector contains a large amount of data with high speed. This huge volume of data needs novel BDA framework where conventional machine learning tools cannot be applied directly. In [42], BDA framework was proposed to develop risk adjustment model of patient expenditures. Random forest regression algorithm was employed to enhance the accuracy of the predictive model. This paper exhibits the efficacy of predictive analytics using random forest algorithm.

BDA and deep learning are two important techniques as several organizations have been aggregating a huge amount of data [43]. The paper in [43] was discussing the significance of deep learning in BDA and its ability to extract useful information from a huge volume of data.

In [44], the authors were discussing that deep learning plays a significant role in predictive analytics and it can be used in analyzing medical images and diagnosis of diseases.

In [45], a voice pathology detection system using deep learning on the mobile healthcare framework was proposed. A convolutional neural network has been used. The obtained accuracy was 97.5%.

Measuring hospital's performance is a significant process. However, it is not an easy task. BDA can be used to measure the performance of the hospitals in order to enhance the quality of the healthcare. In [46], the performance of US hospitals has been measured using machine learning.

In [47], BDA framework to analyze ten billion health records has been proposed. To build BDA platform, changing the configurations of MapReduce and the index-ing of HBASE are required. This work has exhibited that the presented BDA pro-cess and configuration fulfilled security requirements. Also, the performance was satisfied.

In [48], BDA techniques in healthcare, applications, and challenges have been reviewed. It was found that BDA increases the treatment efficiency. In addition, it can be used to predict diseases. Also, deep learning can provide advanced BDA in the area of medical images.

Health forecasting is very significant. Many researchers have worked on this area in order to provide effective predictive analytics model which can forecast the future health situation using machine learning. In [49], BDA model was proposed for disease forecasting using Naive Bayes Technique (BPA-NB). This technique is an appropriate huge dataset. Heart disease data was used to train the model. The obtained accuracy was 97.12%. Hadoop-spark was employed as a computing tool.

Cancer diagnosis at early stages is very crucial for effective treatment. Each single patient record produces a huge amount of data. Various machine learning methods were proposed to classify cancer [50]. In [50], BDA algorithm was proposed to diagnose cancer. HDFS was used to classify EHRs and EMRs. Also, National Language Processing (NLP) was utilized for the analysis and classification of cancer patient data.

Mining is an approach to explore a huge amount of data and extract the hidden patterns in order to understand the medical data and prevent heart diseases. There are various data mining techniques including Naïve Bayes, Decision tree, Neural network, genetic algorithm and clustering algorithms like KNN, and Support vector machine. In [51], data mining models for predicting heart disease are reviewed.

2.7 Significance of Big Data in Healthcare

It is significant to extract worthy information and get rid of useless parts from Big Data. Big Data in healthcare can achieve economic advantages using BDA such as saving money in the healthcare industry. In addition, it can be employed in clinical diagnosis, medical research, and hospital management [1]. Research institutions can benefit from BDA in developing drugs. For instance, cancer data can also be reprocessed to produce new cancer medicines. Thus, clinical trials can be improved with the help of statistical tools. So, BDA can provide effective drugs and it reduces the cost for patients [1, 37]. BDA assures that patients get the suitable treatment [23]. Also, doctors can made best decision based on these analytics, leading to improving care of patients. BDA can assist in predicting disease in an early stage before spreading. Thus, spreading can be prevented [37]. Using BDA governments can monitor the quality of the hospitals and can take the required procedures against the disqualified hospitals [37]. Health data can be stored, managed, and shared by the patients easily using smart phone apps and online websites. With the help of BDA, the diseases can be detected earlier than before and patients can get their cure in an early stage. Patients can monitor their health and enhance their lives using information mining and make the right decision about their health such as choosing the best diet and exercises [1, 23]. Via BDA, insurance companies can make the best policies [29].

2.8   Challenges of BDA

There is a massive amount of data available in healthcare industry, so it is difficult to know which data can be employed and why. Also, there is another issue, which is the lack of suitable IT infrastructure. Furthermore, there is a need to employ distributed data processing instead of paper records [52]. It is predicted that Big Data of healthcare will be nearly 40 ZB by the end of 2020. Healthcare Big Data consists of a huge amount of unstructured data which makes data analysis a difficult task [1]. In addition, BDA systems which can be employed for real-time cases are required [52]. Also, there is a difficulty in storing large amounts of medical data owing to the high cost of storage process. Healthcare industry generates huge data such as medical images and the outcomes of diagnostic tests. These medical data are growing continuously and they require to be maintained for a long time which is over fifty years in order to track the patient's health [1, 5]. Medical data are the most sensitive one in the Big Data and patient's data need to be protected to maintain the privacy of the patient. Data sharing between hospitals and health organization increases the concern of the issue of Big Data privacy in the healthcare sector. Moreover, one of the problems that governments face in BDA for healthcare is that there isn't much data protocols and standards [1, 5, 52]. Another issue is that EHRs data depend on the team that enter the patient's data and this team may enter wrong data and this will affect the outcome [9]. Also, there are a few companies in the word which are professional in the field of BDA, So, there is an urgent need for well-trained data analysts who have a good knowledge for visualizing the data using best tools and they can interpret the Big Data results [1, 52].

Moreover, a healthcare professional charges their service fees by meeting face to face with the patient. This generates serious prejudice against permitting new technology which reduces human interaction [53].

The data in several healthcare organizations, especially hospitals, are usually fragmented. For example, cost information is employed by the financial team. Clinical data like patient history, vital signs, progress notes, and the outcomes of diagnostic tests are stored in the EHR. These data are available to the physicians and nurses and are employed for tracking patient care and making cure plan [5, 53]. The solution for fragmentation problem is collecting data from different sources

Then this data should be normalized into a consistent structure. So, organizations will not need data bridges. Also, AI will have the ability to perform well in real time [53].

Imbalanced data is another challenge in Big Data. Recently, this issue has gained big attention [11]. Sometimes there are two classes with unequal distributions. Also, imbalanced multi-classes are another issue [11].

Also, monitor systems generate continuous data streams such as electrocardiogram which is hard to store. In addition, storing all these Big Data is too expensive, leading to incompleteness of data [1].

2.9   IoT

IoT can develop our life and save time. Recently, there are many research studies on IoT. So, IoT is a hot topic and there are many investments on it. IoT is composed of billions (even trillions) of connected objects which share data between each other. These objects are called smart objects (SOs) [54–59]. Security and privacy are the main challenges in IoT. In the healthcare sector, there are huge concerns about privacy due to the sensitivity of patient's data [60]. IoT devices produce continuous streams of data. So, it is significant to develop tools for analyzing IoT data [33]. Wearable devices are very significant devices in IoT. Wearable sensors can be utilized for measuring different types of signals. These sensors play a crucial role for patients by measuring different parameters of them. There are different types of sensors with various functions to take care of patients or assist patients to prohibit the risks. These sensors assist doctors to put more attention to patients [61, 62]. There are many types of sensors such as electrocardiogram sensor (ECG) which is utilized for monitoring heart muscles activity [63, 64]. ECG is one of the easiest tests utilized for determining vital data about the cardiovascular system of a patients [64]. Electromyography sensor is employed for monitoring muscle function activity [63]. This measurement is employed for detecting neuromuscular abnormalities [65]. Electroencephalogram is utilized for monitoring brain electrical activity via electrodes at various locations on the scalp [63, 64]. An electroencephalogram machine is composed of electrodes, amplifiers, filters, and recording unit [64]. Blood pressure sensor is used for measuring the force exerted by circulating blood on the walls of blood vessels [63]. The device employed for measuring blood pressure is named sphygmomanometer. The blood pressure is usually expressed in terms of systolic pressure (when the heart beats) over diastolic pressure (when the heart is at rest between two heartbeats) in the cardiac cycle [64]. Breathing sensor monitors respiration [63]. Motion sensors are employed for estimating the level of activity [63]. The normal body temperature of an individual relies upon gender, time of measurement, and recent activities. The typical range for body temperature is from $36.5\ C°$ to $37.2\ C°$ for a healthy individual [61]. A high body temperature is a sign that a person has an infection or fever [64]. Temperature sensor gathers data about temperature from a source and changes it into a form that can be understood by any other device or individual. It is one of the most commonly used sensors in healthcare sector. There are two essential sorts of temperature sensors: contact sensors and non-contact sensors. Contact sensors differ from non-contact sensors in that they need direct physical contact with the object that is being sensed [61]. The level of oxygen in blood is a very significant factor. Pulse oximeter is employed for monitoring a person's oxygen saturation [64]. Wearable devices are usually networked in order to perform powerful tasks. Wireless Sensor Networks (WSN) have potential applications in many industries such as healthcare monitoring application. This application is aimed at guaranteeing continuous monitoring of patients' status in a way that enables patients to have freedom of movement [66, 67]. Body Sensor Network (BSN) is a network which is composed of wireless wearable (programmable) sensor nodes that communicate with a local personal device. The essential elements of this emerging technology are sensors, communication protocols, and coordinators [62, 68]. There are many applications of BSN such as healthcare, fitness, smart cities, and many other IoT applications. BSN is considered as a branch of WSN. However, there are many differences between these two networks. WSN has a larger number of nodes than BSN. In addition, it covers larger geographical range. BSN uses the least number of nodes with high accuracy. Moreover, batteries of BSN nodes can be recharged or replaced [69]. BSN applications need more sensors sampling, data transmission rate, and continuous monitoring [69].

2.10   Sensors Challenges

Careful studies are being carried out by researchers to design intelligent body sensors for continuous monitoring for patients with good accuracy. However, they face many challenges. The first challenge is fabricating and implementations. Second, there are both hardware and software limitations. There are many factors that should be taken into account when designing these sensors such as weight, cost, size, energy consumption, and safety. Another challenge that sensors network may face is loss of packets or fading during data transmission process which will lead to latency issue. So, the solution for this issue is allocating the bandwidth in medium access control (Mac) layer [70]. Also, Wireless Body Area Networks (WBANs) face many challenges such as physical layer, MAC layer, network layer, transport layer, and application layer challenges. Physical layer faces various challenges during the implementation of WBANs such as bandwidth limitations, receiver complexity, and Power consumption [66]. For health monitoring applications, Quality of Service (QoS) needs for emergency traffic should be taken into account [66]. Also, one of the hot topics of wireless healthcare observing networks is the ability of these systems to diminish the energy consumption of computing and communication infrastructure [66]. Moreover, dependable data transmission is a significant requirement of a wireless healthcare network. So, frames or packets loss may lead to a latency of information problem [66]. The application layer is at the head of the stack. Thus, it is anticipated to have a coordination role. In this case, data management is important and needs an effective machine learning algorithm to permit autonomous system replacing [66].

2.11   Integrating IoT with BDA Challenges

1. *Privacy*
   Privacy is the most significant challenge in BDA due to the unwillingness of many users to work on the same system which doesn't provide any agreement to protect their personal data. There some temporary strategies which are used to protect the personal information of the user but these techniques are not related

to privacy. In IoT analysis, security issue is owing to heterogeneous of the devices which interact and share data between them [19, 20]. So, appropriate authentication is needed [19].

2. *Security*
   There are concerns about the safety of the devices due to the possibility of physical damage. So, these devices need to be protected [15].
3. *Data Mining*
   Analysis of huge amount of data which is produced by IoT faces many challenges such as information extraction, data visualization, and integration [19].
4. *Energy Consumption*
   The energy consumption by the devices would be large. So, solutions are needed to reduce this consumption [15].
5. *Integration*
   Data which is aggregated from several devices can be of structured, unstructured, and semi-structured data. Integration of these data is a complex process [19].

2.12 Recent Advances in IoT-Based Big Data

IoT plays a significant role in the healthcare sector by aggregating and analyzing the medical information to minimize the medical errors [71]. The emerging BDA techniques can be used to improve the health sector. BDA can assist in analyzing a massive amount of health data [18]. IoT is one of the most significant Big Data sources which is based on connecting several intelligent devices to the internet [72]. In [18], real-time big medical data were aggregated from patients using sensors. Then these data are transferred to the cloud server in order to be analyzed. Then the analyzed data will be transferred to the associated individuals. This research has merged the technologies of Big Data, IoT and cloud computing. Figure 2.2 illustrates the methodology that has been used.

The authors in [73] have confirmed the significance of Big Data in the healthcare sector. It was found that body sensors produce huge volumes of health data. Two tasks were performed: merging these Big Data points with EHR and displaying these data to supervising doctors in real time. This work has proposed a sensor integration framework which presents a scalable cloud architecture that offer a holistic approach to the EHR sensor system. Apache Kafka and Spark was employed for processing the real-time Big Data. Using this system, a patient's health can be visualized in real time which can assist in detecting urgent cases.

Cardiovascular disease is becoming a major concern worldwide. Many people all over the world have several chronic heart diseases. The number of deaths due to heart diseases also increases constantly. So, there is an urgent need for ECG monitoring system to monitor the patient continuously and remotely [74]. The work in [74] has proposed a system which merges the concept of Nanoelectronics, Internet of Things (IoT), and Big Data. The nanomaterial reduces the cost of ECG sensors.

Fig. 2.2 The used
methodology

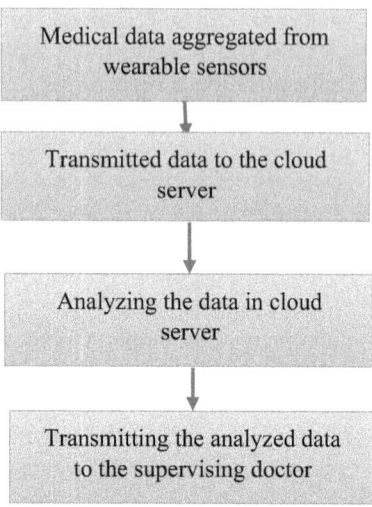

IoT assists the ECG signals to be sent through the sensor via a gateway using communication protocols such as Bluetooth, Zigbee, 3G/4G, Wi-Fi, and LAN. Then the data is transmitted to the doctor's end or the cloud storage to analyze or process the data. The patient's data can be displayed on several intelligent devices. Then urgent situations can be detected. BDA plays a significant role in analyzing data and extracting useful information.

In [75], BDA-based IoT Healthcare system was proposed. This system contains several sensors to monitor patients' health. It is difficult to handle the massive amount of medical data which is generated from sensors. So, Intel Galileo Gen 2 was worked as an IoT agent and was employed for deploying the health information of patients into the Thinspeak Cloud and then these Big Data was analyzed by Hadoop framework. The system can alert doctors in case of emergencies.

Obtrusive sleep apnea (OSA) is a sleep disorder that has a negative effect on the patient's life. So, systems which can detect OSA are needed. In [76], an effective system which can assist in detecting OSA and supporting treatment is proposed. This system monitors several factors like sleep environment, sleep condition, physical activities, and physiological parameters. This system has the capability to perform two kinds of processing, which are preprocessing and batch data processing. Preprocessing is done at the edge of the network which leads to an improvement in the efficiency of the system. The proposed system has demonstrated a 93.3% of effectivity in the air quality index prediction for guiding the OSA cure.

Wearable devices are uncomfortable especially when they are used for a long time. So, another solution is needed [77]. In [77], Smart clothes were designed for health monitoring purpose. The visualization of wearable sensor data is performed using a mobile application. These data are also stored on a "health cloud," which is merged with a machine learning library for diagnostic and predictive analytics purposes [77, 78].

Due to the increased number of the elder and disabled individuals, there is a significant need for efficient systems for health monitoring. In [79], the authors proposed an IoT-based health monitoring system. ECG and other health data which are collected from wearable devices and sensors are sent to the cloud and can be accessed by professionals. Signal improvement, watermarking, and analytics were employed for avoiding identity theft [78, 79].

IoT has proved its significance in remote health organizations [80]. The authors in [80] were discussing about that IoT in healthcare produces a massive amount of data. This paper also demonstrates the architecture of IoT which is composed of five layers: physical layer, network layer, application layer, middleware layer, and business layer. The physical layer composes of sensors which are employed to aggregate data. Network layer is the interface between the sensors and the servers. Application layer is employed for providing services to the users using defining several applications of IoT. Middleware Layer is employed to store and process the data. Business layer deals with system management.

Recently there are concerns about sleep apnea (SA) owing to the increasing number of patients and deaths, as well as the high costs of patient care. Some solutions were proposed to support treatment of elderly people. However, these solutions have some defects. In [81], an effective system to support SA patients was introduced. This system combines fog computing, cloud computing, IoT platform, and Big Data platform. IoT Big Data is analyzed using Big Data analyzer. This system is tested using a dataset with a size of 30 GB and questionnaire which was filled by specialists. The outcomes exhibit that data analytics help specialists to take the right decision and guide patients in treatment which will affect elderly life positively.

In [82], the significance of IoT and BDA in support of precision medicine was discussed. The computational flow of in silico knowledge data discovery was introduced and analyzed and the useful results for the case study of genome mapping dependent on computer model of RNA have been revealed.

There is an urgent need to provide better healthcare services. IoT and BDA can significantly improve the healthcare sector, which is one of the biggest sectors. Thus, better services can be provided. BDA for IoT health data can assist in detecting the diseases at an early stage and making the suitable decisions. In [83], the recent trends in healthcare systems were discussed. The authors focused on cloud computing, fog computing, BDA, and IoT. In addition, the challenges in providing enhanced healthcare systems are discussed. It was clarified that the biggest challenges in the healthcare systems are privacy and security problems.

IoT can be employed in many applications such as smart home, smart farming, and smart healthcare. The massive amount of data produced by deployed sensors needs to be analyzed to make the appropriate decision and improve the accuracy. Deep learning plays a crucial role in making intelligent IoT [84]. In [85], the role of deep learning analytics in IoT has been investigated. In this paper an IoT platform was implemented to analyze and classify the real-time ECG data using Convolutional Neural Network. In [2], IoT architecture was proposed for storing and processing big sensor data of healthcare applications. MapReduce-based logistic regression has been implemented with the assist of Apache Mahout to develop a model for predicting heart diseases.

2.13 Conclusion

IoT means several objects which are connected to each other and has the capability to share data between them. The large amount of data produced by sensors and healthcare applications is continuously increased. These data can be structured, unstructured, or semi-structured data. This massive data is called Big Data. There is a difficulty in storing, processing, and analyzing these data using conventional methods. So, new technologies are needed to extract the useful information for the analysis purpose. There is an increased demand for BDA in healthcare field owing to its crucial role. BDA provides an overview of patient data which has been collected from several sources. Using BDA, decision can be made correctly at the right time. BDA can be employed to manage and control the large datasets. Thus, BDA can enhance the quality of our life. The advancement of Big Data and IoT has a significant impact in all fields including healthcare sector. Integrating IoT and BDA can improve the healthcare field. In this chapter, Big Data characteristics, Big Data sources, and sources of Big Data in healthcare are reviewed. BDA-related work and significance of Big Data in healthcare are highlighted. Reviewing BDA challenges, Big Data platforms and tools, sensors, and integrating BDA with IoT challenges were other parts of this chapter. Finally, the recent advances in IoT-based Big Data are highlighted.

2.14 Future Scope

More efforts are needed for developing machine learning approaches for BDA in healthcare and integrating them with the hardware. Also, future research is required for solving IoT challenges such as security and privacy. Also, most of the research studies on BDA in healthcare sector were from the developed countries. So, it is significant to encourage the researches on BDA in healthcare in the developing countries in order to deliver better quality of care. In addition, future research is required to solve sensors challenges.

References

1. L. Hong et al., Big Data in health care: Applications and challenges. Data Inform. Manag **1**(2), 122–135 (2018)

2. R.M. Stuppia, E. Ferone, L. Manzoli, A. Pitasi, *Innovative Healthcare Systems for the 21st Century* (Springer, Cham, 2017), pp. 15–70
3. I.A. Ajah, H.F. Nweke, Big Data and business analytics: Trends, platforms, success factors and applications. Big Data Cogn. Comput. **3**(2), 32 (2019)
4. G. Chen, M. Islam, Big Data analytics in healthcare, Proceedings of 2019 2nd international conference safe production informatization IICSPI 2019, vol. 2015, pp. 227–230, 2019
5. D. Press, A review of Big Data in health care: Challenges and opportunities. Open Access Bioinform **2014**, 13 (2014)
6. G. Kapil, A. Agrawal, R.A. Khan, A study of Big Data characteristics, Proceedings of international conference on communication and electronic system. ICCES 2016, September 2018, 2016
7. H.B. Patel, S. Gandhi, A review on Big Data analytics in healthcare using machine learning approaches, in *Proceedings of the 2nd International Conference on Trends in Electronics and Informatics, ICOEI 2018*, (2018, no. ICOEI), pp. 84–90
8. J.A. Rodger, Informatics in medicine unlocked discovery of medical Big Data analytics: Improving the prediction of traumatic brain injury survival rates by data mining patient informatics processing software hybrid Hadoop Hive. Inform. Med. Unlocked **1**(2015), 17–26 (2016)
9. B. Ristevski, M. Chen, Big Data analytics in medicine and healthcare. J. Integr. Bioinform. **15**(3), 1–5 (2018)
10. M.M.H. Onik, S. Aich, J. Yang, C.-S. Kim, H. Kim, Blockchain in healthcare: Challenges and solutions, in *Big Data Analytics for Intelligent Healthcare Management*, (Elsevier Inc., London, 2019), pp. 197–226
11. A. Oussous, F. Benjelloun, A. Ait, S. Belfkih, Big Data technologies: A survey. J. King Saud Univ. - Comput. Inf. Sci. **30**(4), 431–448 (2018)
12. K. Padmavathi, C. Deepa, P. Prabhakaran, Internet of Things (IoT) and Big Data. Int. J. Manag. Technol. Eng **8**(Xii), 217–246 (2020)
13. R. Priyanka, M. Reji, IoT based health monitoring system using machine learning. Int. J. Eng. Adv. Technol. **8**(6), 78–81 (2019)
14. M.D. Lytras, K.T. Chui, A. Visvizi, Data analytics in smart healthcare: The recent developments and beyond. Appl. Sci. **9**(14), 2812 (2019)
15. T. Bomatpalli, Blending Iot and Big Data analytics. Int. J. Eng. Res. Technol **4**, 1 (2018)
16. K.R. Kundhavai, S. Sridevi, IoT and Big Data-the current and future technologies: A review. Int. J. Comput. Sci. Mob. Comput. **5**(1), 10–14 (2016)
17. Y. Simmhan, Big Data analytics platforms for real-time applications in IoT, in *Big Data Analytics*, (Springer, New Delhi, 2016)
18. A.P. Plageras et al., Efficient large-scale medical data (eHealth Big Data) analytics in Internet of Things, 2017
19. H. Kaur, A.S. Kushwaha, A review on integration of Big Data and IoT, in *Proceedings - 4th International Conference on Computing Sciences, ICCS 2018*, (2019), pp. 200–203
20. M.J. Bharathi, V.N. Rajavarman, A survey on Big Data management in health care using IOT. Int. J. Recent Technol. Eng. **7**(5), 196–198 (2019)
21. A. Gandomi, M. Haider, International Journal of Information Management Beyond the hype: Big Data concepts, methods, and analytics. Int. J. Inf. Manag. **35**(2), 137–144 (2015)
22. https://www.cloudmoyo.com/blog/data-architecture/what-is-big-data-and-where-it-comes-from/?fbclid=IwAR3vhpxLIhxnJerGXMosUgeQZ8VvGYYHoEgyvAlMa7rasn6w6jNP1xsZ85I
23. S. Kumar, M. Singh, Big Data analytics for healthcare industry: Impact, applications, and tools. Big Data Min. Anal. **2**(1), 48–57 (2018)
24. A. Rghioui, J. Lloret, A. Oumnad, Big Data classification and internet of things in healthcare. Int. J. E-Health Med. Commun. **11**(2), 20–37 (2020)
25. N. Nalini, P. Suvithavani, A study on data analytics: Internet of Things & health-care. Int. J. Comput. Sci. Mobile. Comput **6**, 20 (2017)

26. I.K. Subagja et al., Evaluation of Big Data analytics in medical science. Int. J. Eng. Adv. Technol **8**(6 Special Issue 3), 717–720 (2019)
27. P. Saranya, P. Asha, Survey on Big Data analytics in health care, Proceedings of 2nd international conference on smart systems and inventive technology, no. Icssit, pp. 46–51, 2019
28. S. Mishra, B.K. Mishra, H.K. Tripathy, A. Dutta, Analysis of the role and scope of Big Data analytics with IoT in health care domain, in *Handbook of Data Science Approaches for Biomedical Engineering*, (Elsevier Inc., London, 2020)
29. E. Ahmed et al., The role of Big Data analytics in Internet of Things. Comput. Netw. **129**, 459 (2017)
30. S. Mishra, Appl and undefined 2018, A review on Big Data analytics in medical imaging. IJCEA. Com **XII**(I), 31–37 (2013)
31. T.L. Coelho Da Silva et al., Big Data analytics technologies and platforms: A brief review, in *CEUR Workshop Proceedings*, vol. 2170, (2018, Aug), pp. 25–32
32. S.S.R.D. Reddy, U.K. Ramanadham, Big Data analytics for healthcare organization, BDA process, benefits and challenges of BDA: A review. Adv. Sci. Technol. Eng. Syst. **2**(4), 189–196 (2017)
33. R.S.K. Althaf, R.K. Sai, R.K. Girija, Challenging tools on research issues in Big Data analytics. Int. J. Eng. Dev. Res. **6**(1), 637–644 (2018)
34. M. Marjani et al., Big IoT data analytics: Architecture, opportunities, and open research challenges. IEEE Access **5**, 5247–5261 (2017)
35. L. Elezabeth, V.P. Mishra, J. Dsouza, The role of Big Data mining in healthcare applications, in *2018 7th International Conference on Reliability, Infocom Technologies and Optimization: Trends and Future Directions, ICRITO 2018*, (2018, Aug), pp. 256–260
36. J. Antony Basco, N.C. Senthilkumar, Real-time analysis of healthcare using Big Data analytics, in *IOP Conference Series: Materials Science and Engineering*, vol. 263, no. 4, (2017)
37. J. Archenaa, E.A.M. Anita, A survey of Big Data analytics in healthcare and government. Procedia Comput. Sci. **50**, 408–413 (2015)
38. G. Chen, M. Islam, Big Data analytics in healthcare, Proc. - 2019 2nd international conference safe production informatization. IICSPI 2019, no. May 2015, pp. 227–230, 2019
39. T.W. Kim, K.H. Park, S.H. Yi, H.C. Kim, A Big Data framework for u-healthcare systems utilizing vital signs, in *Proceedings - 2014 International Symposium on Computer, Consumer and Control, IS3C 2014*, (2014), pp. 494–497
40. C.A. Alexander, L. Wang, Big Data analytics in heart attack prediction. J. Nurs. Care **06**(02), 393 (2017)
41. B. Shaikh, M. Bagwan, K. Shah, P. Jain, B.K. Bodkhe, HUMAN - Hadoop used medical ANalytics: A survey, in *Proceedings of the 2017 International Conference on Big Data Analytics and Computational Intelligence, ICBDACI 2017*, (2017), pp. 122–127
42. L. Li, S. Bagheri, H. Goote, A. Hasan, G. Hazard, Risk adjustment of patient expenditures: A Big Data analytics approach, in *Proceedings - 2013 IEEE International Conference on Big Data, Big Data 2013*, (2013), pp. 12–14
43. M.M. Najafabadi, F. Villanustre, T.M. Khoshgoftaar, N. Seliya, R. Wald, E. Muharemagic, Deep learning applications and challenges in Big Data analytics. J. Big Data **2**(1), 1–21 (2015)
44. B. Jeyakumar, Big Data deep learning in healthcare for electronic health records. Int. Sci. Res. Organ. J. **02**(02), 31–35 (2017)
45. M. Alhussein, G. Muhammad, Voice pathology detection using deep learning on mobile healthcare framework. IEEE Access **6**, 41034–41041 (2018)
46. N.S. Downing et al., Describing the performance of U.S. hospitals by applying Big Data analytics. PLoS One **12**(6), 1–14 (2017)
47. M.H. Kuo, D. Chrimes, B. Moa, W. Hu, Design and construction of a Big Data analytics framework for health applications, in *Proceedings - 2015 IEEE International Conference on Smart City, SmartCity 2015, Held Jointly with 8th IEEE International Conference on Social Computing and Networking, SocialCom 2015, 5th IEEE International Conference on Sustainable Computing and Communic*, (2015), pp. 631–636

48. N.C. Onyemachi, O.F. Nonyelum, Big Data analytics in healthcare: A review, in *2019 15th International Conference on Electronics, Computer and Computation, ICECCO 2019*, (2019, no. ICECCO), pp. 2–6
49. R. Venkatesh, C. Balasubramanian, M. Kaliappan, Development of Big Data predictive analytics model for disease prediction using machine learning technique. J. Med. Syst. **43**(8), 272 (2019)
50. K. Sivakumar, N.S. Nithya, O. Revathy, Phenotype algorithm based Big Data analytics for cancer diagnose. J. Med. Syst. **43**(8), 264 (2019)
51. N.K. Salma Banu, S. Swamy, Prediction of heart disease at early stage using data mining and Big Data analytics: A survey, in *2016 International Conference on Electrical, Electronics, Communication, Computer and Optimization Techniques, ICEECCOT 2016*, (2017), pp. 256–261
52. N. Mehta, A. Pandit, International Journal of Medical Informatics Concurrence of Big Data analytics and healthcare: A systematic review. Int. J. Med. Inform. **114**, 57–65 (2018)
53. D.V. Dimitrov, Medical Internet of Things and Big Data in healthcare. Healthcare Inform. Res **22**(3), 156–163 (2016)
54. M.S. Mahdavinejad, M. Rezvan, M. Barekatain, P. Adibi, P. Barnaghi, A.P. Sheth, Machine learning for internet of things data analysis: A survey. Digit. Commun. Netw **4**(3) Elsevier Ltd, 161–175 (2018)
55. G. Akash, C. Chinmay, G. Bharat, Medical information processing using smartphone under IoT framework, in *Energy Conservation for IoT Devices, Studies in Systems, Decision and Control*, vol. 206, (Springer, Singapore, 2019), pp. 283–308
56. G. Fortino, P. Trunfio, *Internet of Things Based on Smart Objects: Technology, Middleware and Applications* (Springer Science & Business Media)
57. C. Savaglio, M. Ganzha, M. Paprzycki, C. Bădică, M. Ivanović, G. Fortino, Agent-based Internet of Things: State-of-the-art and research challenges. Futur. Gener. Comput. Syst. **102**, 1038–1053 (2020)
58. G. Fortino, W. Russo, C. Savaglio, W. Shen, M. Zhou, Agent-oriented cooperative smart objects: From IoT system design to implementation. IEEE Trans. Syst. Man Cybern. Syst **48**(11), 1939–1956 (2018)
59. Akash G, Chinmay C., Bharat G, Sensing and Monitoring of Epileptical Seizure under IoT Platform, IGI: Smart Medical Data Sensing and IoT Systems Design in Healthcare, 201–223, **2019**. 10.4018/978-1-7998-0261-7.ch009
60. W. Sun, Z. Cai, Y. Li, F. Liu, S. Fang, G. Wang, Security and privacy in the medical Internet of Things: A review. Secur. Commun. Netw **2018**, 5978636 (2018)
61. S. Gawade, M. Studies, Overview of different types of sensors used in eHealth environment. Int. J. Infin. Innov. Technol, 5, 2017 (2014)
62. M. Zheng, P.X. Liu, R. Gravina, G. Fortino, An emerging wearable world: New gadgetry produces a rising tide of changes and challenges. IEEE Syst. Man Cybern. Mag **4**(4), 6–14 (2018)
63. C. Chakraborty, B. Gupta, S.K. Ghosh, A review on telemedicine-based WBAN framework for patient monitoring. Int. J. Telemed. e-Health, Mary Ann Libert inc. **19**(8), 619–626 (2013)
64. P.K.D. Pramanik, B.K. Upadhyaya, S. Pal, T. Pal, Internet of Things, smart sensors, and pervasive systems: Enabling connected and pervasive healthcare, in *Healthcare Data Analytics and Management*, (Elsevier Inc, London, 2019)
65. H. Hasni, N. Yahya, V. Asirvadam, M. Jatoi, Analysis of Electromyogram (EMG) for detection of neuromuscular disorders. International conference on intelligent and advanced system (ICIAS), 2018
66. H. Elayan, R.M. Shubair, A. Kiourti, Wireless sensors for medical applications: Current status and future challenges, in *2017 11th European Conference on Antennas and Propagation, EUCAP 2017*, (2017), pp. 2478–2482
67. G. Fortino, R. Giannantonio, R. Gravina, P. Kuryloski, R. Jafari, Enabling effective programming and flexible management of efficient body sensor network applications. IEEE Trans. Human-Machine Syst 43(1), 115–133 (2013)

68. R. Venkatesh, C. Balasubramanian, M. Kaliappan, Development of Big Data Predictive Analytics Model for Disease Prediction using Machine learning Technique, J. Med. Syst., vol. 43, no. 8, 2019
69. R. Gravina, P. Alinia, H. Ghasemzadeh, G. Fortino, Multi-sensor fusion in body sensor networks: State-of-the-art and research challenges. Inf. Fusion **35**, 68–80 (2017)
70. S. Sharma, Survey paper on sensors for body area network in health care. 2017 international conference on emerging trends in computing and communication technologies (ICETCCT), 2017
71. M. Ge, H. Bangui, B. Buhnova, Big Data for Internet of Things: A survey. Futur. Gener. Comput. Syst. **87**, 601–614 (2018)
72. M. Mohammadi, G.S. Member, A. Al-fuqaha, S. Member, Deep learning for IoT Big Data and streaming analytics: A survey. IEEE Commun. Surv. Tutor **X**(X), 1–40 (2018)
73. C. Vuppalapati, A. Ilapakurti, S. Kedari, The role of Big Data in creating sense EHR, an integrated approach to create next generation mobile sensor and wearable data driven Electronic Health Record (EHR), Proceeding of 2016 IEEE 2nd international conference on Big Data computing service and application BigDataService 2016, pp. 293–296, 2016
74. M. Bansal, B. Gandhi, IoT Big Data in smart healthcare (ECG Monitoring), Proceedings of international conference machine learning Big Data, cloud parallel computing trends, prespectives prospects com. 2019, no. ii, pp. 390–396, 2019
75. P. Dineshkumar, R. Senthilkumar, K. Sujatha, R.S. Ponmagal, V.N. Rajavarman, Big Data analytics of IoT based health care monitoring system, in *2016 IEEE Uttar Pradesh Section International Conference on Electrical, Computer and Electronics Engineering, UPCON 2016*, (2017), pp. 55–60
76. D.C. Yacchirema, D. Sarabia-Jacome, C.E. Palau, M. Esteve, A smart system for sleep monitoring by integrating IoT with Big Data analytics. IEEE Access **6**, 35988–36001 (2018)
77. M. Chen, Y. Ma, J. Song, C.F. Lai, B. Hu, Smart clothing: Connecting human with clouds and Big Data for sustainable health monitoring. Mob. Networks Appl. **21**(5), 825–845 (2016)
78. E. Siow, T. Tiropanis, W. Hall, Analytics for the internet of things: A survey. ACM Comput. Surv. **51**(4), 74 (2018)
79. M.S. Hossain, G. Muhammad, Cloud-assisted Industrial Internet of Things (IIoT) - enabled framework for health monitoring. Comput. Netw. **101**, 192–202 (2016)
80. E. Laxmi Lydia, A.S.D. Murthy, C.U. Kumari, N.A. Vignesh, T. Padma, Health care protection and empowerment of Internet of Things (IoT) through Big Data. Test Eng. Manag. **82**(1–2), 1187–1196 (2020)
81. D. Yacchirema, D. Sarabia-Jácome, C.E. Palau, M. Esteve, System for monitoring and supporting the treatment of sleep apnea using IoT and Big Data. Pervasive Mob. Comput. **50**, 25–40 (2018)
82. P. Borovska, Big Data analytics and Internet of medical Things make precision medicine a reality. Int. J. Internet Things Web Serv. **3**, 24–31 (2018)
83. V. Jagadeeswari, V. Subramaniyaswamy, R. Logesh, V. Vijayakumar, A study on medical Internet of Things and Big Data in personalized healthcare system. Heal. Inf. Sci. Syst. **6**(1), 1–20 (2018)
84. T.J. Saleem, M.A. Chishti, Deep learning for Internet of Things data analytics. Procedia Comput. Sci. **163**, 381–390 (2019)
85. J. Granados, T. Westerlund, L. Zheng, Z. Zou, IoT platform for real-time multichannel ECG monitoring and classification, in *Research and Practical Issues of Enterprise Information Systems*, vol. 1, (Springer International Publishing, New York, 2018)

Chapter 3
Big Medical Data Analytics Using Sensor Technology

Shweta Kaushik

3.1 Introduction

3.1.1 Big Data

As the title recommends, 'big data' signifies giant volumes of information, which is incontrollable victimization ancient software package or internet-based stands. It exceeds the historically castoff quantity of loading, process, and systematic power. Despite the fact that a variety of definitions for large knowledge exist, the foremost in style and well-accepted definition were specified by political leader Laney. He determined that huge knowledge was rising in 3 completely dissimilar magnitudes specifically, volume, velocity, and variety [1]. The 'big,' a part of massive knowledge, is symbolic of the giant volume. In addition to capacity, the massive knowledge portrayal includes rapidity and variability. Velocity specifies the speed or frequency of information assortment, making it reachable for any investigation, whereas variation annotations are obtained on the various kinds of systematized and disorderly knowledge that any system will collect and appreciate transaction-level knowledge, text or log files, and audio or video. All the 3 Vs became the quality description of huge knowledge. Even though others have additional many other Vs to the current definition [2], the foremost accepted fourth V remains 'veracity' as shown in Fig. 3.1.

This tenure "big data" has developed tremendously fashionable crossways the world in recent scenario. Nearly each segment of analysis, whether or not it relates to business or lecturers, is producing and analyzing massive knowledge for numerous functions. The foremost difficult mission relating to this immense heap of information that may be ordered or disordered is its organization. Agreeing the very

S. Kaushik (✉)
ABES Engineering College, Ghaziabad, India

© The Author(s), under exclusive license to Springer Nature Switzerland AG 2021
C. Chakraborty et al. (eds.), *Efficient Data Handling for Massive Internet of Medical Things*, Internet of Things,
https://doi.org/10.1007/978-3-030-66633-0_3

Fig. 3.1 Big data
magnitude

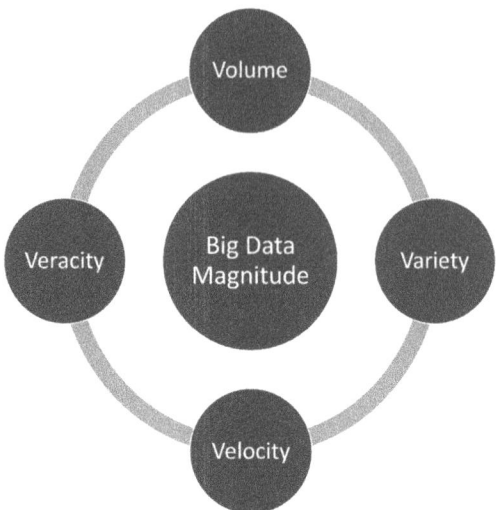

statistic that massive knowledge is uncontrollable victimization of the normal software package, we want technically progressive submissions and software package
that may exploit quick and well-organized high-end machine control for such
responsibilities. Application of Artificial Intelligence (AI) algorithms and new synthesis algorithms would be essential to create sense from this huge quantity of information. Indeed, it'd be a good exploitation to realize machine-driven supervisory by
the employment of machine learning (ML) ways like Neural networks and different
AI approaches.

3.1.2 Healthcare as a Repository

Medicinal offerings may be a multidimensional framework constructed up with the
principle real attention at the counteraction, determination, and remedy of well-
being allied difficulties or stumbling blocks in people. The enormous portions of an
attention framework are the well-being specialists (medical researchers, doctors, or
followers), well-being offices (amenities, hospitals for conveying prescriptions, and
one of a kind project or remedy innovations), and a subsidizing basis assisting
beyond 2. The well-being specialists have an area with diverse well-being elements
like medication, medication, birthing assistance, nursing, mind science, remedy,
and masses of others. Attention is needed at several stages wagering at the despera-
tion of the case. Experts fill it in mild of the reality that the primary discussion is
needed for crucial attention, extreme attention requiring overall specialists (auxiliary attention), propelled medical exam and remedy (tertiary attention), and distinctly splendid analytic or surgeries (quaternary attention). Withinside the littlest
recognition of those stages, the well-being specialists are answerable for very

sudden styles of statistics taking after affected person's medical history (locating and answers related to statistics), medical and medical statistics (like statistics from imaging and studies facility assessments), and numerous men or women or man or woman medical statistics.

Beforehand, the everyday see to keep such medical statistics for an affected person turned into in the form of both composed notes or typewritten reports [3]. With the arrival of laptop frameworks and their latent capacity, the transformation of each unmarried medical check and medical statistics in the attention frameworks has emerged as a widespread and largely acquired watch nowadays. In 2003, a department of the National Academies of Sciences, Engineering, and medicines alluded to as Institute of medicines selected the expression "digital well-being statistics" to talk to statistics saved up for up the social coverage section closer to the useful issue approximately sufferers and clinicians. Electronic well-being statistics (EHR) as illustrated by way of means of Murphy, Hanken, and Waters are treated as medical statistics for sufferers of any statistics regarding the beyond, blessing, or destiny physical/emotional health or nation of an man or woman who dwells in the digital system(s) acclimated catch, transmit, get, keep, recover, interface, and manage media framework statistics for the number one motive for giving medicinal offerings and well-being-associated administrations [4].

Recent improvements in sensor innovation, wearable processing, Internet of Things (IoT), and remote correspondence have offered to ascend to look into omnipresent medicinal services and remote checking of human well-being and exercises. Well-being observing frameworks include preparing and investigation of information recovered from cell phones, savvy watches, keen armbands, just as different sensors and wearable gadgets. Such frameworks empower ceaseless checking of patient's mental and well-being conditions by detecting and transmitting estimations, for example, pulse, electrocardiogram, internal heat level, respiratory rate, chest sounds, or circulatory strain. Inescapable human services, as a pertinent application area in this unique situation, target changing the conveyance of clinical administrations through a clinical assistive condition and encourage the free living of patients.

Big Data are large measures of facts that may perform a little exquisite thing. It has turned out to be a topic of unusual enthusiasm for as some distance again as a long time in view of a first rate capacity, this is included up in it. Different open and personal vicinity firms produce, store, and dissect big facts with an intend to enhance the administrations they give. In the medicinal offering industry, specific hotspots for good sized facts include emergency hospital facts, scientific facts of patients, effects of scientific assessments, and devices that might be a chunk of net of things. Biomedical studies likewise create a noteworthy part of good sized facts pertinent to open medicinal offerings. These facts call for valid management and examination for you to decide tremendous facts. Something else, looking for arrangement by breaking down large information rapidly gets tantamount to finding a needle in the bundle. There are different difficulties related to each progression of dealing with enormous information, which must be outperformed by utilizing top of the line registering answers for huge information investigation. This is the reason, to give significant answers for improving general well-being, human service suppliers are required to be completely outfitted with suitable framework to methodically create and dissect enormous information. A proficient administration, examination, and understanding of enormous information can revolutionize the disposed by opening new roads for current social insurance. That is actually why different ventures, including the humanoid service manufacturing, are finding a way to change over this potential into better administrations and money-related points of interest. With a solid reconciliation of biomedical and social insurance information, present day human service associations can reform the clinical treatments and customized medication.

This section studies Big Data by presenting the enormous evidence examination in medication and medicinal services. Enormous information attributes, esteem, volume, speed, assortment, veracity, and fluctuation, are portrayed. Huge information investigation in medicine and humanoid facilities covers reconciliation and examination of enormous measure of complex heterogeneous information, for example, different omics information, biomedical information, and electronic well-being record information. We emphasize the tough problems about enormous information fortification and safety. Concerning information attributes, a few bearings of utilizing reasonable and promising open-source disseminated information preparing programming stage are given.

Big Data investigation has been of late applied toward helping the procedure of care conveyance and sickness investigation. In any case, the gathering rate and exploration improvement in this space are as yet steamed at some significant issues normal in the tremendous data perspective. In this area, we talk about a segment of these critical challenges with an accentuation on three best-in-class and promising regions of clinical exploration: picture, signal, and genomics-based examination, as shown in Fig. 3.2. Late examination, which targets utilization of gigantic volumes of clinical data while joining multimodal data from various sources, is discussed. Possible zones of exploration in this field, which can have significant impact on human administration transport, are investigated in a similar manner.

Fig. 3.2 Big data: region of clinical exploration

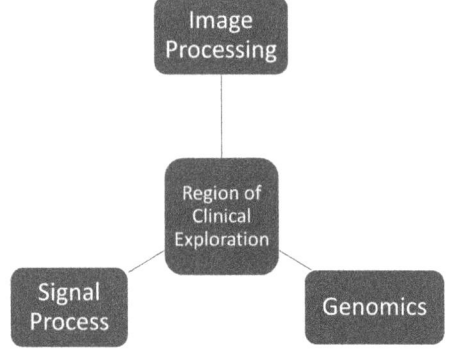

Medical Image Processing Medical pictures are an essential gracefully of information oft utilized for recognizable proof, clinical guide appraisal, and planning. CT, atomic imaging, X-beam, photoacoustic imaging, ultrasound, radiology, anti-electron outflow envisioning processed tomography (PET-CT), and indicative strategy are some of the examples of imaging strategies that are entrenched at clinical settings. Clinical picture information will differ wherever from numerous megabytes for one examination (e.g., infinitesimal life structures pictures) to numerous megabytes per study (e.g., dainty cut CT contemplates including up to 2500+ outputs per study [5]). Such information needs goliath stockpiling limits if saved for what's to come. It moreover requests speedy and right calculations if any call helping mechanization was to be performed to abuse the data. Furthermore, if various wellsprings of information nonheritable for each patient additionally are utilized all through the conclusions, forecast, and treatment forms, at that point, the matter of giving durable stockpiling and creating affordable ways equipped for embodying the wide fluctuation of information turns into a test.

Signal Procedure Sort of similar clinical pictures, clinical signals moreover cause volume and speed impediments especially all through constant, high-goal securing, and capacity from an enormous number of screens associated with each patient. Be that as it may, moreover to the data size issues, physiological signals furthermore cause the intricacy of a spatiotemporal sort. Investigation of physiological signs is normally extra significant once given close by situational setting mindfulness that must be inserted into the occasion of constant recognition and prophetical frameworks to ensure its viability and quality.

As of now, care frameworks utilize different unique and constant recognition gadgets that use solitary physiological wave shape information or discretized significant data to flexibly caution components just if there should be an occurrence of flagrant occasions. Be that as it may, such uncombine approaches toward the occasion and execution of alert frameworks will in general be questionable and their sheer numbers may cause "caution weakness" for each guardian and patient [6]. During this setting, the adaptability to discover new clinical data is stressed by past information that has generally fallen with the need to maximally use high-dimensional measurement information. The clarification that these alert components will in general fall flat is fundamental that these frameworks will in general concede single wellsprings of information, though inadequate with regard to the setting of the patients' actual physiological conditions from a more extensive and extra far reaching perspective. In this manner, there's a prerequisite to create improved and extra far reaching approaches toward learning connections and relationships among multimodal clinical time-arrangement information. This is regularly fundamental because of studies despite everything showing that people are poor in thinking with respect to changes moving very 2 signs [7].

Genomics The motivation to grouping the human request (inclusive of 30,000–35,000 qualities) is recoil sever decreasing with the event of high-throughput sequencing innovation. With tips for modern widespread health preparations and conveyance of care [8], investigating genome-scale facts for developing uncalled proposals in a great manner will be a widespread take a look at the circle of system science. Really well worth and time to bring tips are crucial in an incredibly scientific setting. Activities adapting to this propelled downside encapsulate following a 100,000 topics extra than 20–30 years abuse of the prophetical, preventive, regulation primarily based totally, and custom-designed health, named P4, drug worldview [9, 10], further as AN integrative man or woman omics profile. The P4 hobby is utilizing a framework technique for (i) breaking down genome-scale datasets to work out unwellness states, (ii) transferring toward blood, primarily based totally analytic apparatuses for steady reputation of an issue, (iii) investigating new approaches to address sedate goal revelation, developing contraptions to cope with big fact problems of catching, approving, setting away, mining, and coordination, and finally (iv) showing facts for every person. The integrative man or woman omics profile (iPOP) consolidates physiological reputation and special high-throughput approaches for request sequencing to think about defined health and unwellness situations of an issue. At last, acknowledging unfair tips on the scientific stage remains an incredible take a look at for this field [11]. Using such high-thickness facts for investigation, disclosure, and scientific interpretation requests novel big facts that attract close to and examination.

3.2 Openings with Big Data in Healthcare

Because of digitization and interconnection of medicinal services information, huge advantages (openings) are accomplished today. The potential points of interest incorporate quality organization, decrease of remaining burden, investment funds of counsel time, recognizing infections at prior stages to treat it more easily and adequately with diminished cost, identifying social insurance extortion (that includes the documenting of deceptive medicinal service claims) all the more rapidly and effectively, overseeing specific individual and populace well-being appropriately, and so forth. A portion of the significant advantages (principally accomplished through examination) are itemized underneath, however, much as could be expected for demonstrating increasingly functional bits of knowledge, as shown in Fig. 3.3.

3.2.1 Advantages to Patients

Healthcare information can help patients in settling on right choice at perfect time. Actually, investigation of patient information carries out this responsibility. Furthermore, investigation might be applied to distinguish the people who need "proactive consideration"or changes in their way of life to stay away from debasement of well-being condition. In this way, it brings about improving the well-being of patients while diminishing the expense of care. A solid model in this regard is the Virginia well-being framework Carilion Clinic venture, which utilizes prescient models for early mediations.

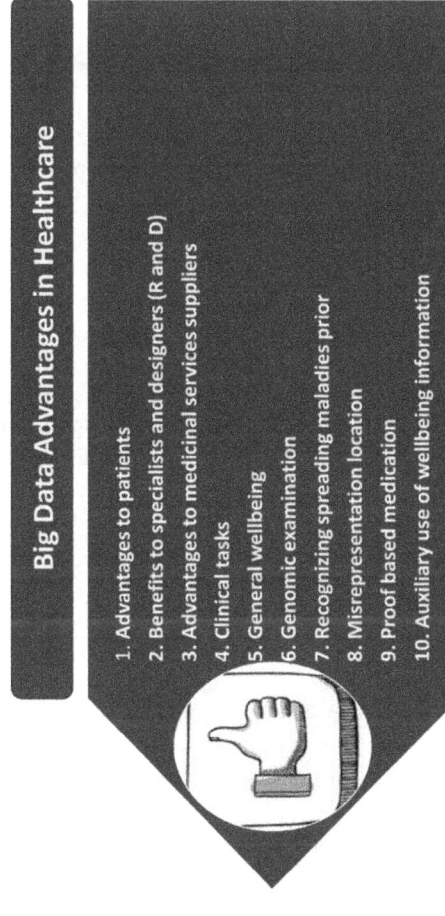

Fig. 3.3 Big data advantages in health care

3.2.2   Benefits to Specialists and Designers (R and D)

Patient information gathered from various sources help innovative work to improve nature of exploration about new sicknesses and treatments. As a matter of fact, R and D may propose new calculations (particularly identified with information mining and AI) to recognize new infections that may cause pandemics. In this regard, one may allude the examinations.

3.2.3   Advantages to Medicinal Service Suppliers

Healthcare information helps the suppliers to outline preventive acts. Furthermore, the suppliers can structure new systems to take care of patients. As needs be, it decreases the quantity of pointless hospitalizations.

3.2.4   Clinical Tasks

The well-being informational collection is able to give relative adequacy examination to choose progressively down to earth and clinically significant methodologies. It likewise recommends the financially savvy approaches to analyze and treat patients.

3.2.5   General Well-Being

On breaking down infection designs, following illness episode and its transmission guarantee to improve general well-being observation and speed reaction. Model incorporates quicker improvement of all the more precisely focused antibodies, e.g., picking the yearly flu strains. In this unique situation, Lazer et al. express that transforming enormous measure of information into noteworthy data can be utilized to distinguish the requirements, particularly to serve populaces. Also, it offers types of assistance, predicts, and forestalls emergencies for the people.

3.2.6   Genomic Examination

It helps to execute quality sequencing all the more proficiently and cost adequately. Ohlhorst states that genomic examination must be a piece of the normal clinical consideration choice procedure and the developing patient clinical record.

3.2.7 Recognizing Spreading Maladies Prior

Healthcare investigation has capacity of early forecast of viral sicknesses before their spreading. Without a doubt, this may not be conceivable by breaking down the social logs of the patients experiencing a malady in a particular geoarea. All things are considered; investigation causes the medicinal service experts to exhort the casualties by taking basic preventive measures.

3.2.8 Misrepresentation Location

Misuse of an individual's clinical personality to improperly get social insurance merchandise, administrations, or assets might be identified from medicinal service examination. Without a doubt, misrepresentation in clinical cases can build the weight on the general public. Critically, prescient models like choice tree, neural systems, straight relapse, and so on can be utilized to anticipate and forestall misrepresentation at the purpose of exchanges.

3.2.9 Proof-Based Medication

It includes the utilization of measurable examinations and evaluated research by specialists to perform determination. This training empowers specialists to settle on choices dependent on their own recognitions as well as from the best accessible confirmations. It is, to be sure, a successful bit of leeway got from social insurance information.

3.2.10 Auxiliary Use of Well-Being Information

The optional utilization of well-being information manages conglomeration of clinical information from fund, tolerant consideration, managerial records to discover significant bits of knowledge like recognizable proof of patients with uncommon malady, treatment decisions, clinical execution estimation, and so forth.

3.3 Healthcare Monitoring System

Personal satisfaction in many nations has been expanding loads over the numerous couples of decades on account of crucial upgrades in medications and general social insurance. Thus, there's tremendous interest for the occasion of cost-effective far off well-being recognition, which might be relaxed to usage for more seasoned persons. The distant medicinal service recognition incorporates sensors, actuators, and propelled correspondence advancements and offers the prospect for the persistent to visit at his/her contented location as an alternative of modest social insurance offices. These frameworks screen the physiological indications of the patients in timeframe, will evaluate some well-being conditions, and offer criticism to the specialists. Why these frameworks are consequently relaxed and important to utilize? The essential explanation is that they're transportable, easy to use, of minuscule sizes, and light-weight. A normal model could be a Healthcare Monitoring System (HMS) [12] that basically utilizes a microcontroller, which trails and processes well-being information and directs an SMS to a specialist's versatile or any companion who may give crisis help (Fig. 3.4). The most preferred position of this strategy is that somebody may convey it all over because the gadget is pretty much nothing, light, and remote. Another preferred position of those frameworks is that they'll screen well-being conditions in timespan and each one the stretch. People use HMS in clinics, for home consideration, and to follow the organ of competitors (pulse, pressure level, and internal heat level). These data can be prepared by changed sensors incorporated into the frameworks.

Well-being recognition frameworks will utilize wearable sensors, a microcontroller, or FPGA. A source gets corporeal signs of the heart rate of any human and arrangements of the information and sends through Wi-Fi to the ZigBee. At that point, the statistics is moved by the recipient to the PC or server. The source utilizes a microcontroller that distinguishes the heartbeat of patient and changes over it to a power signal so showed. The idea is that with the equivalent HMS with wearable sensors, the qualification goes in close vicinity to the evident truth that here the sensors that watch crucial sign and pressure level/heartbeat rate are arranged on the patient's body without any wires. For remote data transmission in word separation

Fig. 3.4 Healthcare monitoring system (HMS)

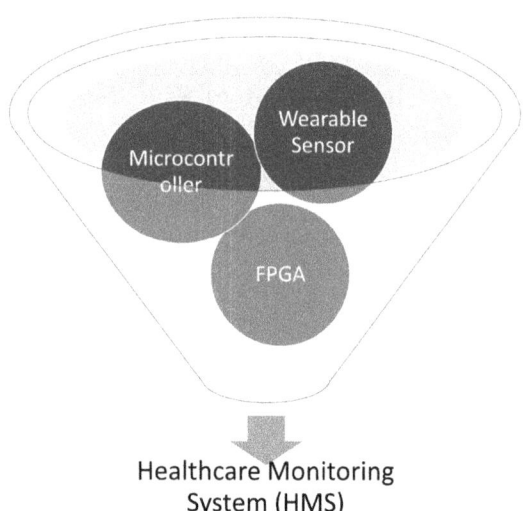

Healthcare Monitoring
System (HMS)

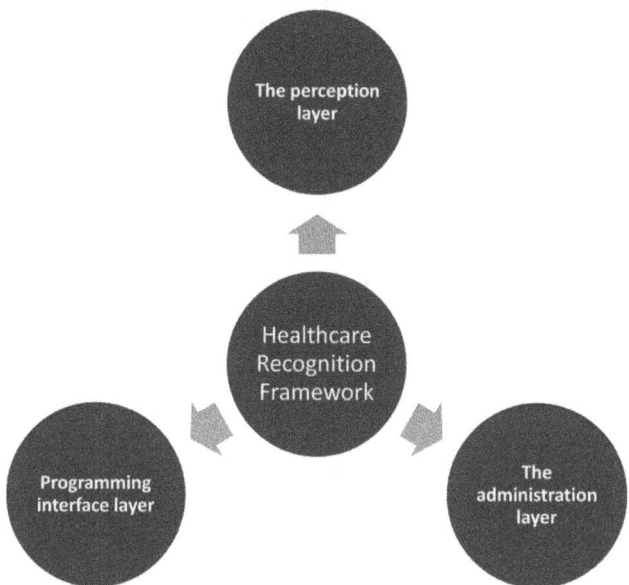

Fig. 3.5   Healthcare recognition framework

conventions, worship Bluetooth or ZigBee is utilized. The remote detecting component gadget contains a breath sensor, electrodermal action detecting component
(EDA sensor), and indicative system detecting component (EMG sensor). FPGA
proposes a field-programmable entryway cluster that might be modified once created
through HDL (equipment depiction language). A Healthcare recognition framework
abusing this innovation contains a modest, information converter. Digitization
licenses clients to append the FPGA to the total framework. E-well-being recognition configurations are regularly isolated into 3 principle layers, as shown in Fig. 3.5.

3.3.1   The Perception Layer

This contains entirely unexpected clinical and ecological devices (sensors) that are
gathering the information in timeframe. Clinical sensors observe a patient's significant signs through ecological one's measure markers, which affect a patient's health
condition and revere the compound component level or temperature.

3.3.2   Programming Interface Layer

This incorporates changed Application Programming Interfaces (APIs). The information gives finished cloud advances giving access to patient's well-being information and current well-being records. The API layer could be a layer that stores newly

admitted patient well-being data by creating a profile abusing one API and presentations prevailing clinical information for a previously enrolled persistent data abusing another API.

3.3.3 The Administration Layer

This contains AN e-well-being application, where examinations provide data and propose methodologies to improve the patient's condition or give a solution. The data are dissected by the incorporated algorithmic program and might be contrasted with various patient's encounters or past well-being statuses of indistinguishable patient. This layer is responsible for disturbing the clinical laborers just if there should arise an occurrence of crisis.

HMS is a prudent instrument that may spare human lives. It's good and might be sorted out looking on the patient's needs, which make it cost-productive and accommodating not only for clinics but also conjointly for home use.

3.4 Sensor Techniques

The development of semiconductor VSLI advancements has prompted the presence of low-power processors and sensors just as keen remote systems combined with Big Data investigation. These are the essential structure squares of the wealthy idea of the Internet of Things (IoT) in which setting emerges the advancement of distinguishing proof and detecting advances. At its center, the IoT is tied in with associated gadgets letting them speak with different gadgets and applications. Subsequently, the IoT worldview requires system administration and detecting abilities [13]. At present, the goal is to transduce (sense), get (gather), and examine (process) data from different articles around us so as to guarantee ideal asset utilization. The answer for this solicitation is the Internet of Things, which speaks to the ability of associating each pertinent gadget with the Internet. The enormous measure of created information could be prepared by utilizing cloud administrations, i.e., effective, and available information structures that can give figuring as a help. Contemporary innovation headways, including hardware, advanced installed frameworks, remote correspondences, and sign preparing, have made it conceivable to create sensor hubs with detecting, control, information handling, and system administration highlights. Associating these sensor hubs in systems empowers the spine for the IoT and Big Data period, as shown in Fig. 3.6.

Fig. 3.6 Sensor technologies

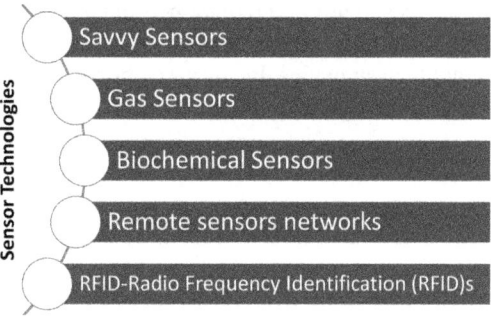

3.4.1   A Savvy Device

It is a type of sensor that exemplifies alerts obtained from the bodily situation and techniques with its inherent registering property earlier than passing them to an introduced collectively sensor middle point. Savvy sensors are key crucial additives of the IoT concept. One execution of eager sensors is as segments of faraway sensor systems (WSNs) whose hubs can have variety in thousands, each certainly considered one among that are related to distinctive sensors and with the included middle points. Brilliant sensors have numerous packages together with logical, military, common, and domestic packages.

3.4.2   Gas Sensors

They are a category of compound sensors. These sensors determine the centralization of fuel online in its neighborhood. Gas detecting frameworks are regularly tested for packages in ecological checking (air nice manage and hearthplace recognition), automobile industry (gasoline ignition staring at and dirtying gases of vehicles), present day creation (technique managing mechanization, vicinity of gases in mines, and discovery of fuelline spillages in strength stations), scientific packages (example, digital noses and liquor breath tests), kettle manage, domestic security, and so on. Various styles of fuel line sensors exist, for instance, optical, floor acoustic wave, capacitive, reactant, electrochemical, and semiconductor fuel line sensors. Gas detecting strategies may be element into classes: in mild of the form of electric residences and depending on the form of different residences [3]. The strategies for fuel line detecting that depend on lots of nonelectric residences include optical, calorimetric, fuel line chromatograph, and acoustic detecting. Optical sensors depend on spectroscopy, which makes use of discharge spectrometry and ingestion. The guiding principle of assimilation spectrometry relies on the ingestion of the photons at express fuel line frequencies; the retention is based on the convergence of photons. Infrared fuel line sensors paintings on the guideline of thumb of atomic ingestion spectrometry; every fuel line has its very own particular assimilation residences to infrared radiation with numerous frequencies. In general, optical sensors should gain higher selectivity, affectability, and soundness in comparison with nonoptical strategies. In any case, their packages are restrained due to their typically great fee and the requirement for small scale sizes.

3.4.3 Biochemical Sensors

They can extrude over an herbal or compound sum into an electrical signal. The biosensor carries a receptor (commonly a biocomponent, for instance, an analyte particle that performs out the real sub-atomic discovery of the targeted on component), artificially sensitive layer, transducer, and digital signal processor. We may also type biochemical sensors in some viewpoints. Thinking approximately the watched boundary, sensors may be categorized as substance or biochemical, and thinking about their shape, they may be expendable, reversible, irreversible, or reusable. As for his or her outer shape, they may be delegated planar or circulation cells. Biochemical sensors predicted for vicinity of electrical signal both straightforwardly experience the electrical charges (aerometric sensors) or experience the electrical subject initiated with the aid of using electric powered charges. Another elegance of biochemical sensors transduces the artificial integrating with mechanical misshaping. Synthetic responses incite mechanical disfigurement disciple to the concept of nanotechnology, for instance, the particle diverts in a molecular layer are proteins that manage ionic porousness on lipid bilayer movie and the motion of this protein is overseen with the aid of using the mechanical floor stress instigated with the aid of using compound response.

3.4.4 Remote Sensor Networks

Current improvements of MicroElectroMechanical Systems (MEMS) innovation and interchanges took into account the approach of minimal effort, low-power sensor hubs having numerous capacities in a conservative structure factor. They are the premise of remote sensor systems. Remote Sensor Networks (WSNs) include countless sensor hubs (additionally called bits) that are spatially dispersed self-ruling gadgets that can acknowledge input data from the associated sensor(s), process the data, and transmit the yield to different gadgets by means of a remote system. WSNs were driven at first by military applications (for example, combat zone observation), yet now they are changed in common applications motivated by the IoT idea, for example, home and building computerization, traffic signal, transport and coordination, mechanical robotization, condition checking, healthcare checking [13], horticultural and creature checking, and so forth. These days, remote sensor systems are permitting a degree of incorporation among PCs and the physical world that has been incomprehensible previously. Advances in microelectronics and corresponding ventures have been a key empowering agent of the improvement of gigantic systems of sensors. By and by, remote availability of sensors may be viewed as an application facilitator as opposed to an element of the sensors. This is because of the way that wired sensor systems on the scale that is required would be too costly to even think about setting up and keep up, which implies they are unusable for applications, for example, observing nature, well-being, military, and so forth.

3.4.5   RFID-Radio Frequency Identification (RFID)

RFID is a strikingly advancing innovation for computerized ID dependent on close-field electromagnetic labeling. It is a remote technique for sending and getting information for different distinguishing proof applications. In contrast to other recognizable proof frameworks (for example, savvy cards, biometrics, optical character acknowledgment frameworks, standardized identification frameworks, and so on), RFID has numerous focal points since it is cost and force effective, withstands serious physical conditions, licenses simultaneous recognizable proof, and doesn't require view (LoS) for correspondence. An RFID can transform basic day by day protests into portable system hubs that may be followed and checked and can react to activity demands. All these totally fit the thought of the Internet of Things.

An RFID framework commonly comprises 3 significant parts: (1) an application, which gives the interface to encode and interpret the ID information from information peruse into a PC or a centralized computer, (2) an RFID tag, which stores the distinguishing proof data or code, and (3) a label peruse or label integrator, which imparts surveying signs to an RFID transponder (transmitter-responder) or to a label that ought to be recognized. RFID frameworks are essentially utilized for the distinguishing proof of articles or following their area without conveying data about the item and its state of being. In various applications, the area or the character of an article isn't sufficient and extra data are required – it very well may be extricated from different boundaries describing the ecological conditions. Sensor systems could help in such cases. WSNs are frameworks comprising little sensor hubs that can gather and convey data by distinguishing natural conditions, for instance, temperature, mugginess, light, stable, pressure, vibration, and so on [14]. In any case, the personality and area of an item are as yet crucial data and they tend to be separated by RFID procedures. In these circumstances, the perfect game plan is to join the two advancements so as to guarantee broadened capacities, transportability, and adaptability [15].

3.4.6   Wearable Sensor

Wearable sensors can screen and record constant data about one's physiological condition and movement exercises. Wearable sensor-based well-being checking frameworks may include various sorts of adaptable sensors that can be incorporated into material fiber, garments, and flexible groups or straightforwardly connected to the human body. The sensors are equipped for estimating physiological signs, for example, electrocardiogram (ECG), electromyogram (EMG), pulse (HR), internal heat level, electrodermal action (EDA), blood vessel oxygen immersion (SpO$_2$), circulatory strain (BP), and breath rate (RR) [16]. Wearable sensors, being dynamically more agreeable and less prominent, are proper for checking a person's well-being or health without intruding on their everyday exercises. The sensors can quantify a few physiological signs/boundaries just as action and development of a person by setting them at various areas of the body. The headway in low-power, smaller wearables (sensors, actuators, receiving wires, and shrewd materials), economical processing, and capacity gadgets combined with current correspondence advancements may provide minimal effort, subtle, and long-haul well-being checking framework.

3.4.7 Body Sensor Network (BSN)

On account of short-range correspondence, the sensors can impart to the door legitimately over a remote medium. On the other hand, the sensors can frame a body sensor organization (BSN) [16–18] and a star network geography and send information to the focal BSN hub. The BSN hub can send information to the door in the wake of playing out some handling. The on-body sensors and the BSN hub could convey by utilizing wired or remote medium. In any case, wired associations can impede the clients' versatility and may cause incessant bombed associations. Consequently, they are not appropriate for wearable and long-haul observing frameworks. A decent choice is to utilize conductive texture yarns as the option conductive medium. These textures can be handily incorporated into garments to speak with material inserted sensors. The equipment and calculation asset for the on-body focal hub of a multisensor BSN framework can be a restricting variable for consistent network and information taking care of. The focal handling hub of the BSN network trades information with the on-body sensors just as the home entryway, and some of the time performs restricted preparing. Hence, a strong and proficient calculation is needed for the focal BSN hub to upgrade its presentation. Notwithstanding that, an effective information pressure calculation should be actualized in the focal hub so as to manage a huge volume of information and send them to the closest door.

3.5 Big Data Analytics in Healthcare

3.5.1 Patient Predictions

For our first case of massive facts in social coverage, we are able to take a gander at one exemplary problem that any pass manager faces: how many people do I place on team of workers at a few random timeframes? Too slightly any professionals, you may have helpless patron care outcomes, which may be lethal for sufferers in that industry.

Enormous facts are supporting by looking after this problem, in any occasion at more than one emergency clinics in Paris. A Forbes article subtlety how 4 emergency clinics which can be a bit of the Assistance Publique-Hôpitaux de Paris were making use of facts from a collection of reasserts to consider each day and hourly forecasts of how many sufferers are required to be at each clinical health center.

One of the key informational indexes is 10 years of clinical health center affirmation records, which facts researchers crunched making use of of "time association research" methods. These investigations authorized the scientists to look relevant examples in affirmation costs. At that factor, they may make use of AI to find the maximum specific calculations that expected destiny affirmation styles. Summarizing the end result of this paintings, Forbes states, "The final results is a web browser-primarily based totally interface meant to be used by professionals, clinical caretakers and health center employer team of workers – undeveloped in facts science – to estimate go to and confirmation costs for the subsequent 15 days. Additional team of workers may be drafted in whilst excessive portions of visitors are normal, prompting dwindled sitting tight activities for sufferers and higher nature of care."

3.5.2 Electronic Health Records (EHRs)

It's the maximum way of accomplishing usage of massive facts in medicine. Each affected person has his personal automatic report that includes socioeconomics, scientific history, hypersensitivities, studies middle take a look at consequences, and so on. Records are shared by way of stable fact frameworks and are available for providers from each open and personal section. Each report contains one modifiable document, which means that professionals can execute modifications after a while without an administrative painting and no risk of fact replication.

EHRs can likewise cause signals and updates, while an affected person should get any other lab take a look at or tune drugs to test whether or not an affected person has been following physicians' instructions [19, 20]. In spite of the truth that EHR is a great idea, several countries no matter the entirety warfare absolutely execute them. United States has made an extensive soar with 94% of emergency clinics receiving EHRs as in line with this HITECH studies, but the EU no matter the entirety falls behind. Be that because it may, a keen order drafted via way of European Commission ought to remodel it: via way of 2020 delivered collectively European well-being report framework ought to change into a reality. Kaiser Permanente is using the route withinside the United States and will supply a version to the EU to follow. They've absolutely performed a framework referred to as Health Connect that stocks facts over the whole thing in their places of work and makes it less complicated to make use of EHRs. A McKinsey record on big fact human offerings expresses that "The included framework has progressed outcomes in cardiovascular infection and achieved an expected $1 billion in reserve price range from reduced workplace visits and lab exams."

3.5.3   Real-Time Alerting

Different times of big facts exam in medicinal offerings percentage one extensive usefulness – steady alarming. In emergency clinics, Clinical Decision Support (CDS) programming examines scientific facts at the spot, furnishing well-being experts with suggestions as they determine prescriptive choices. Notwithstanding, professionals want sufferers to keep away from clinical clinics to avoid exorbitant in-residence drugs. Examination, formerly drifting as one of the commercial enterprise perception modern expressions in 2019, can probably come to be a bit of any other methodology. Wearables will collect sufferers' well-being facts continuously and ship these facts to the cloud.

Moreover, these facts may be gotten to the database at the situation of power of the general population, if you want to allow professionals to reflect on consideration of these facts in monetary placing and adjust the conveyance methodologies as desires be. Establishments and care administrators will make use of complicated gadgets to display screen these vast facts circulate and reply every time the consequences may be upsetting. For instance, if an affected person's circulatory pressure increments alarmingly, the framework will ship a warning step by step to the professional who will at that factor make a pass to reach on the affected person and oversee measures to carry down the weight.

Another version is that of Asthma polis, which has started to make use of inhalers with GPS-empowered trackers with a purpose of distinguishing bronchial allergy styles each on a character stage and taking a gander at larger populaces. This fact is being applied associated with facts from the CDC with a purpose of developing higher remedy plans for asthmatics.

3.5.4   Enhancing Patient Engagement

Numerous purchasers – and subsequently, probable sufferers – as of now have an enthusiasm for intelligent devices that report every development they take, their pulses, resting propensities, and so on, consistently. This vital fact may be blended with different identifiable facts to understand capacity well-being risk sneaking. An incessant and slumbering disease and a raised pulse can flag a risk for destiny coronary infection, for example. Patients are straightforwardly engaged with the watching in their personal well-being, and motivators from clinical coverages can push them to steer a strong manner of life (e.g., giving coins lower back to people making use of intelligent watches).

Another method to accomplish that accompanies new wearables a piece in development, following express well-being styles and handing-off them to the cloud in which medical doctors can display screen them. Patients experiencing bronchial allergies or circulatory pressure ought to income via way of it, end up greater loss, and reduce superfluous visits to the professional.

3.5.5   Prevent Opioid Abuse

In the United States, our fourth case of massive facts' social coverage is dealing with a hard problem. Here's a relaxing actuality: as of this present day year, overdoses from abused narcotics have triggered an increasing number of unintended passing withinside the United States. Than road accidents, which had been ahead the most extreme broadly recognized reason for unintentional downfall. Examination grasp Bernard Marr expounds on the problem in a Forbes article. The situation has gotten so vital that Canada has mentioned narcotic maltreatment to be a "country-wide well-being emergency," and President Obama reserved $1.1 billion greenbacks for developing solutions for the problem at the same time as he changed workplace.

By and by way of, a usage of vast facts research in human offerings can be an appropriate reaction everyone is looking for: facts researchers at Blue Cross Blue Shield have started operating with exam professionals at Fuzzy Logix to address the problem. Utilizing lengthy stretches of safety and drug keep facts, Fuzzy Logix specialists have had the choice to differentiate 742 risk elements that foresee with an extreme quantity of exactness whether or not someone is in risk of mishandling narcotics. As Blue Cross Blue Shield facts researcher Brandon Cosley states withinside the Forbes piece, "dislike a sure something – 'he went to the professional to an extreme' – is prescient … it resembles 'nicely you hit a restrict of placing off to the professional and you've got precise kinds of situations and also you visit a couple of professional and stay in a particular postal district… ' Those matters include."

To be reasonable, contacting people identified as "excessive risk" and preserving them from constructing up a medicine problem is a delicate endeavor. In any case, this assignment no matter the entirety gives a ton of expectation closer to moderating a problem that is annihilating the lives of several people and costing the framework an extremely good deal of coins.

3.5.6   Using Health Data for Informed Strategic Planning

The usage of massive facts in social coverage considers crucial arranging as a consequence of higher bits of know-how into people inspirations. Care troughs can check out registration outcomes among people in numerous section gatherings and understand what variables demoralize people from taking on remedy.

College of Florida applied Google Maps and loose preferred well-being facts to get geared up warm temperature maps targeted at numerous issues, for example, population improvement and steady infections. Along those lines, scholastics contrasted this fact and the accessibility of scientific administrations in maximum warmed zones. The reviews accrued from this and authorized them to audit their conveyance method and upload greater attention gadgets to maximum volatile territories.

3.5.7 Big Data Might Just Cure Cancer

Another fascinating case of the usage of big facts in human offerings is the Cancer Moonshot software. Prior to the furthest restrict of his next term, President Obama's idea of this software had the goal of attaining 10 years of development closer to relieving malignant boom into identical elements that time.

Clinical analysts can make use of a number of facts on remedy plans and restoration paces of malignant boom sufferers with a purpose of finding out styles and drugs that have the maximum noteworthy paces of feat in reality. For instance, analysts can examine tumor exams in biobanks, which can be linked up with knowledge remedy records. Utilizing these facts, professionals can see things such as how sure modifications and sickness proteins accomplice with numerous drugs and find out styles in an effort to activate higher affected person outcomes. These facts can likewise activate unexpected advantages, for example, locating that Desipramine, which is a stimulant, can assist repair unique kinds of lung malignant boom.

Be that because it may, with a purpose of making those kinds of reviews step by step available, chronic databases from numerous foundations, for example, clinics, colleges, and charities, ought to be linked up. At that factor, for instance, professionals ought to get to quiet biopsy reviews from extraordinary agencies. Another capacity use case might be hereditarily sequencing malignant boom tissue exams from scientific initial sufferers and making those facts available to the greater great sickness database.

Be that because it may, there are a ton of obstructions withinside the manner, including: (1) Contradictory facts frameworks. This is perhaps the best specialized take a look at, as making those informational collections geared up to interface with each other is an extreme accomplishment. (2) Persistence privatizes issues. There are differentiating lawful rules nation by means of method of nation which supervise what information realities might be released without or with consent, and those should be explored. Basically, agencies have placed an extremely good deal of time.

3.6 Challenges in Healthcare Big Data

3.6.1 Storage

Storing giant quantity of facts is one of the vital problems, but several institutions are OK with facts stockpiling on their very own premises. It has some factors of hobby like command over protection, get to, and up-time. Be that because it might also additionally, an on-area server device may be steeply priced proportional and difficult to hold up. Apparent with diminishing costs and increasing unwavering great, the cloud-basically based absolutely capacity utilizing IT premise is a high level longing, which the tremendous majority of social coverage institutions have settled on. Associations should choose cloud accomplices that recognize the importance of human offerings expressing consistence and protection problems. Furthermore, dispensed garage gives decrease earlier charges, agile fiasco recuperation, and less complicated improvement. Associations can likewise have a 1/2 of breed manner to address their facts stockpiling packages, which is probably the maximum adaptable and beneficial technique for providers with moving facts getting admission and ability desires.

3.6.2 Cleaning

The facts desire to purged or wiped clean to assure the precision, accuracy, consistency, importance, and distinctive feature after obtaining. This cleansing process may be guided or automatized making use of reason regulations to assure extended stages of exactness and uprightness. Increasingly complicated and precise gadgets use AI techniques to lower time and charges and to save your foul facts from crashing massive fact ventures.

3.6.3 Unified Association

Patients produce a huge quantity of facts that is not something however hard to seize with traditional EHR design, as it's miles knotty and now no longer efficaciously reasonable. It is just too difficult to even consider dealing with massive facts especially when it comes without a great facts' affiliation to the social coverage providers. A want to set up all of the clinically critical statistics surfaced with the quite intention of cases, charging purposes, and scientific examination. In this manner, scientific coding frameworks like Momentum Procedural Terminology (CPT) and International Classification of Diseases (ICD) code units had been created to talk to the middle scientific thoughts. Be that because it might also additionally, those code units have their very own confinements.

3.6.4 Accuracy

Some examinations have shown that the unveiling of affected person facts into EMRs or EHRs is not definitely precise yet [21, 22], probably as a consequence of negative EHR utility, complicated painting procedures, and a wrecked comprehension of why massive facts are terrifically vital to seize well. Every any such additives can upload to the great problems for giant facts up and down its lifecycle. The EHRs anticipate to enhance the great and correspondence of facts in scientific paintings procedures, but reviews exhibit inconsistencies in those specific situations. The great documentation might also additionally enhance through making use of self-file polls from sufferers for his or her facet effects.

3.6.5 Image Preprocessing

Studies have watched distinctive bodily factors that could set off changed facts great and misinterpretations from current scientific records [23]. Clinical photos regularly bear specialized stumbling blocks that consist of diverse varieties of clamor and curios. Inappropriate remedy of scientific photos can likewise reason changing of photos as an instance might also additionally set off defined anatomical structures, for instance, veins that are noncorrelative with proper case scenario. Reduction of commotion, clearing historic rarities, converting differentiation of acquired photos, and imaging great change put-up misusing are a part of the measures that may be performed to increase the motive.

3.6.6 Security

There were several protection breaks, hackings, phishing assaults, and ransomware scenes that fact protection is a want for social coverage institutions. Subsequent to seeing a whole lot of weaknesses, a rundown of specialized shields became created for the secured well-being statistics (PHI). These guidelines, named HIPAA Security Rules, assist direct institutions with placing away, transmission, verification conventions, and powers over get admission to, honesty, and examining. Regular protection efforts like making use of round date antivirus programming, firewalls, encoding sensitive facts, and multifaceted affirmation can spare a remarkable deal of difficulty.

3.6.7 Meta-Statistics

To have a powerful fact management plan, it's miles compulsory to have total, precise, and modern metadata to appreciate all of the positioned away facts. The metadata could be constituted of statistics like time of advent, motive, and character responsible for the facts, beyond use (through who, why, how, and while) for scientists and facts investigators. This could allow investigators to mimic beyond questions and assist later logical examinations and precise benchmarking. This builds the handiness of facts and stops advent of "fact dumpsters" of low or no utilization.

3.6.8 Querying

Metadata could make it less complicated for institutions to inquiry their facts and discover a few solutions. Be that because it might also additionally, without valid interoperability among datasets, the query gadgets might not get to an entire vault of facts. Additionally, diverse components of a dataset should be all round interconnected or linked and efficaciously to be had anyhow a complete image of a character affected person's well-being might not be created. Clinical coding frameworks like ICD-10, SNOMED-CT, or LOINC should be performed to lower freestyle thoughts right into a mutual metaphysics. In the occasion that the exactness, fulfillment, and normalization of the facts aren't being referred to, at that factor, Structured Query Language (SQL) may be applied to impeach giant datasets and social databases.

3.6.9 Visualization

A spotless and drawing in illustration of facts with outlines, warmness guides, and histograms to reveal differentiating figures and proper marking of statistics to reduce anticipated disarray could make it plenty less complicated for us to assimilate statistics and use it suitably. Different fashions comprise bar graphs, pie outlines, and scatterplots with their very own unique techniques to skip at the facts.

3.6.10 Data Sharing

Patients would possibly get their attention at diverse areas. In the preceding case, supplying facts to different medicinal offering institutions could be basic. During such sharing, withinside the occasion that the facts are not interoperable, at that factor facts, improvement among specific institutions can be significantly abridged. This can be due to specialized and hierarchical boundaries. This may likewise also disappear clinicians without key insights for choosing determinations concerning subsequent meet-ups what is more, cure strategies for victims. Arrangements are like Fast Healthcare Interoperability Resource (FHIR) and open APIs.

3.7 Conclusion

Nowadays, numerous biomedical and social coverage gadgets, for example, transportable sensors, genomics and molecular telecall smartphone packages, form a core degree of facts. Accordingly, it's far compulsory for us to reflect on consideration and survey that may be achieved using these facts. For instance, the examination of such facts can provide similar bits of know-how concerning procedural, specialized, scientific, and specific styles of upgrades in social coverage. After a survey of those medicinal offering's strategies, reputedly the most capability of patient-express scientific declare to repute or custom-designed remedy is in progress. The combination of massive fact exams of EHRs, EMRs, and different scientific facts is incessantly supporting manufacture of an advanced prognostic system. The groups imparting aid for human offering exam and scientific alternate are surely contributing to higher and effective result. Shared goals of those groups comprise lessening price of research, growing a hit Clinical Decision Support (CDS) framework, charitable ranges to higher remedy dealings, and spotting and forestalling misrepresentation associated with massive facts. Nevertheless, nearly each one in all them faces problems on authorities' problems like how nonpublic facts are allocated with, collective and persisted careful. The consolidated pool of facts from hominoid offering institutions and biomedical scientists have delivered approximately an advanced standpoint, assurance, and remedy of various sicknesses. This has likewise facilitated in creating an advanced and greater useful convention calculated social coverage system. Present day human offering membership has provided understanding of the functionality of massive facts and, alongside those lines, have actualized massive facts research in social coverage and scientific practices.

3.8 Future Scope

Enormous information examination influences the hole inside organized and unstructured information sources. The move to an incorporated information condition is a notable obstacle to survive. Sufficiently exciting, the standard of large information intensely depends on the possibility of the more the information, the more the experiences one can pick up from these data and can make forecasts for future occasions. It is legitimately extended by different solid counseling firms and medical service organizations that the enormous information medical service market is ready to develop at an exponential rate. In any case, in a limited ability to focus, we have seen a range of examination presently being used that have demonstrated critical effects on the dynamic and execution of medical services industry. The exponential development of clinical information from different spaces has constrained computational specialists to plan imaginative methodologies to examine and decipher such a massive measure of information inside a given time period. The mix of computational frameworks for signal handling from both exploration and rehearsing clinical professionals has seen development. The continual ascent in accessible genomic information including natural concealed mistakes from explored and diagnostic practices needs further consideration.

Notwithstanding, there are openings in each progression of this broad cycle to present foundational upgrades inside the medical care research. High volume of clinical information gathered across heterogeneous stages has put a test to information researchers for cautious joining and usage. It is subsequently proposed that unrest in medical care is additionally expected to aggregate bioinformatics, health informatics, and examination to advance customized and more viable therapies. One can obviously observe the advances of medical care market from a more extensive volume base to customized or singular explicit space. Thus, it is fundamental for technologists and experts to comprehend this advancing circumstance. In the coming year, it tends to be extended that huge information investigation will walk toward a prescient framework. This would mean expectation of advanced results in a person's well-being state dependent on current or existing information.

References

1. D. Laney, *3D Data Management: Controlling Data Volume, Velocity, and Variety, Application Delivery Strategies* (META Group Inc, Stamford, 2001)
2. A.D. Mauro, M. Greco, M. Grimaldi, A formal definition of big data based on its essential features. Libr. Rev. **65**(3), 122–135 (2016)
3. S. Doyle-Lindrud, The evolution of the electronic health record. Clin. J. Oncol. Nurs. **19**(2), 153–154 (2015)
4. M. Reisman, EHRs: The challenge of making electronic data usable and interoperable. Pharm. Ther. **42**(9), 572–575 (2017)
5. K. Shameer et al., Translational bioinformatics in the era of real-time biomedical, health care and wellness datastreams. Brief. Bioinform. **18**(1), 105–124 (2017)
6. Y. Yin et al., The internet of things in healthcare: An overview. J. Ind. Inf. Integr. **1**, 3–13 (2016)
7. Apple, ResearchKit/ResearchKit: ResearchKit 1.5.3 (2017)
8. M. Zaharia et al., Apache spark: A unified engine for big data processing. Commun. ACM **59**(11), 56–65 (2016)
9. H. Ahmed et al., Performance comparison of spark clusters configured conventionally and a cloud servicE. Procedia Comput. Sci. **82**, 99–106 (2016)
10. M. Saouabi, A. Ezzati, A comparative between hadoop mapreduce and apache Spark on HDFS, in *Proceedings of the 1st International Conference on Internet of Things and Machine Learning*, (ACM, Liverpool, 2017), pp. 1–4
11. L. Li et al., Identification of type 2 diabetes subgroups through topological analysis of patient similarity. Sci Transl. Med. **7**(311), 311ra174 (2015)
12. G.V. Angelov et al., Healthcare sensing and monitoring, in *Enhanced Living Environments*, (Springer, Cham, 2019), pp. 226–262
13. A. Banerjee, C. Chakraborty, A. Kumar, D. Biswas, Emerging trends in IoT and big data analytics for biomedical and health care technologies, in *Handbook of Data Science Approaches for Biomedical Engineering*, (Academic Press, London, 2020), pp. 121–152
14. A. Mitrokotsa, C. Douligeris, Integrated RFID and sensor networks: Architectures and applications, in *RFID and Sensor Networks: Architectures, Protocols, Security, and Integrations*, (CRC Press, Taylor & Francis Group, Boca Raton, 2010), pp. 511–536
15. A. Mason, A. Shaw, A.I. Al-Shamma'a, T. Welsby, RFID and wireless sensor integration for intelligent tracking systems, in *Proceedings of 2nd GERI Annual Research Symposium GARS*, (Liverpool, 2006)
16. M. Zheng et al., An emerging wearable world: New gadgetry produces a rising tide of changes and challenges. IEEE Syst. Man Cybern. Mag. **4**(4), 6–14 (2018)
17. R. Gravina et al., Multi-sensor fusion in body sensor networks: State-of-the-art and research challenges. Inform. Fusion **35**, 68–80 (2017)
18. G. Fortino et al., Enabling effective programming and flexible management of efficient body sensor network applications. IEEE Trans. Human Mach. Syst. **43**(1), 115–133 (2012)

19. N.G. Valikodath et al., Agreement of ocular symptom reporting between patient-reported outcomes and medicalrecords. JAMA Ophthalmol. **135**(3), 225–231 (2017)
20. J.F. Echaiz et al., Low correlation between self-report and medical record documentation of urinary tract infectionsymptoms. Am. J. Infect. Control **43**(9), 983–986 (2015)
21. A. Belle et al., Big data analytics in healthcare. Biomed. Res. Int. **2015**, 370194 (2015)
22. C. Chakrabarty, B. Gupta, S.K. Ghosh. A Review on Telemedicine-Based WBAN Framework for Patient Monitoring, Int. Journal of Telemedicine and e-Health, Mary Ann Libert inc., 19(8), 619-626, 2013. ISSN: 1530–5627, 10.1089/tmj.2012.0215
23. S. Vitabile et al. Medical data processing and analysis for remote health and activities monitoring. *High-Performance Modelling and Simulation for Big Data Applications*. Springer, Cham, 2019. 186–220

Chapter 4
Smart Healthcare Technologies for Massive Internet of Medical Things

Vijayakumar Ponnusamy, J. Christopher Clement, K. C. Sriharipriya, and Sowmya Natarajan

4.1 Introduction to smart Healthcare

The next-generation health care system is focusing on Patient-centric. The next-generation health care system is trying to utilize the ICT technology effectively in the direction of efficient, quick diagnosis of diseases, remote monitoring, remote diagnosis and treatments, robotic-based surgery, machine learning-based disease prediction, and artificial intelligent-based decision support system. It is going to utilize the mobile phone for image-based diagnosis and recommendation of treatment.

Next-generation healthcare targets give on-time access to medical services, enhancing the quality services for a large volume of the population, enable to disease prevention, effectively managing diseases with an affordable low cost. In earlier days, the health care system uses ICT for getting and storing patients' data, enabling remote-diagnosing diseases and monitoring and proving medical care without internet technology is called telemedicine, telehealth.

When internet technology is integrated with telehealth, it is called as eHealth. After the integration of the internet in the medical system, there are many technologies of internet incorporated in the health care system like cloud-based solutions, IoT medical devices, Blockchain technology, etc. [1].

In the eHealth systems, different healthcare institutions like the hospital, diagnosis center, and health insurance companies are interconnected to share medical data.

V. Ponnusamy (✉) · S. Natarajan
ECE Department, SRM IST, Chennai, Tamil Nadu, India
e-mail: vijayakp@srmist.edu.in

J. Christopher Clement · K. C. Sriharipriya
VIT, Vellore, Tamil Nadu, India

© The Author(s), under exclusive license to Springer Nature
Switzerland AG 2021
C. Chakraborty et al. (eds.), *Efficient Data Handling for Massive Internet of Medical Things*, Internet of Things,
https://doi.org/10.1007/978-3-030-66633-0_4

It enables us to collaborate in real-time to avoid delays in the process and decision making. The eHealth system growing ever and reached the fourth generation now.

The first generation of the eHealth system is given in Fig. 4.1. The first generation of eHealth consists of the interconnection of independent hospital networks, which has the data center for storage locally within the local hospital network.

Figure 4.2 shows the second generation of eHealth where all medical devices store the data in the cloud and the physician can access them remotely. It also includes cloud and IoT technologies. This made the eHealth system as cloud-centric instead of hospital-centric. But, this cloud-based solution introduced the safety/security issue and privacy of the patients' details. In that respect, introduced second-generation eHealth maintains cost, and power consumption is significantly less because of shared resources in the cloud. The IoT medical devices in this generation enable remote monitoring and data collection with better comfort and reduce the cost of the patient for the diagnosis of the diseases and enabled real-time tracking in a nonstop manner by 24 × 7, which also reduced the risk of getting severe problem to the patient.

In the eHealth system, a single big shot is the safety and privacy of the data. Next, the Third generation of eHealth systems incorporated the blockchain technology to label the security and privacy issue. Figure 4.3 shows the third generation eHealth system with blockchain technology added on the top of the second-generation system.

Even though there are many security and authentication mechanisms proposed for protecting patient medical data, blockchain technology will be the promising one for medical data security and privacy because of its scalability and distributive nature of the solution. The self-viable Smart contracts can be implemented on the Blockchain, which enables to examine credentials of the users, to change authorization privileges and roles, and also allow to modify the extent of control based on

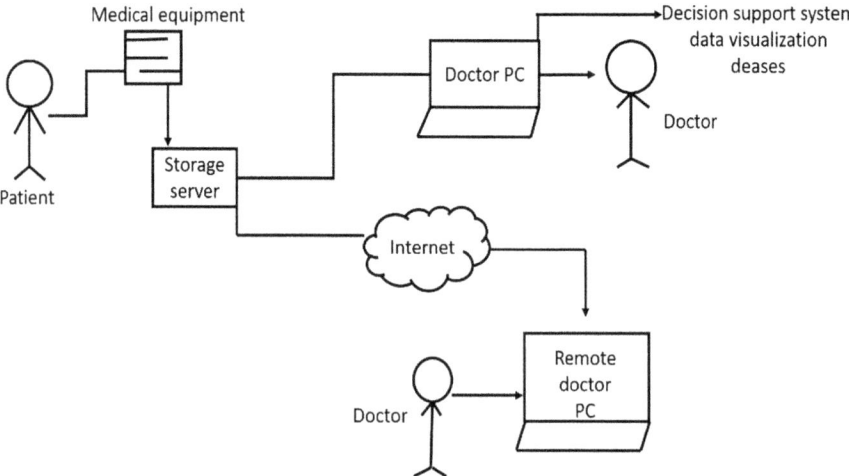

Fig. 4.1 First generation eHealth care system

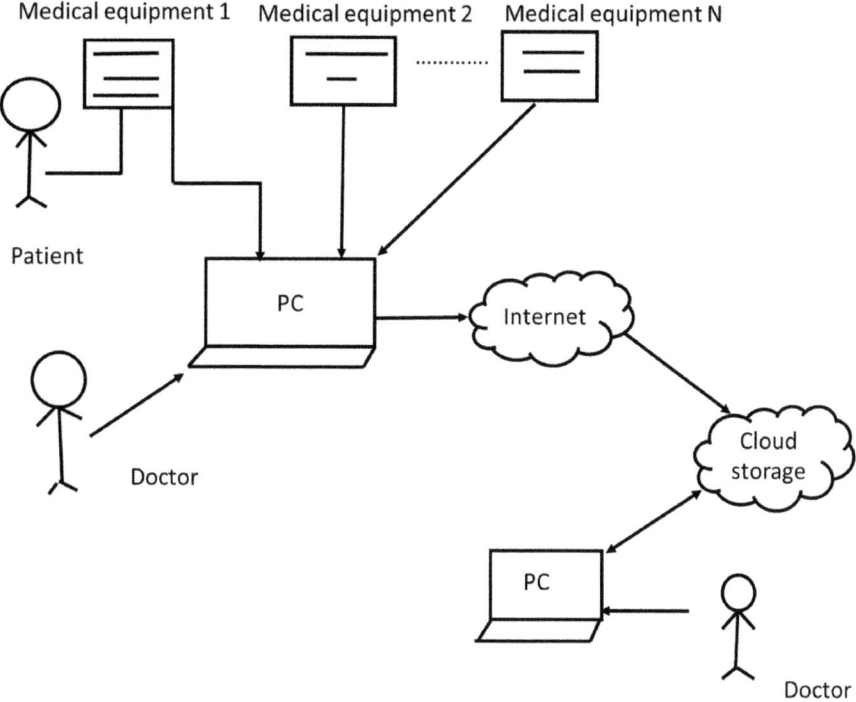

Fig. 4.2 Second generation eHealth care system

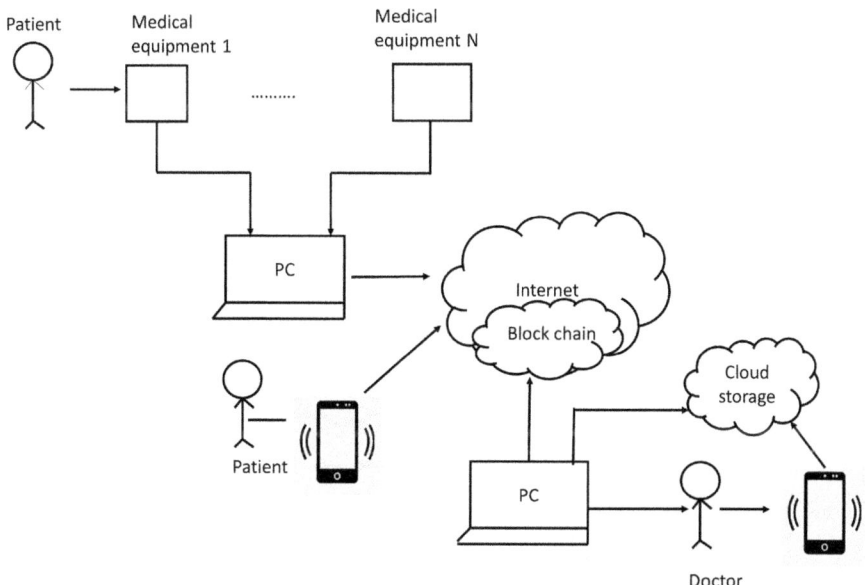

Fig. 4.3 Third generation eHealth care system

patients' requirements. The Blockchain ledger will able to store all patient medical data, roles, and privileges of data used for access management. This kind of blockchain-based implementation of automatic Smart contracts will open another new opening called machine-to-machine communications, where the medical devices or machines can communicate themselves automatically to exchange the patient medical information, which automates the proper diagnosis of diseases.

Health care services are introduced based on mobile applications, which are called as mHealth services. This mobile phone-based mHealth services enabled the patients to grand permission and to authenticate the access of their medical data in the blockchain-based distributed system.

Figure 4.4 shows the fourth generation of the eHealth system. The fourth-generation focused on medical service availability and patient-centric services with predictive analysis using Artificial Intelligence (AI) agents. The AI agents are software entity which may be running on the cloud service and enable community health diagnosis. Continuous monitoring of health via wireless communication is a primary component in the next-generation health care. This wireless-based monitoring enables in a residence-custody service, which reduces the expenses of patient spent on continual visits to hospitals and provides excellent relief for the aged and disabled patients by reducing travel difficulties. The Wireless Body Area Network (WBAN) enables this kind of in-home care medical services [2]. Miniaturization of the medical IoT devices to make them Implantable and wearable is also introduced in this generation for closely monitoring the health parameters. The external entity, like pharmaceutical companies, insurance companies allowed to access the medical data to enhance the services.

Beyond the fourth generation, Wearable 2.0 technology introduced Human-Cloud Integration for the following Generation of Healthcare Systems [3]. Wearable

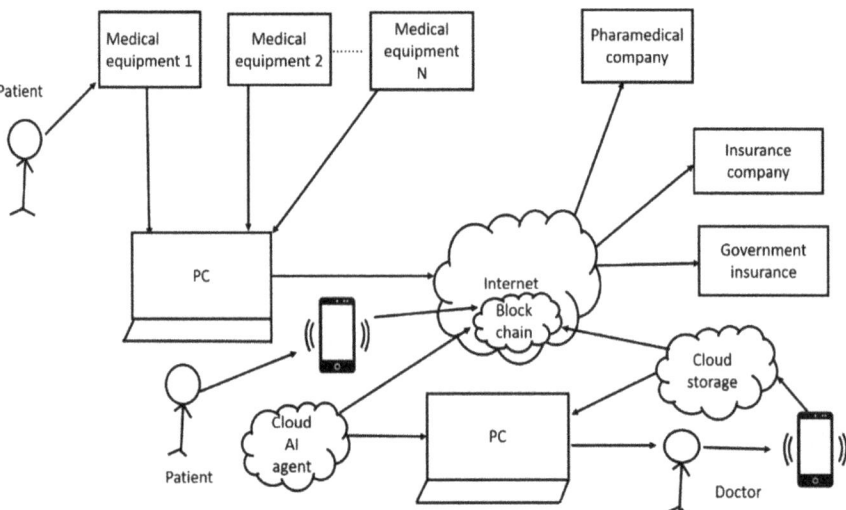

Fig. 4.4 Fourth generation eHealth care system

2.0 aims to enhance the Quality of Service (QoS) and Quality of Experience (QoE) of the upcoming generation healthcare system. In this system, washable smart clothing is introduced, which is fabricated with tiny sensors, electrodes, and connecting wires to collect physiological data for health and emotional monitoring with the help of cloud-based machine learning.

With the ever-increasing number of Internet of medical devices, cloud computing may not be the right solution for smart health. Since the centralized approach in the cloud system may not be able to provide the required level of scalability, it may not be able to offer a required response time in the case of a large-scale system, which introduces heavy communication traffic. Multi-access Edge Computing (MEC) will be the correct solution to overcome the above problem [4]. The MEC can process and reserve data at the boundary of the network, which is located near to the data sources, which provides quick response time, decreases in energy consumption, reduces network bandwidth, and maintains data privacy.

In a nutshell, machine learning, IoT, augmented reality, cloud technology, and mHealth technology are going to innovate and impact the next generation of the health care system, which is further delineated. The remaining part of the present chapter is organized as follows: Sect. 4.2 will explain the use of machine learning and deep learning for health care, Sect. 4.3 will be analyzing how the IoT medical device will automate the health care services, Sect. 4.4 deals with the use of Augmented reality for smart healthcare, Sect. 4.5 discusses how cloud technology is utilized in intelligent healthcare, Sect. 4.6 deals with the mobile phone-based mHealth system and the data analytic, and finally, the chapter ends with a summary of the entire chapter in the conclusion section.

4.2 Machine Learning and Deep Learning for Smart Healthcare

Deep Learning (DL) and Machine Learning (ML) in healthcare provide game-changing impact, which reduces the error in decision making and time for decision making. It automated the entire health care system with very minimal participation of the stack holder, which increases the availability of the health care services for everyone with less cost. It helps the service availability even for the largely populated countries where available physicians, experts, and resources are very limited comparing to that of the population size. This section discusses the following area of ML. (1) ML-based auto diagnosis, (2) ML-based recommender or decision support system development, (3) AI-based treatment system.

4.2.1 Machine Learning and Deep Learning for Disease Diagnosis

Earlier diagnosis of diseases is an important one for preventing severe diseases. But many people are not carrying out the earlier diagnosis because the traditional diagnosis involves a blood test and imaging [5]. Those testing are costlier, which may not be affordable by large communities of people and also time-consuming. But employing machines and deep learning for the diagnosis will automate the process and reduce the cost and time delay. There are various machine and deep learning approaches proposed in the literature to carried out the diagnosis.

The deep-learning mechanism can extract hidden disease symbolic data called feature set, which may not be possible by human analysis. This extracted feature data set able to provide information on molecular status, prognosis, and also can provide the level of treatment sensitivity. This type of inherent automatic feature extraction and selection capability makes deep-learning mechanisms to automate the diagnosis process without much involvement of experts [6].

Figure 4.5 shows a DL-based diagnosis system, where the necessary patient particulars are, the medical device measured data, basic information of the patient, and also his/her historical data are applied as an input. There are many diagnosis systems proposed using the DL mechanism; among them, diabetic diagnosis is given more attention. Diabetes is a more widely available common health problem nowadays because of improper lifestyle and food habits.

Ophthalmic diagnosis using retinal fungus images can be made using ML [7]. Deep-learning mechanisms are used for the segmentation of essential diagnostic optical elements in the eye images. The primary optical element which needs to be segmented using deep learning is (1) optic disk, (2) optic cup, (3) blood vessels, (4) lesions cell. Deep learning is employed to detect glaucoma and diabetic retinopathy, etc., by considering them as a classification problem.

Cardio-Vascular Disease (CVD) is the primary origin of death worldwide. Earlier stage detection of Coronary Artery Disease (CAD) is required because it may result in Myocardial Infarction (MI) and Congestive Heart Failure (CHF).

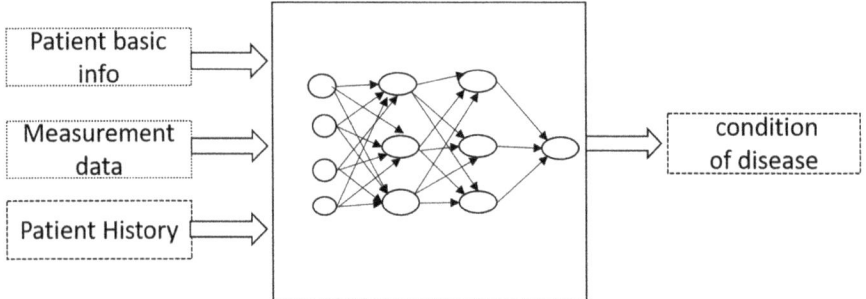

Fig. 4.5 Disease diagnosis using deep learning

Electrocardiography (ECG) signals are widely used for early diagnosis of CAD. There is more chance of misclassification of the ECG signal by manual inter-pretation. The Convolutional Neural Network (CNN) is an efficient deep-learning architecture because of its automatic feature detection and selection. But the ECG signal is time serial data, which is handled efficiently by Long Short-Term Memory (LSTM) models. So combined architecture of CNN and LSTM will be highly prom-ising architecture for the ECG signal analysis. CNN, combined with Long Short-Term Memory (LSTM) models, is used for cardiovascular disease analysis using ECG. A 16-layer LSTM model-based cardiovascular disease diagnosis system can achieve a classification accuracy of 98.5% [8].

The deep-ensemble learning can enable us to integrate multisource data and tap the "wisdom of experts." An Alzheimer's disease classification based on deep-ensemble learning is employed with improved accuracy [9]. A voting layer is employed for feature learning with two sparse autoencoders and decreases the cor-relation of the feature to diversify the base classifiers. A nonlinear feature-weighted vast reliance network is used as the collecting layer for ranking the base classifiers. The neural network is employed as a mega classifier.

Automatic diagnosis of unipolar depression is required in this era because many people suffer such kind of disorders. It results in severe mental health issues. The electroencephalographic (EEG) signal, which is recorded from the human brain, is used to diagnose such kind of disorder [10]. Deep-learning mechanisms are used to automatic detection of such type of unipolar depression successfully. Since the EEG signals are time serial signals, LSTM will be a promising solution for the classifica-tion of EEG signals. A 1-Dimensional Convolutional Neural Network (1DCNN), accompanied by Long Short-Term Memory (LSTM) architecture, is employed to detect the patterns in the EEG data and to classify depressed ones.

A deep transfer-learning technique applied to classify healthy children kidneys and those with Congenital Abnormalities Kidney and Urinary Tract CAKUT [11]. Features of kidneys are extracted from ultrasound images of 50 children with CAKUT and with 50 control samples.

4.2.2 Recommender System/Decision Support System Using Machine and Deep Learning

The recommended/decision support system is used by the physician to get a hidden diagnosis parameter, which may not be extracted manually. The recommend system also acts as an initial screening system for the rural community, where the accessing of medical services are difficult. The decision support system reduces diagnosis time and increases diagnosis accuracy. There are many recommended systems reported using ML and DL. A cloud-supported clinical decision support system accompanied by IoT was designed for the prediction of Chronic Kidney Disease (CKD) [12]. IoT devices are attached to patients who acquire data and store them in the cloud. Deep Neural Network (DNN) classifier is used for the anticipation of CKD with the intensity of severity. A Particle Swarm Optimization (PSO) algorithm is used for best feature selection.

The prediction of Mental disorders is complex, which can be handled by ML. One of the major kinds of mental disorders is Social Anxiety Disorder (SAD), which induces severe fear of embarrassment in social situations. An intelligent decision support system for a SAD diagnosis is carried out with the help of an Adaptive neuro-fuzzy inference system (ANFIS) technique [13]. The system is designed with stages of the procedure of preprocessing, classification, and evaluation. In the preprocessing stage, feature selection, anomaly detection, and normalization using the Self-Organizing Map (SOM) clustering are made.

A generalized decision support system which can detect multiple diseases with deep-learning network is proposed with a name of Health Quest [14]. It clutches the patient's medical information records and family history as input. It works on natural language processing to convert this medical data into organized text. The system is evaluated with 5000 EHR records with multiple diseases.

4.2.3 AI-Based Treatments Using Machine and Deep Learning

Applying machine learning and deep learning for the treatment process is an emerging trend in health care. It helps to derive the best treatment policy by the systematic analysis from various treatment options available for the given disease, which is usually a very challenging task for a human. Figure 4.6 shows the framework of

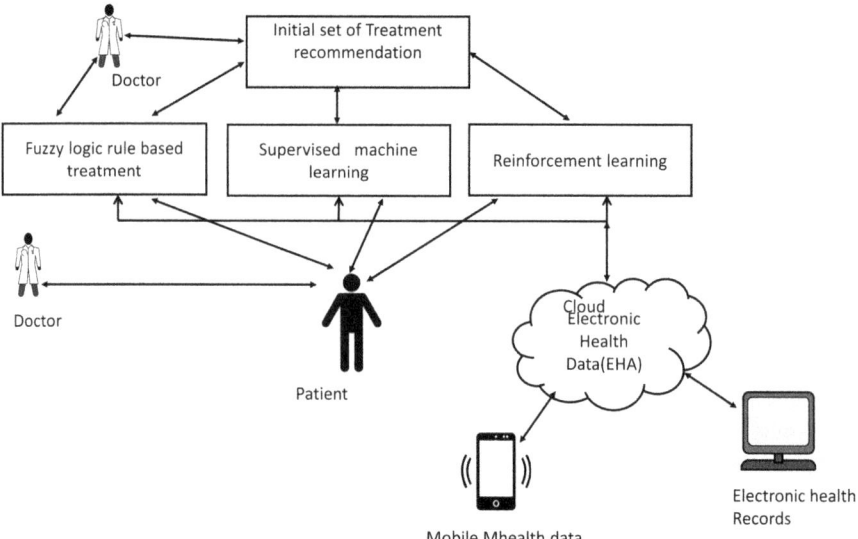

Fig. 4.6 Treatment of diseases using machine learning and deep learning

ML- and DL-based treatment systems. In this framework, supervised learning, Reinforcement Learning (RL), fuzzy decision system [5], and cloud technology are utilized.

Reinforcement Learning is widely used for the treatment purpose since it can learn from the observation of the given environment [15]. The fundamental principle behind reinforcement learning is provided in Fig. 4.7.

In Fig. 4.7, an Agent applies a set of action and observes the impact of those actions in the environment through the collected data. It also estimates the state and a reward value for the given action sets. Here, the reward value indicates the effeteness of the applied action numerically. The Agent adjusts the action such a way the selected action set will increase the reward value. Even though we can deploy the reinforcement-based treatment system very quickly, and we can only make the Agent become experts on the progress of time. But there are still many challenges for applying reinforcement learning for the treatments. The challenges are:

- Getting a real-time observational environment and data are difficult because it makes ethical issues.
- The time to complete the training may be taking some years and which makes the system costlier.
- Evolution of rewards in real-time is not possible due to ethical issues.
- The amount of data needed for training is not definable under RL.
- Viruses, and infections are mostly rapidly changing and evolve dramatically. Such rapid dynamics may not be observed in the training data, which reduces accuracy.
- We are not able to observe everything going on the body; only partial data are available for the training. The agent has to estimate the state of the condition using it.
- Defining reward function is a challenging task with a balance of short-term improvement and overall long-term success.

Despite the above challenges, there are many attempts made to adopt RL for the treatment of the diseases; a small review of such attempts is discussed below.

Treatment planning in radiotherapy is a transposed optimization problem with limitations on a lay of treatment planning parameters (TPPs). The current treatment planning system (TPS) is inadequate of quality because of human solving it. Solving such treatment problems are monotonous and tiresome. A mathematical model of the diseases simulates virtual patients for automatic treatment planning for efficient TPS.

Fig. 4.7 Reinforcement learning

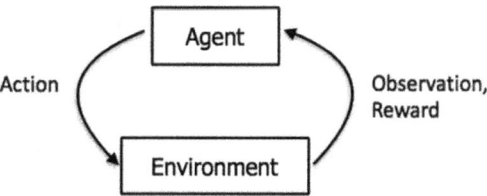

Simulation of such virtual patient and diseases are efficiently carried out by ML, RL, and DL mechanism. RL is a data-driven method to solve consecutive decision-making problems, which can be used for efficient treatment. Finding optimal drug levels for chronic diseases and schedule is naturally a future decision-making problem to find the best sequence of drug dosage.

Proper optimal scheduling of chemotherapy will be one of the promising solutions to treat the cancer patient. A Reinforcement Learning based on a closed-loop controller for drug dosage control of chemotherapy will give an accurate treatment [16].

The antiangiogenic drug is the molecular level-targeted treatment for a tumor. The reinforcement learning framework is used for closed-loop control of antiangiogenic drug dosing. A mathematical model-based virtual tumor growth in the existence of an antiangiogenic inhibitor is created, which is used to interact with the RL model. The tumor size is controlled to the minimal volume within 84 days with the utmost drug of 30 mg/kg/day [17].

Patient-specific treatment is the main focus of the fourth generation and beyond the health care system. The patient-specific model of optimal chemotherapy agents for the treatment of Glioblastoma multiforme (GBM) patients is proposed [18]. Glioblastoma multiforme (GBM) is one of the widely affected brain tumors in adults. A chemotherapeutic agent called Temozolomide (TMZ) is an effective treatment agent for a GBM brain tumor. A modified Q-learning agent is used to interact with a virtual GBM for treatment, and the target is given as to minimizing tumor size. Spatiotemporal dynamics growth of GBM and curing reaction to TMZ agents are replicated on a three-dimensional hybrid cellular automation. The reward value is calculated based on the reaction of the TMZ agent, which is used for learning of Q learning, and an optimal chemotherapy schedule is obtained based on patient-specific parameters like body weight, tumor size, and its position in the brain. The results prove that the RL-based chemotherapy schedule is minimizing tumor growth.

Anemia is another common disease because of an imbalanced diet and lifestyle. The optimal dosing of Erythropoiesis-Stimulating Agents (ESAs) can treat this disease [19]. This ESAs dosing is usually done by clinical protocol manually without considering the individual patient variability for responding to the agent. Since the protocol is not patient-centric, the hemoglobin intensity of patients swings around the target value. This oscillation will result in multiple risks and side-effects. To avoid the above problem, a patient's-centric dosing of ESAs using reinforcement learning (RL) will be the better solution. It is possible to achieve an improvement of 27.6% within their targeted range of hemoglobin, and the drug required can be decreased by 5.13% [20].

Deep Reinforcement Learning (DRL) is a fusion of reinforcement learning and deep-learning algorithms. It is a promising one for auto diagnosis and treatment. A Virtual Treatment Plan (VTP) using a DRL-based framework with Q-learning is presented [21]. A deep neural network perceives the histogram of dose-volume with the constraints of TPPs and generates a magnitude to adjust TPPs. Two VTPs models are designed for cervical cancer High-Dose-Rate Brachy-Therapy (HDRBT), and next is for external beam Intensity-Modulated Radiation Therapy (IMRT). The quality score of the Virtual Treatment Plans 10.7% higher than that of physician-assigned plans. Deep reinforcement learning can be applied for lung cancer detection [22].

Diabetic is another significant disease that almost affected every human being. RL algorithms-based controllers are designed for personalized insulin dosage to control the Blood Glucose (BG) level. But, there are still some issues in using the RL for blood glucose control; (1) the model needs to take care of the influence factor on BG levels like meal intakes and patient physical activity, (2) Clinical validation is required to evaluate the model [23].

4.3 IoT and Healthcare

IoT is an idea of a connected set of everything, anytime, everywhere, and every service. In other words, IoT is an interconnection of all smart, unique devices through internet facilitation with some add-on benefits. This section describes the advancement in IoT-based healthcare technologies and its applications.

4.3.1 Overview of IoT in Healthcare

IoT will have a benefit of advanced connection between the devices for some dedicated applications and services [24]. Fitness program, remote health monitoring, chronic disease analysis, and elderly care are the few critical areas in medical care in which IoT is effectively used. It is useful in-home medication and treatment. Healthcare based on IoT increases one's life quality, and it reduces the cost because of its customizing capacity. Figure 4.8 depicts the IoT-based healthcare networked system. The IoT architecture, including gateways, databases, and medical packages, plays an essential role in making records related to patients' health and providing its services to on-demand to authorized users. The vital features achieved by IoT-based smart healthcare can be of 7Ps, including personalized, persuasive, predictive, participatory, preventative, perpetual, and programmable [25, 26].

Narrowband IoT is the thinner version of IoT communication technology in healthcare [27]. It utilizes a narrow band of the frequency of 180 kHz for the operation. In clinical care, the physiological status of patients' needs to be taken much care, which can be done through the narrowband IoT.

This requires the collection of physiological data using sensors, and the data stored in the gateways, then in the clouds. Stored data are then given to the caretakers so that the periodical health checking by a medical professional is reduced.

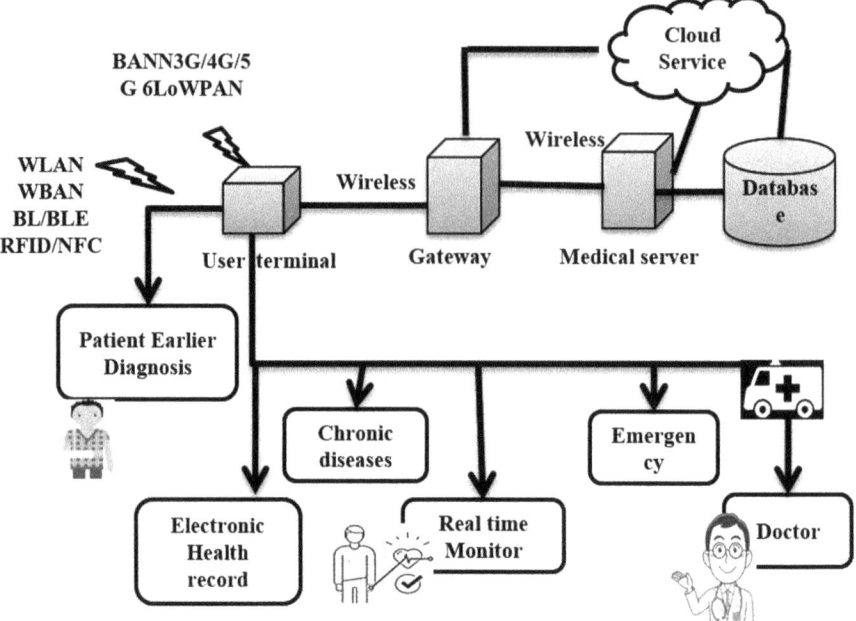

Fig. 4.8 IoT-based networked healthcare system

4.3.2   IoT Healthcare Applications

IoT healthcare can be applied in various applications ranging from pediatric to geriatric, including the monitoring of chronic disease, private health, and fitness. The forthcoming sections illustrate the services and applications of IoT healthcare in detail.

4.3.2.1   Ambient-Assisted Living

A smart home is expected to support the geriatric patients who are aged and sick in such a way that they can live a self-supported and confident life. Artificial intelligence, in association with IoT, can help older adults. This technology is called Ambient-Assisted Living (AAL). It offers an independent life to the elderly. Neural network models for analysis and 6LoWPAN for data communication can be used for implementing AAL [28, 29].

4.3.2.2 Adverse Drug Reaction

Adverse Drug Reaction refers to an effect because of proceeding medication or a group of medications either wrongly or exceeding the limit. IoT-based healthcare can able to help in checking the medication profile of a patient and initiate the proper medication based on the allergy profile of the patients [28].

4.3.2.3 Community Healthcare

IoT healthcare for a group of people is called community healthcare [28]. A dedicated IoT network module can be assigned to a group of hospitals. This structure is called a cooperative healthcare structure. A cooperative platform is proposed [30] in which a distinct authentication mechanism is used for authorization to ensure security. This structure can be viewed as a virtual hospital.

4.3.2.4 Children Health Information

The behavioral, emotional, and mental problems associated with the children are not usual nowadays. In a pediatric ward of a hospital, an interactive IoT totem is placed to offer a "children health information," which is used to educate, amuse, and to empower the children.

4.3.2.5 Wearable Device Access

Sensors can be embedded into the wearable, and IoT services can be used to implement a loyal wearable device access. Fusing wearable devices into IoT is mentioned in [21], which introduces a prototype system that can be used in a wide variety of healthcare applications. Wearable technology provides multimodal interfacing, sensing, and observing capabilities. Basic sensor networks (BSNs) developed more wearable sensory instruments [31] which are helpful to measure various signals such as images, movements, sounds, physiological cues, and forces. Sensor network technology introduces creativity in sports, health care, fitness, and various industries. Sensor fusion, is a state of art of the techniques [32] at different levels, is discussed. A comparison framework and systematic categorization are provided from the feature-level, data-level, and decision-level. This work identifies various properties and the parameters influencing fusion design options at every level. Wireless body sensor networks face issues in programming systems due to high-level abstractions in software and the wearable hardware difficulties. To overcome the flaws, a rapid signal processing in node environment (SPINE) with an open source domain-specific framework programming designed for Body sensor network applications with distinctive characteristics and also based on requirements [33]. SPINE enables environment free from losing the connectivity problems with the system even human beings without carrying personal device.

SPINE2 environment [34] developed with better independent platform and raising the used level of task-related programming model. The developed model enables simultaneous task scheduling and collaborative task execution and for the resource-constrained areas. Although many effective applications are developed for the body sensor area networks related to specific sensor platforms [35]. But still platform-independent body sensor network applications are not implemented. SPINE2 focused on designing the platform-independent programming extraction by giving the task-oriented programming model. The body sensor network application develops a framework [36] which allows signal processing control, dynamic configuration, and monitoring functions of sensor nodes. The designed framework helps to sense the healthcare applications in physical therapy and for defining posture recognition.

4.3.2.6   Other Applications

IoT application can be extended electrocardiogram monitoring, glucose quantity testing, body temperature monitoring, oxygen saturation monitoring, blood pressure monitoring, rehabilitation system, medication management, immediate healthcare solutions, and wheelchair management. There are many more applications of IoT in healthcare [37] like

- Fall Detection: Ensures the independent living of older adults.
- Sportsmen Care: measurement of sleep disorder, weight, blood pressure.
- Patient Surveillance: Remote monitoring of patients' health.
- Chronic Disease Management: Takes care of monitoring and medication for chronic disease.
- Ultraviolet Radiation Alert: Alarms people about ultraviolet radiation in a particular region.
- Sleep Control: Devices like hand watch connected with the mobile phone to keep a note of the sleep profile.

4.4   Augmented Reality for Smart Healthcare

AR provides real-time augmentation to the physician by computer-generated data, 3D images, which makes the diagnosis, treatment, and surgery task very easy and more precise. A basic introduction and application of AR in health care are provided here.

4.4.1 Introduction to Augmented Reality

Augmented reality binds the 3D objects to the real world, which makes humans link the real world so interactively. Even in education, it has so many applications that texts and images can be inserted into the real world, enabling people to get a clarity of understanding in education. Furthermore, it is used in translating applications that can translate one language to another [38, 39]. AR strengthens the interaction between humans and the virtual world.

4.4.2 Healthcare Applications of Augmented Reality

AR holds a lot of applications from healthcare, entertainment, education, defense, rehabilitation, navigation, and maintenance. Among all applications, healthcare is an important application, which we will look at in this section. Using AR, doctors can visualize any part of the human body, and then they can diagnose, perform surgery, use artificial intelligence along with AR for improved prediction and accuracy.

4.4.2.1 AR for Medical Student Education

Patients' body state and the state of the human body organs can be brought into reality for study, diagnosis, and surgery purposes [38]. Students of medical courses require a lot of real-time training, in which AR's application is inevitable. Using computer vision technology, AR helps medical students to have virtual human organs into reality for better understanding.

The development of augmented reality for medical training systems is shown in Fig. 4.9 [40]. The medical training system includes 3D anatomical objects and some

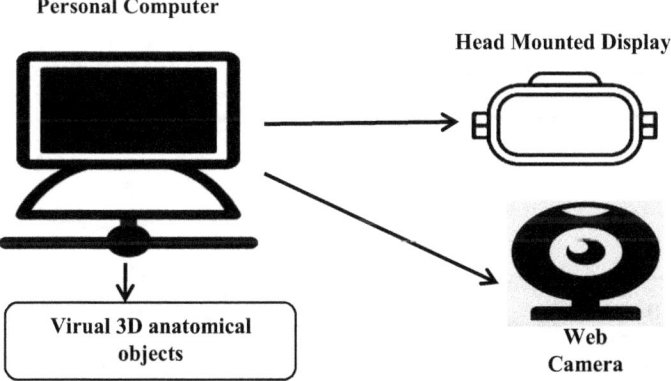

Fig. 4.9 AR setup for generating virtual 3D anatomical objects for training medical students

calculable intuitive interface. When the video is captured using the web camera, the system recognizes it as a marker, then overlays a computer-generated mapping layer over the real-time image. This is how the AR unveils digital components into the recognizable real-world object [41].

4.4.2.2 AR for Electronic Record Generation

An electronically manageable record includes the patient's age, health profile, medication details, etc. AR provides a way to generate an electronic medical form that can be accessed from anywhere within the hospital network, which is a connected computer environment [42]. With the development of AR and VR, technicians can improve in view of electronic medical records so that it can be in a more interactive manner.

In this section, we are going to look at how the AR-based 3D model of lungs or any other organs can be used in surgery [42].

4.4.2.3 AR for Surgery Application

AR system makes surgery very easy and makes precision by the electronics data augmenting during the surgery. A model electronic medical record-based Surgery system in association with AR is illustrated in Fig. 4.10, in which a data glove, server, and Android devices are in interactions for performing the surgery. The hospital's integrated system not only diagnoses but also projects the 3D model of a lung image or any other organ to the surgeon through the segmentation and reconstruction process. So, a surgeon can be able to connect to the server through an Android device and using a gesture, through wearing a headset, he/she performs surgery.

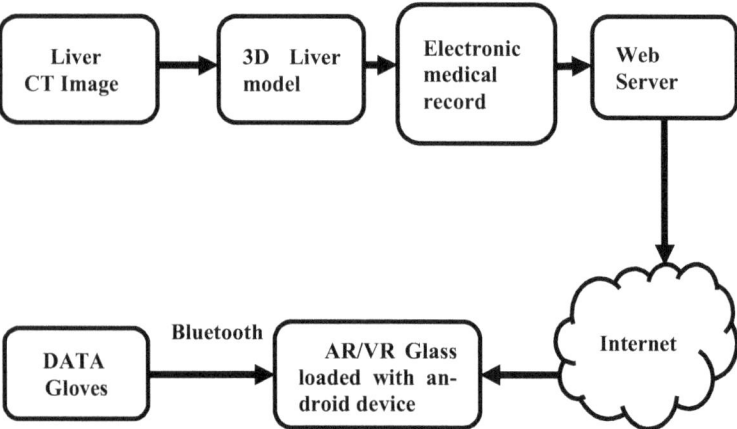

Fig. 4.10 Augmented reality-based remote liver surgery setup

Separate algorithms for segmentation of organ of interest, reconstruction, and gesture recognition are implemented in the server [42].

When surgery in tissues and bones is considered, its success rate is not that high. The employing of AR, VR, and MR bring down the complexity of tissue and bone surgery to its ease. This technology is called Virtual and Augmented Surgical Intelligence (VASI), which involves deep learning, and machine learning provides better accuracy of prediction and diagnosis [43].

A speech and gesture can control AR devices. It makes the possibility of merging 3D image on the patient's organ when the surgeon wears the headset. It even sends accurate anatomical information of the patient. The surgeon can more clearly explain the surgery details to his coworkers or patients themselves with the VASI headset, as shown in Fig. 4.11. This process can let the patients mentally prepare for the surgery. VASI includes all the technologies on one smart device, namely, artificial intelligence, IoT, and machine learning, which will enclose all the required functionalities. It helps to reduce the anesthetic time of the patients and further reduces the rate of error.

VASI converts MRI and CT images into 3D images so that doctors with their headsets can diagnose the problem well and carry out the surgery without any distractions [43].

Though it serves better virtual communication, few limitations exist of using the VASI Headset are short battery life, weight, comfortableness, mobility, and durability of the headset or glove.

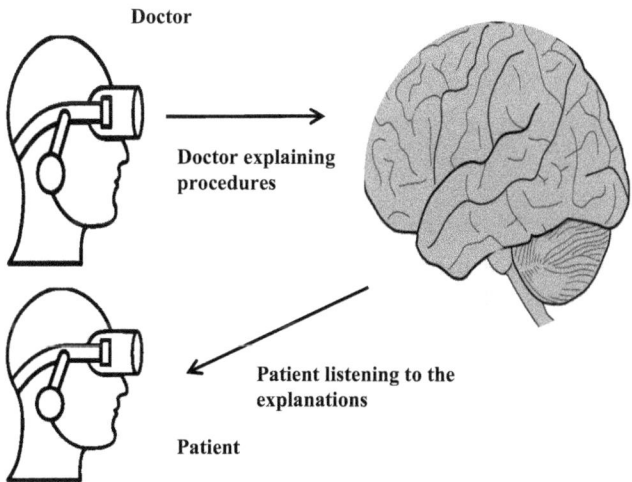

Fig. 4.11 AR-based surgery procedures knowledge creation to patients

4.4.2.4   AR for Knowledge Transfer to Patient

The virtual reality experience increases patient medical education, engagement, and knowledge to enhance patient comfort level to the treatment. The authors of [44] proposed a new virtual reality technology called Health Voyager, which helps facilitate the knowledge pass on between patients and physicians. It uses a smartphone to visually captivate the families of patients with an animation of their anatomy [44]. The platform connects any smart mobile phone or tablet to display digital Medical images through virtual reality and multimedia technology. The technology also enables patients to provide feedback about their condition.

4.4.2.5   Wound Management System

Authors [45] have developed a wound management system using an augmented reality. Chronic wounds require treatment for more than 8 weeks. During the treatment, physicians are required to give accurate documentation for the wound treatment process. The documentation improves the outcome of wound treatment. It enables healthcare physicians to check how wound behavior changes during medication progress [46].

At present, the wound documentation process is cumbersome. If a camera or some devices are used for capturing the wound, then there is a possibility that the germs can go inside the wound. The authors have developed an application along with the smart glass, which receives a command from a gesture or eye blinking, and voice. They used an onboard voice command library of the Microsoft HoloLens to provide voice command, by simulating different wounds and delivering printed pictures for each type of treatment. After that, participants are allowed to do the experimental version of the treatment, and the feedback will be collected from them. After this experimental treatment, real clinical care will be imposed [45].

4.5   Role of Cloud in Smart Healthcare

Cloud technology reduces the cost of equipment, maintenance cost, provides the security of data, reliability by backup mechanism, and offers scalable service anywhere at any time. The above feature attacked the health care industry to deploy their service with less effort.

In the following section, an introduction of cloud technology, how the cloud technology fulfills the requirements of health care services, how it makes it easy to deploy AI-based health care service, and the application of it in health care, is presented.

4.5.1   Introduction to Cloud Technology

In recent days, cloud computing is inspected to be the most promising technology. Cloud authorizes to access the stored information from any place, any time, and any device, which is the need of many companies around the globe.

Cloud is simply a metaphor for the internet. Cloud computing utilizes the computing resources on both software and hardware, delivering the service over the network, as shown in Fig. 4.12.

Three service models are available in a cloud, namely Platform as a Service (PaaS), Infrastructure as a Service (IaaS), and Software as a Service (SaaS) [47]. IaaS model offers processing, networks, computing infrastructure resources, and storage to the users. The PaaS model permits consumers to deploy implementations on the developed programming languages/tools into the Cloud infrastructure. The SaaS model allows the users to gain the applications running on a Cloud infrastructure from different end-user devices.

There are different methods to deploy a cloud [48], namely private, public, hybrid, and community clouds. Individual clouds operate solely for an individual or a single organization. The public clouds are usually possessed and maintained by cloud service providers for the general public and industrial groups.

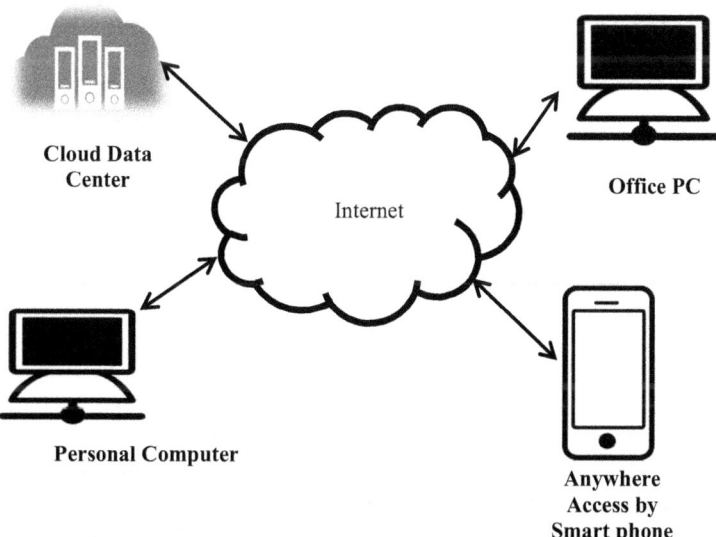

Fig. 4.12 Typical cloud-computing environment

4.5.2   Need of Cloud in Healthcare

Cloud platform serves as a medical record storage center, which acts as an exchange platform for healthcare organizations. The acceptance of cloud in the healthcare field is mainly due to better service to patients and lower cost compared to earlier efforts. BodyCloud, a Cloud-authorized Software [49] as a service architecture proposed for managing the body sensor data cycles and whole life cycle of data analysis. This approach provides intuitive programming model on a less web-based programming group, which permits deploying the community-based body sensor networks applications. Activity aaService enables better BSN-related sensor data collection, high-processing performance and computing, processing at local sensor data, storing and processing the sensor for work flow data analysis, and to update the visualization of results [50]. The performance validation for the developed framework carried out based on the battery consumption, CPU usage, data transmission time, processing load, memory foot print. The most common benefits of cloud computing in healthcare are summarized below.

4.5.2.1   Security and Reliability

The strongest features that a cloud can pay to any of its organization are security and reliability. Even in the case of equipment/technology failure, a healthcare provider will not lose its information.

While talking about a cloud in healthcare, the foremost concern is about its security in the usage of all its applications and data of patients in a third-party server. In recent days, it has been observed that almost all the clouds provide security, monitoring services, and risk management for its users to protect from unauthorized access.

4.5.2.2   Cost

The cost plays a significant role in choosing any application. With cloud computing, the healthcare organization pays only the subscription cost, which is the operating expense, rather than the high price of hardware and capital expenditures.

4.5.2.3   Scalability/Flexibility

Healthcare organizations need to deal with patient portals, medical records, mobile apps, and big data. So, there is a lot of data to be managed, analyzed, and stored. Cloud computing has the flexibility to increase or decrease data storage depending on the flow of patients (example: during flu, the number of patients may increase), and avoid the extra cost in maintaining servers. Further, cloud computing provides the flexibility to adapt to new technology and preventing expensive software and hardware updates.

4.5.2.4   Collaboration

Cloud computing provides an opportunity for the medical service providers to transfer data between each other, thus giving a better treatment by boosting collaboration.

4.5.3   Cloud Computing as a Platform for HealthCare Service

Cloud computing integrates AI and ML in healthcare services, which supports in managing massive data. In recent times, automated decision making has become a mandate in all industries. An AI-based automatic intelligent system must be able to analyze the mixed data generated in multiple sources and identify the fundamental pattern and knowledge that support decision making [51].

The challenges of ML implementation are (1) more execution time required, (2) handling of extensive data. Cloud computing helps to solve those issues.

The cloud platform can impact ML in multiple ways [52, 53]. First, the machine-learning environment from the cloud creates a computer cluster. Its complex libraries working on distributed machine learning setups, which permit the users to use out of box algorithms. It runs the ML algorithm on a collection of parallel implementations over computer clusters.

Cloud Computing provides a scalable, good storage, and efficient infrastructure for processing to perform offline and online analysis of body sensor data streams [54]. For development and management of cloud-assisted body area networks introduced to address the challenges faced by the cloud-assisted BAN architecture.

Cloud offers high-performance data mining and analysis. Platform as a service (PaaS) or SaaS provides machine-learning services, which allow the clients to access ML algorithms through web services [55].

Health organizations can use the cloud for easy deployment of AI-based services with less effort and cost.

4.5.4   Applications of Cloud Computing in Healthcare

The applications of cloud computing in health care have been categorized in many domains, namely teleconsultation/telemedicine, medical imaging, therapy, clinical information systems, and public health.

4.5.4.1   Tele-consulting/Tele-medicine Emergency

Cloud computing-based service is implemented in many Japanese hospitals, where the server environment is built on virtual routers and virtual servers. A peer to peer network to shift medical resources between ambulances and hospitals has been implemented [56], where every hospital has a community cloud on its own to share and upload data with nurses in an ambulance. They termed it as "cloud emergency medical services." It avoids delays during the transportation of patients and reduces the death rate in emergencies by sharing critical patient information with hospitals and ambulances.

4.5.4.2   Medical Imaging

Cloud computing has a notable focus on medical imaging, which includes sharing, intensive computation, and archiving of images.

A distribution framework called Comet Cloud is proposed [57], which is used in image texture analyses. A cloud-based Picture Archiving and Communication Systems (PACS) help in enabling reposting medical images.

Deep learning and Artificial Intelligence are playing a vital role in medical diagnostics [58]. With the medical imaging data, it is possible to provide solutions related to the issues on cardiovascular disease diagnostics. The deep-learning methodology applied to cardiovascular disease diagnostics image classification, segmentation, and identification. Deep learning and Artificial intelligence applications always work efficiently as the training data samples increase [59], and it is necessary to build the optimal neural network to solve the clinical problem. Deep Learning supports second set of eyes in providing integration between smart machines and human beings. Physicians play a supervisor role to sense and exploit the skills that provide them superior to machines.

4.5.4.3   Public Health and Patient's Self-Management System

Telecare Medical Information Systems (TMIS) can assist in providing services like distant monitoring of physiological signals for patients. The user's smartphone needs to have 3-factor authentication based on a dynamic cloud-computing environment to ensure data security and privacy.

An automatic cloud-based Tele-PTSD (Post-Traumatic Stress Disorder) monitor system is developed, which can be accessible through the internet to screen the patients who have PTSD and track their progress during treatment [60].

An expert cloud prototype called iFit is developed [61], which helps in promoting the fitness of older adults by giving fitness suggestions through game activities by receiving physiological data from the user through web services.

4.5.4.4 Hospital Management/Clinical Information Systems

The decision criteria like system ease of use, usefulness, service quality, reliability are identified for the hospital management system using an appraisal model based on the Fuzzy Analytical Hierarchy Process (FAHP) and Fuzzy Delphi Method (FDM) [62].

A private cloud system is developed with virtual desktop infrastructure, 400 virtual machines, and virtual technology support overall and easy access to each hospital information system from every device in the whole hospital.

4.5.4.5 Enhanced Mobile Health Applications

Mobile phone securities and computational power are significantly less. Cloud computing can be used to enhance computation power and security in mHealth applications.

A framework has been developed for implementing security algorithms and complex multimedia on the cloud rather than mobile devices [63]. This work depends on the cloud-computing protocol management model that distributes mobile health services.

4.5.4.6 Therapy

Many applications have been developed for planning, accessing, or managing therapeutic interventions. A web-based application is proposed [64] to model radiation treatment components. It includes the amazon cloud-based model on Monte-Carlo simulation for radiation therapy or dose.

A prototype was developed [65] for a Clinical Decision Support System (CDS) that packets the patient's data and sends it to the rural area.

4.6 mHealth and Data Analytic

Smartphones are a part of human life. So, the utilization of smartphones for health care domain services enables continuous monitoring and patientcare [66]. The utilization of mobile/smartphone for health care services is referred to as mHealth. The typical mHealth system is given in Fig. 4.13.

mHealth uses mobile phone tablets, personal digital assistants (PDAs), and wearable devices such as smartwatches for health services and data collection [67]. There are many mHealth applications: (1) mobile devices-based clinical health and community data collection, (2) proving healthcare data to practitioners and patients in any location, (3) on-field monitoring of the patient, (4) direct provision for health care, (5) Training and collaboration, (6) Healthcare supply chain management, (7)

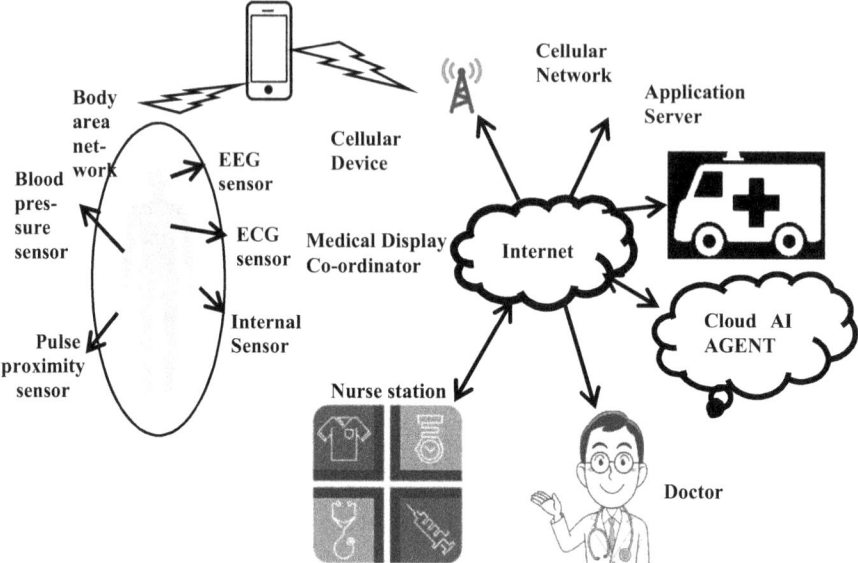

Fig. 4.13 Typical mHealth system setup

Home-based remote patient monitoring, (8) Guidance for chronic care management such as asthma, cancer, and diabetes. This section will describe the application and data analytic aspects of mHealth.

4.6.1 Applications of mHealth

The respiratory disorder diagnosis system, which uses microelectromechanical sensor technology using a mobile phone, is presented. Motion sensors are used to detect the variation in the anterior-posterior diameter of the chest wall during breathing. Novel feature extraction is employed to detect eight different pathological breathing patterns [68].

Night waking is one of the main problems for infants. A research study is carried out for using mobile applications to tackle this issue. The study is dealing with the Customized Sleep Profile (CSP) with 404 infant's age 6–11.9 months. They utilized the freely available behavioral sleep intervention application for smartphone-like Bedtime®, Baby Sleep Application. In the study, it is observed after the application, there is a decrease in the number of night waking. The finding shows that good sleep outcomes can be found in infants within 4 days [69]. Internet of medical things develops many applications in the health care research community. Various automated techniques developed [70] to detect brain tumor with better accuracy in less time. Partial Tree (PART) rule learner, with updated feature set is adopted to identify the brain tumors in terms of grade I through grade IV. The above-mentioned methodology provides better accuracy in detecting the brain tumors with its respective grades.

Various fuzzy and nonfuzzy dissimilarity measures employed to examine the feature wise discrimination [71]. The fuzzy discernibility matrix algorithm uses K parameter for selecting length of the features. It is found that empirical results can identify the most distinctive features. This model employs Convolutional neural network structure to select the health condition and lifestyle pattern-related dataset to analyses and classify the conditions [72]. This model can detect either regular-positive or regular-negative-correlated factors which help to enhance the lifestyle and daily activities. CNN model provides regular health parameters to gain knowledge about the blood pressure, obesity, and diabetes.

4.6.1.1   Effective Self-Management Programs Implementation Using mHealth

Self-management programs are required for an effective treatment for many disease control like asthma and diabetes. But the self-management program implementation in practice is very poor. Current self-management programs are based on symptoms only and suffer from a lack of precision, patients feel uncomfortable, and it consumes more time. The automatic data collection, analysis, and suggestion generation may improve self-management practice and enhance acceptance among patients through mHeath applications.

mHealth system is now able to integrate physiological, behavioral, and environmental information to realize an effective self-management. The mobile application-based effective self-management program offers to the patients: (1) enforce them to use medication and devices correctly, (2) impose them the significance of lifestyle, (3) giving awareness of environmental-influencing factors, (4) help them to recognize aggravating factors, (5) make them understand the value of self-monitoring, (6) Facilitate them to identify worst-case scenarios of the disease and their symptoms; thereby, they can acquire knowledge about when to get urgent medical attention.

A framework called myAirCoach is introduced to study the clinical effectiveness and technological acceptance of the mobile app for self-management practice for asthma patients [73] using inhalation medication. In this study, first applying traditional clinical procedure-based asthma action plans are given to 133 patients for evaluating and managing the symptoms. It is observed that patient adherence to self-management programs seems only 20%. After applying for a mobile application-based self-management program, it is found that there is a significant improvement in managing asthma.

Another study on self-management of asthma is presented with the mHealth and machine learning approach. The work employs machine learning-based prediction for asthma control status. The support vector machine and random forest classifiers algorithms are given an excellent performance for asthma control status prediction [74].

Dementia disease management requires specialized knowledge and training, which makes dementia management is a challenging one. An educational and supportive mHealth/smartphone application is developed to analyze the feasibility of applying it to the dementia functional disability. The study is conducted in three phases; phase 1: an online survey is done to get the needs to the management of functional disability. Experts are involved in developing the mobile application for this need survey. Phase 2: mHealth application is deployed. Phase 3: conduction of a feasibility study with the parameters of usability, adherence, acceptance, and their experiences with the deployed application is carried out [75].

Stress is another significant disease, which impacts many health factors and causes many side-effects. It also affects the treatment and the medication of an existing illness. Accurate detection of stress is one of the requirements for the management of mental health. The current methods are subjective with questionnaires based, which is not accurate. A miniaturized mHealth wireless device that uses a laser-enabled flexible graphene sensor for electrochemical sensing is presented for noninvasively monitor of the level of stress-causing hormones called cortisol [76]. This study can act as a stress monitoring, mHealth application with reliability and accuracy.

The cardiovascular mHealth system is an emerging one for the prevention of cardiac disease, cardiac rehabilitation, and education. mHealth application based on a smartphone with Bluetooth and Global Positioning Systems (GPS) can be used for prevention [77]. The usage of mHeath for cardiac diseases is conducted with a randomized control trial of 120 patients in Australia, which shows that smartphone-based home care service increased to 80% comparing the traditional system, which has only 62%. The adherence analysis proves that 94% of people accepted the system where the conventional center-based system has 68% of acceptance [78].

4.6.2   Data Analytics in mHealth

As the volume of health monitoring data is increasing daily from various sources, the management of such massive data and decision making is a challenging one. The utilization of the big-data analytic will make it easier and able to provide real-time results on the monitoring applications. Through this big-data analysis, a meaningful trend of diseases can be extracted on an extensive community level.

A multiagent system with data analysis is proposed to characterize the physiological conditions of older adults to monitor their behavior [79]. Every ones personal data were collected using Fit bit wristbands and analyzed using the k-means clustering algorithm.

Another smart healthcare system in the IoT environment is developed to monitor the real-time status of the patient using the sensors. Five developed sensors capture the current environmental situation, and it is conveyed to medical staff via a portal, where it can process, analyses the live situation of the patients [80].

A sensor-based biofeedback system is developed as a support model for knee replacement for the patient's healthcare. This model is implemented for the end-user who lacks on exercise rehabilitation. The evaluation is made on 15 patients for 2 weeks. The quality of the developed sensor design is rated as 4.1 out of 5 [81].

4.7 Conclusion

The usage of the latest ICT technologies like ML, DL, IoT, Augmented Reality, and cloud technologies are ever-increasing almost in all the fields. This chapter presented the adoption of those technologies in the health care segment. Overall, all those technologies focus on patient-centric health care solutions at an affordable cost.

In other aspects, those technologies help to automate the entire health care process and try to provide any health service at any place. It also minimizes the human error factors that are involved in the diagnosis and treatment process.

Currently, those technologies are in research and lab level only except one or two implementations. There is a need for standardization of those technologies to adopt. The regulation and policy forming by government agencies to deploy them practically are also another requirement.

Currently, cloud computing has congregated special attention. The healthcare industry has also taken it is call-in using cloud-based platforms to provide better services. Cloud computing-based healthcare is going to be a hugely growing industry shortly.

AR cannot replace the skill of human clinicians; nevertheless, it simplifies and upgrades the complex reconstructive surgery procedures. So, it can complement the process. With an improvement in machine learning and its association with AR can take this technology in healthcare to the next highest level.

References

1. J. Karamachoski, L. Gavrilovska, Framework for next generation of digital healthcare systems, in *International Conference on Future Access Enablers of Ubiquitous and Intelligent Infrastructures*, (Springer, Cham, 2019), pp. 12–24
2. C. Chakraborty, B. Gupta, S.K. Ghosh, A review on telemedicine-based WBAN framework for patient monitoring. Int J. Telemed. e-Health, Mary Ann Libert, Inc. **19**(8), 619–626 (2013). ISSN: 1530-5627). https://doi.org/10.1089/tmj.2012.0215
3. M. Chen, Y. Ma, Y. Li, D. Wu, Y. Zhang, C.-H. Youn, Wearable 2.0: Enabling human-cloud integration in next-generation healthcare systems. IEEE Commun. Mag. **55**(1), 54–61 (2017)
4. A. Awad Abdellatif, A. Mohamed, C. Fabiana Chiasserini, M. Tlili, A. Erbad, Edge computing for smart health: Context-aware approaches, opportunities, and challenges. IEEE Netw. **33**(3), 196–203 (2019)
5. F. Mansourypoor, S. Asadi, Development of a reinforcement learning-based evolutionary fuzzy rule-based system for diabetes diagnosis. Comput. Biol. Med. **91**, 337–352 (2017)

6. A.B. Levine, C. Schlosser, J. Grewal, R. Coope, S.J. Jones, S. Yip, Rise of the machines: Advances in deep learning for cancer diagnosis. Trends Cancer **5**(3), 157–169 (2019)
7. S. Sengupta, A. Singh, H.A. Leopold, T. Gulati, V. Lakshminarayanan, Ophthalmic diagnosis using deep learning with fundus images-a critical review. Artif. Intell. Med. **102**, 101758 (2019)
8. O.S. Lih, V. Jahmunah, T.R. San, E.J. Ciaccio, T. Yamakawa, M. Tanabe, M. Kobayashi, O. Faust, U.R. Acharya, Comprehensive electrocardiographic diagnosis based on deep learning. Artif. Intell. Med. **103**, 101789 (2020)
9. N. An, H. Ding, J. Yang, R. Au, T.F. Ang, Deep ensemble learning for Alzheimer's disease classification. J. Biomed. Inform., 103411 (2020)
10. W. Mumtaz, A. Qayyum, A deep learning framework for automatic diagnosis of unipolar depression. Int. J. Med. Inform. **132**, 103983 (2019)
11. Q. Zheng, S.L. Furth, G.E. Tasian, Y. Fan, Computer-aided diagnosis of congenital abnormalities of the kidney and urinary tract in children based on ultrasound imaging data by integrating texture image features and deep transfer learning image features. J. Pediatr. Urol. **15**(1), 75–e1 (2019)
12. S.K. Lakshmanaprabu, S.N. Mohanty, S. Krishnamoorthy, J. Uthayakumar, K. Shankar, Online clinical decision support system using optimal deep neural networks. Appl. Soft Comput. **81**, 105487 (2019)
13. S. Fathi, M. Ahmadi, B. Birashk, A. Dehnad, Development and use of a clinical decision support system for the diagnosis of social anxiety disorder. Comput. Methods Prog. Biomed. **190**, 105354 (2020)
14. S. Khan, J.A. Shamsi, Health Quest: A generalized clinical decision support system with multi-label classification. J. King Saud Univ. Comput. Inf. Sci. (2018)
15. https://towardsdatascience.com/a-review-of-recent-reinforcment-learning-applications-to-healthcare-1f8357600407
16. R. Padmanabhan, N. Meskin, W.M. Haddad, Reinforcement learning-based control of drug dosing for cancer chemotherapy treatment. Math. Biosci. **293**, 11–20 (2017)
17. P. Yazdjerdi, N. Meskin, M. Al-Naemi, A.E. Al Moustafa, L. Kovács, Reinforcement learning-based control of tumor growth under anti-angiogenic therapy. Comput. Methods Prog. Biomed. **173**, 15–26 (2019)
18. A.E. Zade, H.S. Haghighi, M. Soltani, Reinforcement learning for optimal scheduling of Glioblastoma treatment with Temozolomide. Comput. Methods Prog. Biomed., 105443 (2020)
19. R. Padmanabhan, N. Meskin, W.M. Haddad, Optimal adaptive control of drug dosing using integral reinforcement learning. Math. Biosci. **309**, 131–142 (2019)
20. P. Escandell-Montero, M. Chermisi, J.M. Martinez-Martinez, J. Gomez-Sanchis, C. Barbieri, E. Soria-Olivas, F. Mari, et al., Optimization of anemia treatment in hemodialysis patients via reinforcement learning. Artif. Intell. Med. **62**(1), 47–60 (2014)
21. C. Shen, Y. Gonzalez, L. Chen, D. Nguyen, X. Jia, Automatic treatment planning in a human-like manner: Operating treatment planning systems by a deep reinforcement learning-based virtual treatment planner. Int. J. Radiat. Oncol. Biol. Phys. **105**(1), S256 (2019)
22. Z. Liu, C. Yao, H. Yu, T. Wu, Deep reinforcement learning with its application for lung cancer detection in medical Internet of Things. Futur. Gener. Comput. Syst. **97**, 1–9 (2019)
23. M. Tejedor, A.Z. Woldaregay, F. Godtliebsen, Reinforcement learning application in diabetes blood glucose control: A systematic review. Artif. Intell. Med., 101836 (2020)
24. S.R. Islam, D. Kwak, M.H. Kabir, M. Hossain, K.-S. Kwak, The Internet of Things for health care: A comprehensive survey. IEEE Access **3**, 678–708 (2015)
25. H. Zhu, C.K. Wu, C.H. Koo, Y.T. Tsang, Y. Liu, H.R. Chi, K.-F. Tsang, Smart healthcare in the era of Internet-of-Things. IEEE Consum. Electron. Mag. **8**(5), 26–30 (2019)
26. A.P. Muhammad, M.U. Akram, M.A. Khan, Survey-based analysis of Internet of Things-based architectural framework for hospital management system, in *2015 13th International Conference on Frontiers of Information Technology (FIT)*, (IEEE, 2015), pp. 271–276
27. S.K. Routray, S. Anand, Narrowband IoT for healthcare, in *2017 International Conference on Information Communication and Embedded Systems (ICICES)*, (IEEE, 2017), pp. 1–4

28. H. Rajini, A comprehensive survey on Internet of Things-based healthcare services and its applications, in *Proceedings of the Third International Conference on Computing Methodologies and Communication*, (IEEE, 2019), pp. 483–487

29. S. Durga, R. Nag, E. Daniel, Survey on machine learning and deep learning algorithms used in Internet of Things (IoT) healthcare, in *2019 3rd International Conference on Computing Methodologies and Communication (ICCMC)*, (IEEE, 2019), pp. 1018–1022

30. V.M. Rohokale, N.R. Prasad, R. Prasad, A cooperative Internet of Things (IoT) for rural healthcare monitoring and control, in *2011 2nd International Conference on Wireless Communication, Vehicular Technology, Information Theory and Aerospace & Electronic Systems Technology (Wireless VITAE)*, (IEEE, 2011), pp. 1–6

31. M. Zheng, P.X. Liu, R. Gravina, G. Fortino, An emerging wearable world: New gadgetry produces a rising tide of changes and challenges. IEEE Syst. Man Cybern. Mag. **4**(4), 6–14 (2018)

32. R. Gravina, P. Alinia, H. Ghasemzadeh, G. Fortino, Multi-sensor fusion in body sensor networks: State-of-the-art and research challenges. Inf. Fusion **35**, 68–80 (2017)

33. G. Fortino, R. Giannantonio, R. Gravina, P. Kuryloski, R. Jafari, Enabling effective programming and flexible management of efficient body sensor network applications. IEEE Trans. Human Mach. Syst. **43**(1), 115–133 (2012)

34. G. Fortino, A. Guerrieri, F. Bellifemine, R. Giannantonio, Platform-independent development of collaborative wireless body sensor network applications: SPINE2, in *2009 IEEE International Conference on Systems, Man and Cybernetics*, (IEEE, 2009, October), pp. 3144–3150

35. G. Fortino, A. Guerrieri, F.L. Bellifemine, R. Giannantonio, SPINE2: Developing BSN applications on heterogeneous sensor nodes, in *2009 IEEE International Symposium on Industrial Embedded Systems*, (IEEE, 2009, July), pp. 128–131

36. S. Iyengar, F.T. Bonda, R. Gravina, A. Guerrieri, G. Fortino, A. Sangiovanni-Vincentelli, A framework for creating healthcare monitoring applications using wireless body sensor networks, in *Proceedings of the ICST 3rd International Conference on Body Area Networks*, (2008, March), pp. 1–2

37. Z. Alansari, S. Soomro, M.R. Belgaum, S. Shamshirband, The rise of Internet of Things (IoT) in big healthcare data: Review and open research issues, in *Progress in Advanced Computing and Intelligent Engineering*, (Springer, Singapore, 2018), pp. 675–685

38. V. Mehta, H. Chugh, P. Banerjee, et al., Applications of augmented reality in emerging health diagnostics: A survey, in *2018 International Conference on Automation and Computational Engineering (ICACE)*, (IEEE, 2018), pp. 45–51

39. M. Eckert, J.S. Volmerg, C.M. Friedrich, Augmented reality in medicine: Systematic and bibliographic review. JMIR mHealth uHealth **7**(4), e10967 (2019)

40. R. Umeda, M.A. Seif, H. Higa, Y. Kuniyoshi, A medical training system using augmented reality, in *2017 International Conference on Intelligent Informatics and Biomedical Sciences (ICIIBMS)*, (IEEE, 2017), pp. 146–149

41. Y. Shelke, C. Chakraborty, Augmented reality and virtual reality transforming spinal imaging landscape: A feasibility study. IEEE Comput. Graph. Appl. (2020)

42. M. Weng, L. Huang, C. Feng, F. Gao, H. Lin, Electronic medical record system based on augmented reality, in *2017 12th International Conference on Computer Science and Education (ICCSE)*, (IEEE, 2017), pp. 753–756

43. K. Rahul, V.P.D. Raj, K. Srinivasan, N. Deepa, N.S. Kumar, A study on virtual and augmented reality in real-time surgery, in *2019 IEEE International Conference on Consumer Electronics-Taiwan (ICCE-TW)*, (IEEE, 2019), pp. 1–2

44. A. Palanica, M.J. Docktor, A. Lee, Y. Fossat, Using mobile virtual reality to enhance medical comprehension and satisfaction in patients and their families. Perspect. Med. Educ. **8**(2), 123–127 (2019)

45. K. Klinker, M. Wiesche, H. Krcmar, Digital transformation in health care: Augmented reality for hands-free service innovation. Inf. Syst. Front., 1–13 (2019)

46. T. Ermakova, J. Huenges, K. Erek, R. Zarnekow, Cloud computing in healthcare–a literature review on current state of research, Jan 2013
47. N. Reddy, U. Reddy, Study of cloud computing in healthcare industry, arXiv preprint arXiv:1402.1841, (2014)
48. G. Fortino, D. Parisi, V. Pirrone, G. Di Fatta, BodyCloud: A SaaS approach for community body sensor networks. Futur. Gener. Comput. Syst. **35**, 62–79 (2014)
49. R. Gravina, C. Ma, P. Pace, G. Aloi, W. Russo, W. Li, G. Fortino, Cloud-based activity-aaService cyber–physical framework for human activity monitoring in mobility. Futur. Gener. Comput. Syst. **75**, 158–171 (2017)
50. R. Cioffi, M. Travaglioni, G. Piscitelli, A. Petrillo, F. De Felice, Artificial intelligence and machine learning applications in smart production: Progress, trends, and directions. Sustainability **12**(2), 492 (2020)
51. V. Radhamani, G. Dalin, Significance of artificial intelligence and machine learning techniques in smart-cloud computing: A review. Int. J. Soft Comput. Eng. (2019)
52. D. Pop, Machine learning and cloud computing: Survey of distributed and SaaS solutions, arXiv preprint arXiv:1603.08767, (2016)
53. G. Fortino, G. Di Fatta, M. Pathan, A.V. Vasilakos, Cloud-assisted body area networks: State-of-the-art and future challenges. Wirel. Netw. **20**(7), 1925–1938 (2014)
54. D. Bhamare, T. Salman, M. Samaka, A. Erbad, R. Jain, Feasibility of supervised machine learning for cloud security, in *2016 International Conference on Information Science and Security (ICISS)*, (IEEE, 2016), pp. 1–5
55. V. Koufi, F. Malamateniou, G. Vassilacopoulos, Ubiquitous access to cloud emergency medical services, in *Proceedings of the 10th IEEE International Conference on Information Technology and Applications in Biomedicine*, (IEEE, 2010), pp. 1–4
56. X. Qi, H. Kim, F. Xing, M. Parashar, D.J. Foran, L. Yang, The analysis of image feature robustness using comet cloud. J. Pathol. Inform. **3** (2012)
57. K.K. Wong, G. Fortino, D. Abbott, Deep learning-based cardiovascular image diagnosis: A promising challenge. Futur. Gener. Comput. Syst. **110**, 802–811 (2020)
58. F. Piccialli, V. Di Somma, F. Giampaolo, S. Cuomo, G. Fortino, A survey on deep learning in medicine: Why, how and when? Inf. Fusion **66**, 111–137
59. R. Xu, G. Mei, G. Zhang, P. Gao, A. Pepe, J. Li, Tpm: Cloud-based tele- ptsd monitor using multi-dimensional information. Stud. Health Technol. Inform. **184**, 471–477 (2013)
60. K.C. Tseng, C.-C. Wu, An expert fitness diagnosis system based on elastic cloud computing. Sci. World J. **2014**, 981207 (2014)
61. C. Low, Y.H. Chen, Criteria for the evaluation of a cloud-based hospital information system outsourcing provider. J. Med. Syst. **36**(6), 3543–3553 (2012)
62. M. Nkosi, F. Mekuria, Cloud computing for enhanced mobile health applications, in *2010 IEEE Second International Conference on Cloud Computing Technology and Science*, (IEEE, 2010), pp. 629–633
63. D. Parsons, J.L. Robar, D. Sawkey, A Monte Carlo investigation of low-z target image quality generated in a linear accelerator using Varian's VirtuaLinaca. Med. Phy. **41**(2) (2014)
64. B.E. Dixon, L. Simonaitis, H.S. Goldberg, M.D. Paterno, M. Schaeffer, T. Hongsermeier, A. Wright, B. Middleton, A pilot study of distributed knowledge management and clinical decision support in the cloud. Artif. Intell. Med. **59**(1), 45–53 (2013)
65. G. Karageorgos, I. Andreadis, K. Psychas, G. Mourkousis, A. Kiourti, G. Lazzi, K.S. Nikita, The promise of mobile technologies for the health care system in the developing world: A systematic review. IEEE Rev. Biomed. Eng. **12**, 100–122 (2018)
66. M.Z. Alam, M.R. Hoque, W. Hu, Z. Barua, Factors influencing the adoption of mHealth services in a developing country: A patient-centric study. Int. J. Inf. Manag. **50**, 128–143 (2020)
67. A.R. Fekr, M. Janidarmian, K. Radecka, Z. Zilic, Respiration disorders classification with informative features for m-health applications. IEEE J. Biomed. Health Inform. **20**(3), 733–747 (2015)

68. E.S. Leichman, R.A. Gould, A.A. Williamson, R.M. Walters, J.A. Mindell, Effectiveness of an mHealth intervention for infant sleep disturbances. Behav. Ther. (2020)
69. S.R. Khan, M. Sikandar, A. Almogren, I.U. Din, A. Guerrieri, G. Fortino, IoMT-based computational approach for detecting brain tumor. Futur. Gener. Comput. Syst. **109**, 360–367 (2020)
70. R. Chatterjee, T. Maitra, S.H. Islam, M.M. Hassan, A. Alamri, G. Fortino, A novel machine learning-based feature selection for motor imagery EEG signal classification in Internet of Medical Things environment. Futur. Gener. Comput. Syst. **98**, 419–434 (2019)
71. W.N. Ismail, M.M. Hassan, H.A. Alsalamah, G. Fortino, CNN-based health model for regular health factors analysis in Internet-of-Medical Things environment. IEEE Access **8**, 52541–52549 (2020)
72. R.J. Khusial, P.J. Honkoop, O. Usmani, M. Soares, A. Simpson, M. Biddiscombe, S. Meah, et al., Effectiveness of myAirCoach: A mHealth self-management system in asthma. J. Allergy Clin. Immunol. Pract. (2020)
73. O. Kocsis, A. Lalos, G. Arvanitis, K. Moustakas, Multi-model short-term prediction schema for mHealth empowering asthma self-management. Electron. Notes Theor. Comput. Sci. **343**, 3–17 (2019)
74. R. Sarath, W. Moyle, C.J. Jones, P. Calleja, Development of an mHealth application for family careers of people with dementia: A study protocol. Collegian **26**(2), 295–301 (2019)
75. R.M. Torrente-Rodríguez, J. Tu, Y. Yang, J. Min, M. Wang, Y. Song, Y. Yu, et al., Investigation of cortisol dynamics in human sweat using a graphene-based wireless mHealth system. Matter (2020)
76. C.K. Chow, N. Ariyarathna, S.M. Islam, A. Thiagalingam, J. Redfern, mHealth in cardiovascular health care. Heart Lung Circ. **25**(8), 802–807 (2016)
77. M. Varnfield, M. Karunanithi, C.K. Lee, E. Honeyman, D. Arnold, H. Ding, et al., Smartphone-based home care model improved use of cardiac rehabilitation in postmyocardial infarction patients: Results from a randomised controlled trial. Heart **100**(22), 1770–1779 (2014)
78. S. Mendes, J. Queiroz, P. Leitão, Data driven multi-agent m-health system to characterize the daily activities of elderly people, in *2017 12th Iberian Conference on Information Systems and Technologies (CISTI)*, (IEEE, 2017), pp. 1–6
79. R. Argent, P. Slevin, A. Bevilacqua, M. Neligan, A. Daly, B. Caulfield, Wearable sensor-based exercise biofeedback for orthopedic rehabilitation: A mixed-methods user evaluation of a prototype system. Sensors **19**(2), 432 (2019)
80. C. Chinmay, Mobile Health (m-Health) for Tele-wound Monitoring, IGI: Mobile Health Applications for Quality Healthcare Delivery, Ch. 5, 98-116, (2019) ISBN: 9781522580218 https://doi.org/10.4018/978-1-5225-8021-8.ch005
81. R. Argent, P. Slevin, A. Bevilacqua, M. Neligan, A. Daly, B. Caulfield, Wearable sensor-based exercise biofeedback for orthopedic rehabilitation: a mixed-methods user evaluation of a prototype system. Sensors, **19**(2), 432 (2019)

Chapter 5
Sensor Informatics of IoT, AR/VR, and MR in Healthcare Applications

J. Priya, C. Palanisamy, and C. Vinothini

5.1 Introduction

Invigorating researches are taking place in many fields such as healthcare, networking, information technology, and so on. Amongst all applications, healthcare is the unit where the elitist researchers are concentrating on. Smart healthcare applications instigate the growth in medical sciences. Though adequate medical facilities are there, most of the facilities are not reached to the needy on time. Here the technology comes and paves a way to resolve it. Emerging technologies are nowadays make circumstances topsy-turvy with the help of numerous smart applications. The backbone for all these things is the so-called "Sensors".

A sensor can be of any type, a gadget, a piece of equipment, or simply a device that senses any type of events related to the application for the sensor specifically designed for. Sensor is the backbone of every existing and upcoming technology. Based on sensor information, applications are being designed for any purpose. There are wide-ranging kinds of sensors used everywhere which include temperature and humidity sensor to the flagship of sensor types. The applications of sensors are vast in various fields from the ground to galaxies. It includes Agriculture, Human comfort, Food processing, Building, Medical, Robotics, Remote sensing, and so on.

In today's world, the Emerging technologies include the internet of Things (IoT), Artificial intelligence, Machine Learning, Deep Learning, Augmented Reality,

J. Priya (✉) · C. Palanisamy
Department of Information Technology, Bannari Amman Institute of Technology, Coimbatore, Tamilnadu, India
e-mail: cpalanisamy@bitsathy.ac.in

C. Vinothini
Department of Computer Science and Engineering, Dr. N.G.P Institute of Technology, Coimbatore, Tamilnadu, India

Virtual Reality, and so on. These technologies made human life as ease. Among all those applications of emerging technology, Healthcare domain is being the top most important and needy field of public. Hence, so many researchers are working on the Healthcare domain by integrating all the existing and emerging technologies. Internet of Medical Things (IoMT), one among those technologies, helps in a great manner with the help of medical sensors. IoMT defines the Medical sensors as the sensors used to monitor, diagnose, and treat illness in the medical domain. Another term called Smart Sensors, which can be defined as a sensor package that employs "on-chip signal processing". Therefore, to make the virtual world to be a real one, sensor technology plays a vital role to invent newer applications with the help of emerging technologies in all walks of life.

The short remainder of this chapter falls here; Sect. 5.2 is about the sensors, classification, medical applications. Sensors in great technologies are described in the Sect. 5.3. IoT and sensors, AR, VR, and MR and their corresponding role in health care are given in the Sections 5.4, 5.5, 5.6, and 5.7, respectively. Section 5.8 lists out the existing medical application of emerging technology. A brief about data handling and the summary with future work are explained in Sections 5.8 and 5.9.

5.2 Sensors and Sensor Networks

In general, the term "transducer" is defined as "a device which converts one form of energy into another form" means it provides as output in a readable format of human, with respect to a particular object being measured or a specific quantity that meant to be measured. The definition of the transducer is given here just because it is being a near-synonym of the so-called "Sensor". A sensor can be of any type, a gadget, a piece of equipment, or simply a device or a module defined for a specific purpose or a function that senses the changes or events in an environment and conveys the detected information to further electronic devices connected to the sensor.

Today's digital era moves towards the emerging technologies which include the internet of Things (IoT), Artificial intelligence, Machine Learning, Deep Learning, Augmented Reality, Virtual Reality, and so on. These technologies made human life as easy as possible. There is a well-known saying, "Smart work is better than hard work" which means being smart in work saves time and energy a lot. Because of these technologies exist, the meaning for "smart" becomes more Smarter with the help of the "sensor". Sensor is the backbone of every existing and upcoming technology. Based on sensor information, applications are being designed for any purpose. The new epoch in sensor technology has steered in since there is a demand for new sensors, allowing new approaches for transmitting physical events into an output that would be processed by a processor readily. For specific functions, the sensors can be customized with integrated circuits (IC).

Sensors are commonly used in our day-to-day things that start from touch sensor in smart mobile to MARG sensors in smart automobiles. Also there are so many applications that are being existed still in our lives, but most of them are unaware to common people. The uses and sensor-based applications are expanded to an unimaginable extinct. With advancement in manufacturing technology, sensors are beyond the conventional fields of pressure, humidity, temperature or distance measurements, for instance into gyroscope, magnitude, and altitude sensors, also chemical properties measurement of a material. Besides, conventional sensors like potentiometer, distance measuring sensors are still being used widely in so many fields.

The rate of sensitivity of a sensor can be identified by calculating the changes in output value of a sensor when input value of quantity is being changed. Consider a level sensor is placed in a water tank. If the water level in the tank increased by 1 cm when the intake is increased by 1 L, here the sensitivity of the level sensor is 1 cm/L. Basically, most of the sensors work on linear transfer function model. The sensitivity is simply stated in the form of the slope of the linear characteristics. In case of analog type of measurand, the sensor's analog output or electrical output to be converted to the unit of measurand requires a mathematical operation i.e., dividing the electrical output of the sensor by value of slope. For digital type, an ADC (analog-to-digital converter) is required.

Classification There are a wide-ranging kinds of sensors used everywhere. Certain sensors are intended to measure very simple measurands like temperature and humidity. In other hand, cutting-edge sensors are envisioned to sense accurate information in applications like remote sensing, satellite information, and even to detect the global position of a robot.

Quite a lot of classifications are made for sensor, based on the form of output signal, type of measurand, and means of application and in many ways. First type of classification is done based on the signal as Analog sensor and Digital Sensor. Analog sensor gives output as continuous signal in response to the quantity to be measured whereas Digital sensor deals with the digital data or discrete input devices. Probably analog-to-digital converter would have been used with digital types of sensors.

Next, broad classification is based on the form of signal and the respective measurand. It includes the Thermal sensors for measurands like temperature, heat, and entropy. Similarly, Radiation sensors for gamma rays, ultraviolet, radio waves, etc., and Mechanical sensors for displacement, acceleration, force, flow, and so on. And it extends as Magnetic sensor, Chemical Sensor, Biological sensors for measurands like magnetic permeability, chemical properties, and bio-medical metrics as sugar, antigens in that order.

Another classification is based on the application. In Robotics, sensors are of proprioceptive and exteroceptive sensors. Sensors used to measure the speed of motor, robot joints, voltage of battery used, are called as proprioceptive sensors whereas exteroceptive sensors are used to measure distance, amplitude, and intensity of light, etc. In Remote Sensing, the sensors are grouped into active sensors and passive sensors. Sensors that create its own drive, no need of external power supply (interacts with surface/atmosphere) are known as active sensors. In other hand, passive sensors work with naturally existing energy (solar energy or microwave radiations).

Whatever category the sensor lies on, it should obey the following:

- Precise to the measured stuffs.
- Unaffected by any other metrics probably come across in an application.
- Does not sway the measured things.

If the above-mentioned rules are followed by a sensor, then it is said to be a first-class sensor. And the characteristics of sensors are generally grouped into static and dynamic. Static characteristic includes accuracy, threshold, hysteresis, and nonlinearity while dynamic characteristics comprise instability, drift, noise, repeatability, and step response.

Smart Sensor Since IoT brings out everything as "smart and intelligent", the massive advancement in sensor technology focuses on smart sensor development. The simple principle of smart sensors is that the "*sensor complications must be covered inside and must be translucent to the system*". In the way of presenting as simple aspects to a network by means of a digital interface, the smart sensors are devised. In simple terms, a smart sensor can be defined as a sensor package that employs "on-chip signal processing". In addition, a smart sensor primarily encompasses any type of sensor module, interfacing unit, signal processing circuit, and a power source. Along with these primary portions, sensing element, analog filter, data conversion, digital information and communication processing, and amplification systems are included as subsystems. Nevertheless, the concept "smart-sensing" makes fresh chances for using new innovative materials and compounds for sensor manufacturing. It avoids the constraints of applications on various fields. Possible advantages of smart sensor includes lower down time, lesser maintenance, increased reliability, less weight, minimum cost, fault tolerance, a lesser amount of complexity, and adaptability, etc. At present, the usage of smart sensors appears to be limited to specific applications.

The applications of sensors are vast in various fields from the ground to galaxies. It includes Agriculture, Human comfort, Food processing, Building, Medical, Robotics, Remote sensing, and so on. Different sensors are used in different applications based on certain criteria like environmental condition, range of sensor, calibration, accuracy, and cost of sensor. And based on sensor property too, can be applied in some matters. The focus of this chapter is all about the sensor with emerging technologies in the medical field.

Sensors in Medical Medical sensors are defined as the sensors used to monitor, diagnose, and treat illness in the medical domain. Based on the risk profiles, the medical devices are classified into different classes such as Class-I for lower potential risk, Class-IV for highly potential risk, and it goes on.

The sensors used in medicine have some salient features. Sensors should act in accordance with the safety standard "IEC 60601-1" and statutory conditions including additional enforcement and criteria for quality management, usability, functional safety, and risk management in order to make sure that the prescribed device works properly in response with the given inputs. A good sensor should provide the accurate measurement with high precision, highly stable, and with quick response time. In order to connect with processor and controllers, a sensor must deliver measurements in the form of digital output.

Figure 5.1 represents the different types of sensors used in health care and its functions are briefly given in the Table 5.1.

Advanced Sensor technologies offer leading cutting-edge medical sensors specifically for patient care and critical care applications that provide accurate and reliable sensing information from the medical devices to respective destination to monitor critical patients with chronic diseases.

In patient monitoring and tracking applications, the medical sensors are applied in medical instrumentation, clinical thermometry, blood pressure, drug delivery, respiratory, sleep apnea, and fall detection. Whereas in a critical care environment, high-performance medical sensors meant for their reliability, accuracy, affordable, and compact size are used. Under critical care, the medical sensors are implemented primarily in esophageal stethoscopes, normal thermometers, skin sensors, heart catheters, respiration monitors, blood analyzers, hypodermic needle sensors, and incubators. Also used in drug delivery, surgical temperature assemblies, fluid management and medical instrumentation process.

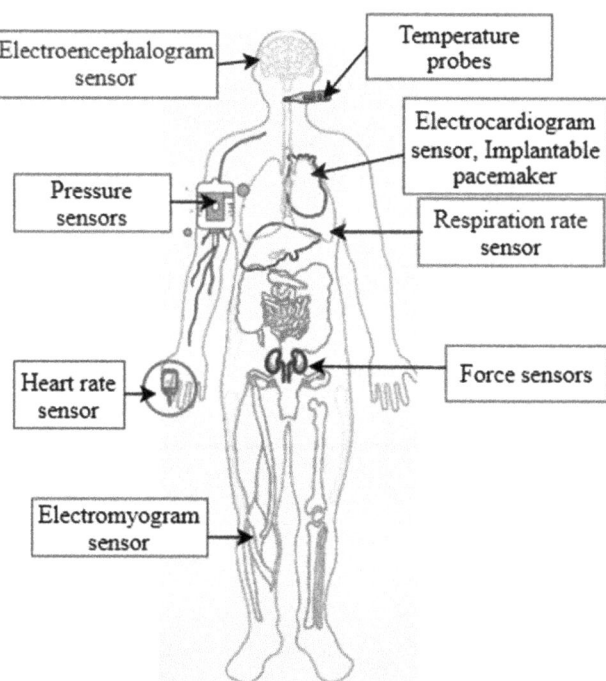

Fig. 5.1 Sensors in Healthcare

Table 5.1 Types of Medical Sensors and Functions

Medical Sensor		Function
	Temperature probes	Body temperature measurement
		gives better treatment and medication for patients
		commonly known as thermometers
	Force sensors	Kidney dialysis machines
	Airflow sensors	Anesthesia delivery systems
		Laparoscopy
		Heart pumps, etc.
	Pressure sensors	Infusion pumps
		Sleep apnea machines
		Most of the pressure sensors are incorporated with embedded systems
		Used for monitoring blood pressure, medical diagnosis
	Implantable pacemaker	A real-time embedded sensor system
		Delivers a harmonized rhythmic electric stimulus to the heart muscle in order to retain active cardiac rhythm.
	Oximeter	Determines the ratio of oxygen-saturated hemoglobin in the blood and the total hemoglobin count in the blood
	Glucometer	Determines rough blood glucose concentration

Medical Sensor		Function
	Magnetometer	Stipulates direction of the user by observing the changes in the earth's magnetic field around the user
	Electrocardiogram sensor	Records the electrical activity of the heart known as ECG sensor
	Heart rate sensor	Counts the amount of heart retrenchments per minute
	Electroencephalogram sensor	Calculates the electrical activity of the brain
	Electromyogram sensor	Measures the electrical activity created by skeletal muscles
	Respiration rate sensor	Counts the chest rises happened in a minute

Wearable Sensors Wearable devices are generally in direct contact with user's skin membrane or implanted in the user's body, therefore the size and physical compatibility of a sensor with human tissues have to be analyzed carefully. This necessity provokes the amalgamation of novel provisions and technologies. Incorporating sensing elements with weaves is a method that a lot many researchers are agreeing and take on to the next level. Few design principles are to be considered before going for wearable devices [1]. They are Comfortable and noninvasive, long-lasting in terms of power, highly accurate, secure, user friendly, customizable, and interoperable that leads to successful user acceptance for wearable devices.

Though sensor by itself as a super good technology grows massively today, it results in very great heights of applications when collaborated with one another great emerging technologies. For instance, finest technologies of today like Internet of Things (IoT), AR/VR, Mixed Reality, Radar, 5G, and goes on. Some technologies where sensors are used copiously are articulated here and moreover how it is helpful in the field of medicine and to what extent it could be benefitted too explained.

5.3   Sensors in Internet of Medical Things (IoMT)

The Internet of Things (IoT), a pulsating word everywhere today. As a technology, it touches an unimaginable zenith by its usages and demand in applications for each and every field than any other technology does [2]. IoT can be related with human for better understanding. Humans having skin, ears, eyes, and nostril as sensing elements for touch and feel habituates. Without these sensing elements, humans could do nothing in day-to-day life. Similarly, deprive of sensors, IoT is nothing. As the brain and nervous system in humans, controllers and actuators are playing their role in IoT. Additional to all above-mentioned hardware, middleware plays an important role especially in communication between devices and applications. It is a type of software which acts between an OS (operating System) and the applications running on the network. Basically functioning as hidden translation layer, the middleware permits communication and data management, data handling for disseminated applications. Middlewares, usually used in conventional distributed systems, are essential tools for the design and implementation of smart objects and smart environment applications. And it provides specific and general abstractions. For example, sensor and actuator interface, knowledge management, interobject communication, etc [3]. This technology is not only about connecting all devices which are capable of getting connected with the help of the internet but also it is about refining the way in all walks of life and also a great impact on the environs. To say stuff simply, with this interconnected devices people can set up their life in the way much more safer, extra productive, super smarter, and well-versed than ever before.

Figure 5.2 represents few sensors that are used frequently in IoT applications and the brief definitions of those sensors are given below:

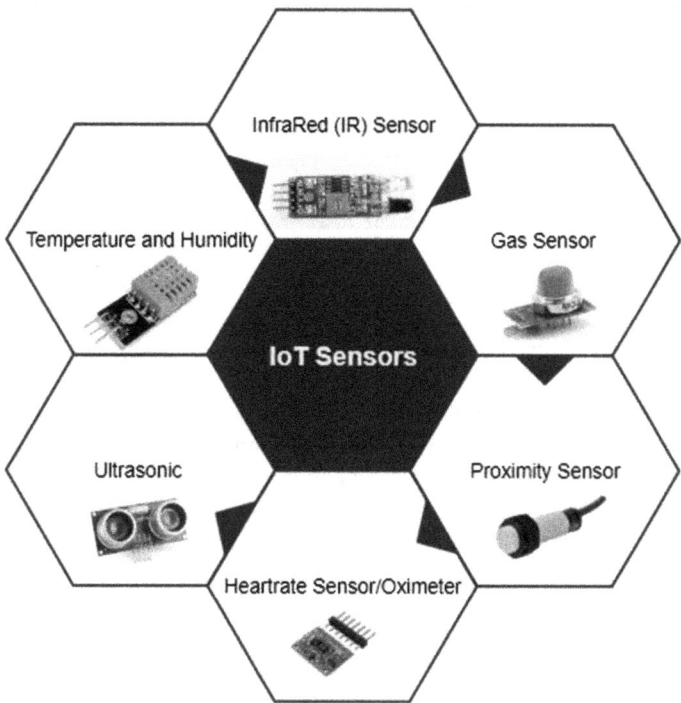

Fig. 5.2 Major IoT Sensors

5.3.1   Gas/Smoke Sensor

One of the commonly used sensors in most of the environment is Gas Sensor. It used to detect gas in an environment, which is more supportive in safety systems. Specifically, this can be implemented in an area to detect leakage of gases and prevents explosions. There are so many readymade sensors available to detect harmful, flammable, and poisonous gases. For instance, MQ7 detects carbon monoxide, most dangerous gas. There are quite a lot of gas sensors are there named as MQ2, MQ3, MQ135, etc.

5.3.2   Temperature and Humidity Sensor

This sensor plays a foremost role almost everywhere. Agriculture, manufacturing industries, and atmosphere are few areas of its application. For example, to measure the machineries temperature in Industries, to detect the value of moisture of soil in agriculture field, temperature and humidity sensors are used. An affordable, basic, ease to use sensor is DHT11, DHT22 available easily in market. No need of analog pins for this category. It is a type of capacitive and digital sensor.

5.3.3 Infrared Sensor

Infrared (IR) sensor works based on the simple principle of emitting and receiving radiation. Here the radiation is infrared. It has been deployed in many more applications. Though it has the capability to detect heat and motion of an object, commonly it is used to detect obstacles. IR detectors are being used for applications as thermal imaging and night vision. IR sensors are also available in market.

5.3.4 Ultrasonic Sensor

Ultrasonic Sensor is a kind of reliable sensor. Similar to infrared sensor, ultrasonic sensor also works based on the principle of transmitting and receiving signal (e.g., SONAR). It transmits sound signal and receives an echo signal of the same. Ultrasonic sensor has the ability to compute the distance covered by the signal from transmitting end to receiving end. Hence, it is used to detect any object or to measure the distance between objects by hitting the signal on an object and receives it back.

5.3.5 Proximity Sensor

Without any physical contact, the sensor has the capability to spot the presence of human or objects nearby. Here, the sensor uses an electromagnetic beam or simply a field of electromagnetic signal and waits for the returning radiation and then it calculates the difference in transmitted and received signal strength. Fall detection and people counting are few common examples. Alarm technique in reversing, a car holds a proximity sensor which detects the obstacles and objects in the pathway. Available in smartphone too, detects human face during a video call. Example for proximity sensor is Si114x, Si1102, etc.

One of the applications of IoT is IoMT. In medical industry, the technology makes things easy, convenient, and secure in a healthcare environment for both professionals and patients. Smart healthcare IoT devices provided with sensors used to monitor and track the patient's condition. For instance, BP, Heart rate can be observed easily today by a smart band that is available with most of the people.

Primary part of IoMT is to sense a patient's health conditions. To make the sensed information useful, the data have to be communicated over internet with people and make it accessible by computers. At the other end, the healthcare people analyses the patient's data and gives medical advice to the corresponding person. This happens only because of the technology so called IoMT.

Nowadays, IoMT-based device manufactures are exponentially increasing and they are using various communication protocols as base for transmitting sensing data between doctor and patient over internet. Since each IoMT equipment has its own unique IP address, the data from applications like in-home glucose monitor, room temperature monitoring, fall detection devices in a room are transmitted first to the neighbor network may be a home wifi connection or hospital IT network. Finally, the data from IoMT devices are available in a database created for each patient by the hospital network, which can be accessed from anywhere by the authorized persons. This phenomenon leads to the development of smart hospitals.

Smart hospital is all about remote-tracking hospital asset, monitoring health condition of in and out patients, and smart medical equipment. Base for this smart hospital is Internet of Things and undoubtedly the soul for IoT is Sensors.

5.4 Sensors in Augmented Reality (AR)

Augmented reality, generally shortened as "AR," is an emerging technology which combines real and virtual worlds. AR is a kind of display environment based on real-time existence and interactive in terms of computer effects includes sound, images, scenes, and text to enrich the user's experience in visualizing the real-virtual worlds. AR enhances the objects in real world by computer-generated modalities and somatosensory information includes touching, sighting, hearing, and even sense of smell. Combination two different worlds, interactive, 3D visualization with accurate information are some features that should be satisfied by the system called Augmented Reality. This type of superimposed sensory modalities and information could be either constructive or destructive means that information may be an additive to the reality or masking of the real-time facts and figures.

The primary intention of AR is to provide a vivid audiovisual treat for users. It works by taking up computer-generated techniques and simulation models such as voice and image recognition, animated characteristics, head-mounted wearable, or handheld standby devices which add virtual presentation overlap with real- world surroundings. AR devices come in various forms as mentioned above as handheld, standby, glasses, or wearable entities. In mere future, advancements in AR technologies lead the user more interactive with the real-time environment and surroundings by integrating smartphone use cases with AR cameras and augmenting computer vision for object recognition like applications. Though many more applications are there, most common and well-known application of AR is video games (e.g., Pokeman go). People are going to stun in forthcoming days with greater advancements in AR applications.

The competence of AR system is getting speeding up day by day because of the immense advancement in IC (Integrated Circuit) manufacturing. Earlier, the technology was relentlessly limited for reasons like weight, size, cost, and power consumption of sensors by which lightweight headsets cannot be constructed. Thanks for vlsi (very large scale integration) and IC manufacturing techniques for optimizing the sensor size and improving the power factor of the same. Nowadays, lightweight headsets are available for AR applications. Since AR is based on computer-generated images as holographs, the system should place the predicted holographs in front of the user. This can be done with the help of computer which detects the motion and location of the user's (headset wearer) head and it can be get completed by a unit of the system known as IMU (Inertial Measurement Unit).

Sensors play role in the Inertial Measurement Unit. IMU comprises of three types of sensors. They are *Accelerometer, Magnetometer, and Gyroscope* given in the Fig. 5.3. The sensed information from these sensors is denoted as 3-dimensional signals of axis x, y, z. Therefore, these three signals return an accurate position of the user's head and help to find the head movement in a precise manner in order to place the holograph. Micro Electro-Mechanical Systems (MEMS) fabrication technology based on IC photolithography mechanism has been employed by most of the sensors. Let us see about these three sensors in brief.

Accelerometer has numerous of functions and applications, but predominantly it is used to determine the direction and orientation where the device is facing. This tiny and sensible devise precisely gives the device positioning details with the pull of gravity in any line among the axis x, y, z, since all the three axes are fixed. For example, on smart phones, the display mode can be varied automatically either landscape or portrait mode by the way the user holds the mobile. This is possible only with the help of accelerometer sensor. The sensor also has the ability to measure the "acceleration" along a specific axis. Any handheld device or wearable holds this sensor, the user can track the speed of any automobile at which the user is journeying. Even Google maps are having this feature. For instance, in an IoT application, vehicle accident detection system or vehicle collision prevention system uses this accelerometer in order to detect the speed of a vehicle and its direction. If collision happens, the controller proceeds with further procedure that fed into the system. Airbag ejecting technology in cars also based on the same technology.

The accelerometer sensors are infinitesimal in size. It is a kind of comb structure, and the generated electrical current from the combs (needle like structures) transformed into acceleration data as soon as the gravity disturbs the combs of the accelerometer. Yet few limitations are there for accelerometer. It may not have the ability

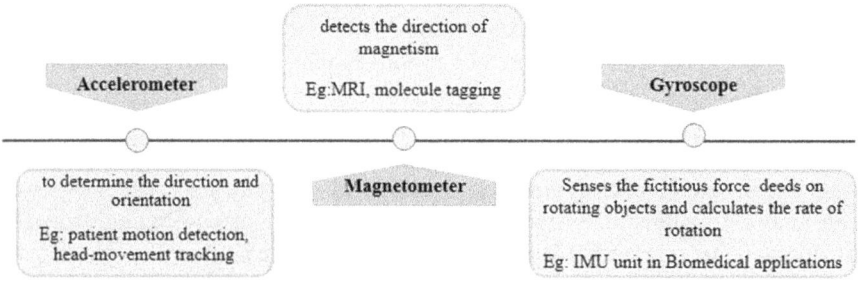

Fig. 5.3 Vital Sensors of Augmented Reality

to produce information to denote the device rotation, when the motion data gathered from the combined readings of all the three axes x, y, z instantaneously. Sometimes, it happens in mobile when playing high-end games. Here the need for gyroscope arises.

The gyroscope is a type of sensor or electronic entity used to determine the orientation of any device. It can be instigated by creating multifingered structure and interdigitized assemblies which, when pulsated at a desired frequencies, are able to sense the fictitious force deeds on rotating objects and calculate the rate of rotation. As said before, IMU has the ability to detect accurate position and orientation is just because of the presence of gyroscope in the IMU unit. A gyroscope is naturally present in smart mobiles too, but typically it is very important in the field of aircraft, helps to find out the flying level of a plane when it is covered by dense cloud and during worst weather conditions.

Just like accelerometer, magnetometer is also a tiny device used to measure magnetic fields. For all intents and purposes the magnetometer acts as a compass and this is essential in the field to detect the magnetic pole north and tells the direction where it is facing. The magnetometer detects the direction of magnetism when it is comes into contact with the magnetic field once the sensor gets powered. It can be worked in various functions, it may use as permanent magnets or as electromagnets. The function of magnetometer can be decided according to the application where it is deployed. Google Cardboard is a best example where this sensor used effectively and cleverly.

Besides measuring the orientation and direction of a device by these abovementioned sensors, the users are being aimed cameras for more precise identification of object in the space direction and orientation at the instant. Former methods of augmented reality entail complex sensors to place the computer-generated models to look as if real in the panoramas. Two dimensional pictures were used as reference by the cameras and headsets to render graphics on the scenes. Nowadays, advances in AR technology changes the AR headsets certainly about one or more distinctive types of cameras. *Time-of-Flight (ToF) Camera, Binocular Depth Sensing sensor, Structured-light sensor* are some extraordinary cameras used in AR technology. The operation ToF based on tempered InfraRed (IR) radiation and to measure the phase delay of reflected radiation to determine the distance between the object and the camera. Marketable examples of this type of high-defined cameras are MLX75023 QVGA Time of Flight sensor and DS325/DS525 from Softkinetic.

Structured Light Sensor technology intends a well-defined array pattern of any type of light or radiation which includes visible as well as IR (IR or visible) onto the computer-generated model. The differences between the pattern emitted and returned are calculated by analyzing the pixel information of a camera. Microsoft's Kinect cameras, Intel F200, Occipital's Structure Sensor are few real time examples of structured-light sensor.

5.5   Sensors in Virtual Reality (VR)

Experiencing and exploring things via a specially designed system that do not exist in real are named as Virtual Reality commonly known as "VR", is a technology similar to Augmented Reality in terms of simulation and projection of two different worlds. AR just combines real and virtual worlds whereas the VR gives the new world which is entirely different from the existence of reality. Here, instead of looking into the screen or the hologram model in front of them, the user actually gets inside the experience which means the user feels they are there on the 3D virtual entity by mentally as well as physically and also users can interact with the artificial world in real.

VR is in essence, computer-generated, believable, interactive, explorable, and particularly more immersive. For instance, in a 3D movie, people can see things which come near to them from the screen, they try to reach out towards it and touch it but the illusion will just fade away. This is an example for submissive environment. In terms of immersive environment, people be able to touch it, sense it, and even reach out; this is possible only in the technology so called virtual reality. It is a two-way communication channel; people can respond to it and get back what they expected. The VR simulation gets adjusted according to the user's head rotation and perspective if they wore a VR headset. The application of VR in various fields includes education, entertainment (games), field of medicine (surgeons), aerospace, and so on. For instance, pilot training in aerospace and military training. In few cases, VR technology takes in augmented reality and mixed reality. A person can interact with the computer-generated virtual 3D environment with the help of extraordinary electronic devices which support VR, as like elite goggles with display, hand gloves with sensors. At present, to generate realistic pictures, acoustics, and other sensations such as haptic, hearing, and viewing are simulated with the help of typical virtual reality-based multiprojected displays or special headsets comprise of head-mounted device with screen in front of eyes. The computer-generated simulation locates the user's eyes position and according to that the simulated environment reacts in real by changing its graphics automatically. By the way, VR creates such an interactive and convincing world for users.

Humans come under chromatic living beings; displaying techniques are easily understandable by humans than any other mode. Hence, display technology makes the huge difference between the standard and artificial user interfaces. VR employs some sensors to detect the movement of user's body and its position. HMD (head-mounted display) is the most commonly used product in VR technology, has two screens for each eyes separately, stereo speakers around in a room, and special gloves were powered by a supercomputer or a workstation. HMD comprises of built-in position sensors, accelerometers to detect the orientation, exact movement of a person, and the accurate position of the person's head, and adjust the VR pictures accordingly. The two screens are used to display stereoscopic images and create a 3D virtual environment in real. Perfect example is the Google's cardboard goggles. It has built-in lenses used to convert a normal smart phone into a type of

HMD that supports VR technology. Google gives this product for low-cost and makes affordable for everyone.

As afore said, HMD plays a vital role in VR technology which comprises of various sensors namely for head-motion monitoring and tracking sensors, eye tracking sensors, and gaming controllers. IMU (Inertial Measurement Unit) included in the VR headsets as a chunk of electronic entity is responsible for projecting the virtual environment on screen in VR immersive headsets. Related to the eye movement and direction and the head position of the user, the computer controls the generated image and stereo information. There is no need for position sensor if and only if the user is static in position. In gaming application, there is need for monitoring and tracking the position and movement of user. Such application needs additional light sources or markers that should be positioned at permanent locations around the gaming environment. Special light sensor or camera ICs are used to sense those light source or markers placed in the gaming space are commonly termed as outside-in tracking.

Most essential sensors for the specialized VR devices in particular for the head-mounted display are *accelerometer, gyroscope, and magnetometer.* These sensors allow user to measure the orientation, movement, direction, and position in the space. A broad explanation for the above-mentioned three sensors was discussed already under the topic augmented reality sensors. At earlier days, hardware and resources for constructing VR technology were very expensive and unmanageable. Due to massive growth in mobile devices and IC manufacturing, the sensors become very tiny and affordable, highly cheap in terms of cost.

The mentioned sensors are responsible for detecting motion and space. The micro electro mechanical systems (MEMS) technology paves the path for building devices like magnetometer and gyroscopes at a small scale. Deprive of this technology, so called smartphones and other electronic entities including AR/VR headsets would become very complex and chunky. Instead it gives smart and slim models by that today, each and every one hold a smartphone as a mini computer in a pocket which comprises of tiny and sophisticated sensors.

A VR device can hold any number of accelerometers, magnetometers and gyroscopes to produce precise and highly accurate information that can be passed to controllers and software to place a rich experience to the people who are incredibly immersive with the technology is all about. Apart from these three sensors, some sensors are used for VR technology. They are, *structured light systems, eye tracking sensors, gaming controllers, and MARG sensors* are precisely described in the Fig. 5.4.

Eye tracking sensors are used to detect the gaze point, which means it makes a computer system or the VR headset display to determine the position of the user's eyes and where they are looking at actually. Gaming controller, simply called as a controller used as an input device in several kind of video games. Primarily it is used to control a character or an object in the video game particularly in VR-based gaming applications. Oculus Rift S and HTC Vive are commercial examples that are available in market.

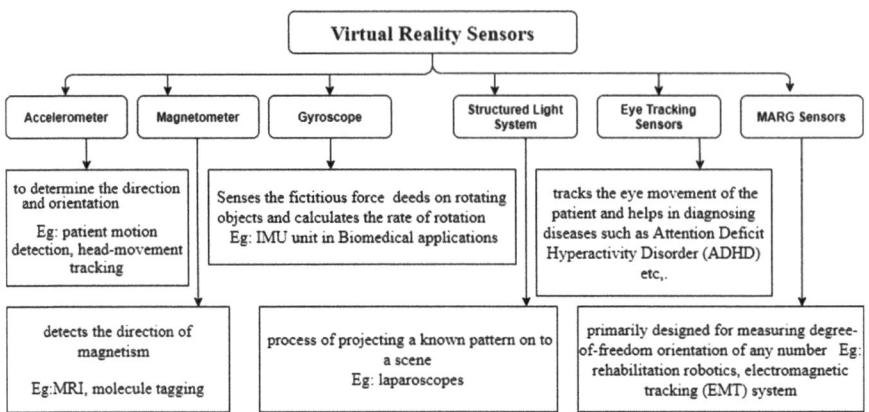

Fig. 5.4 Sensors used in Virtual Reality

MARG (magnetic, angular rate, and gravity) sensor is one of the most dominant sensors in mobile devices and also in AR/VR technologies. Total of nine sensors including orthogonally mounted trios of micromachined rate sensors, magnetometers, and accelerometers are enclosed in every single MARG sensor. This sensor is primarily designed for measuring degree-of-freedom orientation of any number. But the ultimate objective is to attain the 6DoF (six degrees-of-freedom) which gives the freedom for motion within the 3D environment. Six degrees-of-freedom (6DoF) is traditionally defined as the combination of three rotations (pitch, roll, and yaw) and three transformations (up/down, left/right, and forward/backward). MARG sensor is used to measure the movement of person accurately such as user's head and hand gestures in the virtual environment within the 3D space else the illusion may shatter.

Even researches are going to give orientation on 9DoF for better experience. However six degrees-of-freedom is basically essential, if not the 3D environment would not be pleasant. Therefore, modern headsets of VR should offer tracking and monitoring across all 6DoF at the maximum for rich experience.

Here comes the medical application of augmented reality (AR). It is the knack of overlaying computer-generated content over real objects of the world. AR incorporates real objects with the digital data and makes a 3D environment and that is affordable, easily reachable, and accessible for medical training and imaging, nurse training, and dentistry. Examples of AR medical solutions are, AccuVein, ARnatomy, VA-ST. Some of the applications of AR are Dentistry, Training nurses, Medical imaging, Medical education, Pediatric MRI evaluation, Helping the visually impaired, Visualization of peripheral vasculature, Remote surgical expertise, etc.

Apart from the given applications, AR mobile apps are developed for healthcare. It has been illustrated in the Table 5.2.

Virtual Reality along with the surgical training assists and uses in drug design, "telemedicine" is also possible. Telemedicine is defined as monitoring, tracking, examining, and even surgeries on patients from remote location. The real time

Table 5.2 AR mobile application and its description

Mobile AR App	Description
EyeDecide	To simulate the effect of various disorders on a person's vision to train patients with cataracts and macular degeneration using smartphone camera
DoctorMole	Used to detect malignant lesions and helps doctors to detect the suspicious moles on the patient's body and gives feedback instantly
Healthcare App by pixelbug	The working procedure of a medical device or the mechanism of the device can be easily understandable by physicians.
Anatomy 4D	In medical schools, anatomy of human can be easily learnt by students and comfortable for faculties to explain in terms of 4D environment in response to spatial connections of skeleton, muscles, and organs
MEVIS Surgery App	Using the recent technology, 3D printing, reconstruction of real organs is possible and it is established by Fraunhofer MEVIS, Surgeons use this for practical learning. Example, to perform liver resections and helps them to locate blood vessels and tumors
MedicAR	An app by Google developed for surgeons to properly line up the incision points for less patient pains. It is likely to be used in difficult surgeries and MRI examinations

example is daVinci surgical robot, developed in 2009 for doing surgeries by the instruction of surgeons from another remote location even from another continent. This can be possible with VR, consider a surgeon with virtual reality control panel at one location and a robot using knife in another location. After the advancements in VR technology and the successful implementation of the robot daVinci, several robots have been installed in various hospitals across the world. Collaboration of various specialists can be possible now via virtual reality. World's top surgeons are now able to be connected and work together on a particular complex surgery. Till date, VR technology has been treated for various types of psychiatric disorders which include phantom limb pain, agoraphobia, and schizophrenia, and also in stroke patients rehabilitation and for those who are suffering from degenerative illnesses like multiple sclerosis.

5.6 Medical Applications of Emerging Technology

Before all the emerging advancement in healthcare, the foremost technology that has been employed and still in practice is "Telemedicine". Since there are a few notable issues and challenges are incurred in tele-medicine like real-time connectivity, low standardization, QoS (quality of service), cost, and so on [4]. Therefore the field of medicine is in need of a system that takes over all these hassles in practicing methodologies and makes the medicine field outreach.

The corpus of asymmetrical cells inside the brain leads to brain tumor, which can harm the brain and that will be a life-threatening one for all. Thus, detecting brain tumors in initial grade is quite critical for its verdict, prognosis, and cure. To detect accurate brain tumors, smart and secure automated system is required. In [5], the authors implemented a computational method called "PART" identifies correctly the brain tumor with respect to its grade which is nothing but the level of infection. By using advanced feature set, the disease has been identified accurately and facilitated the healthcare supporters in treating the brain tumor.

An application has been proposed by the author Qi An and et al. [6] with the help of Gyro sensor and Accelerometer named as "PocketIMU2". It is a wireless wearable sensor precisely designed for elderly people to detect their motions. It is essential to measure the body state of the patients in particular the elder people who are in need of rehabilitation by any means. Hence the "PocketIMU2" device is helpful for monitoring the human motions.

A very few existing AR and VR applications in medicine are given here in brief. Let us see one after another. In a work "Augmented reality-based upper limb rehabilitation system", the author Wang Ying et al. introduced three different augmented reality games. By playing that, the patient can control the virtual objects in the real-virtual world by any fixed markers in the piece of equipment used. The performance of the patient has been recorded. The therapist from remote location be able to monitor the patient's movement by looking over the training video; hence, the therapist easily gets the data of a patient and guides the patient in a professional manner. The three games are, tea pouring game, simulated driving, and brick breaker [7].

In the tea pouring game, in the virtual environment, the patient be able to see a virtual tea cup and a kettle. As per AR, the patient be able to interact with the virtual objects. Here, the patient views a cup and a kettle. The patient has to hold the virtual kettle by the affected hand. Next, the patient should move the kettle towards the virtual cup and hold the kettle for few moments and then tilt the kettle just like pouring water. The system detects the designated position of the kettle and cup based on its coordinates. As the same process repeats for a while, the ability of the motor in the upper limbs and flexibility of the joints are improved. Similarly, in simulated driving game, patient has to drive virtually whereas in the brick breaker game, the patient moves the virtual reflector to bounce back the virtual balls. So these are some exercises in terms of AR games for rehabilitating the upper limbs.

"Mobile RehApp – AR-based mobile game for ankle sprain rehabilitation" authored by Jaime Andres Garcia et al., proposed a technique that uses Mobile Augmented Reality (MAR) to provide a kind of motion training exercises to patients suffering from an ankle sprain. The game-based system constructs based on AR aspects to permit endless real-time tracking and monitoring of patients movement. The games used in this work are easy to deploy in all type of smart phones. This enhances the interactions between the game controllers and patients. It is based on home-therapy which increases the level of motivation and observance to rehabilitation [8].

A research work related to smart healthcare proposed by Yin Zhang et al. gives an idea about a hybrid ECG feature extraction method that combines standard- and nonstandard-based features to pull out more wide-ranging ECG features and thus increase the endorsement stability. Pattern recognition framework has been used in this application to increase the efficiency in the place of multiple ECG usage [9].

"YouMove" is a novel training system for full-body movement based on AR technology. An AR mirror has been implemented in a real world. The mirror records the full-body movements of a patient and sends to the respective trainer or therapist. Trainer can teach movements via the same mirror to the trainee and the trainer can increase the level of difficulty gradually. This application is based on the video-based learning. "YouMove" approach was proposed by the author Fraser Anderson and et al. to improve the patients' health by doing physical exercise includes yoga, dance, and games with the help of professional trainer from the remote location [10].

"ARTESH – Augmented Reality Tele-Rehabilitation System with Haptics" system facilitated 2D force feedback, enabling synchronous isolated patient's physical assessment with video, audio, and haptic information conveyed alive with the help of internet. The system takes up a few engineering features like a force augmentation algorithm to develop force rendering and choking the existing limitation in it and improved force reparation patient's recuperation [11].

Many more applications are there in medical field with the help of advanced technologies. Spinal Surgery is one of the risky operations. Though advancements are there in medicine, there is a trade-off between the cost of the surgery and in reaching all sorts of people. A study on these stuffs is given in an article [12].

In an another work [13], "Augmented Reality with Application in Physical Rehabilitation" done by the author Yu Jin et al., is an IoS application proposed for the patients who are suffering from strokes. Gait training is one of the insignificant parts of the physical rehabilitation. Augmented Reality (AR) provides a solution for the patients suffered by strokes by giving a proper training and assessment from the specialized trainer or physiotherapists from the remote location. During gait training, the velocity and position of the patient have been recorded by the smart carpet which comprises of capacitive sensors powered by a computation unit with WiFi-based communication strategies. Virtual objects can be added over the head-mounted 3D display to the real world, and the smart sensors in the carpet provide the information about the patients' movement and positioning characteristics.

Limited researches are done on Rehabilitation for hands. One amongst is a system based on AR/VR technology framed by Jia Liu et al. [14] The author designed the framework with four rehabilitation programs that includes trainings for trajectory, shelf, batting, and spile. These trainings and the framework allow patients to interact in real time with virtual environment.

In an article [15], the author Niccolò Butti et al., proposed a system specifically for the patients with a disorder called congenital cerebellar. Rehabilitation for brain functions is essential for these sorts of patients. By the way, the proposed VR-based rehabilitation method has the ability to process on social stimuli of a human and implementing a designed training program over social cognition to improve their ability in predictive social circumstances. This phenomenon is named as "VR-Spirit".

5.7 Sensors in Mixed Reality (MR)

Mixed reality "MR" is a technology that incorporates augmented reality as well as virtual reality with the help of immersive technology. To put it in simple words, MR is the combination of AR and VR. It merges the real and virtual worlds to place a computer-generated simulation in front of the user as like in AR mechanism and by using the immersive technology, MR resembles as VR technology. Therefore, MR produces a fresh environment and 3D visualization where the real (physical) and computer-generated (digital) objects are interacted with each other in real-time. MR will not take place either in physical world or virtual world, instead it is a hybrid of AR and VR which means objects in two different worlds coexist in the environment produced by the mixed reality. During 1992, the first MR project was developed at Armstrong Laboratories of US named as virtual Fixtures platform. It demonstrated that by overlapping virtual objects on top of a real environment of a user's direct gaze point, human performance can be improved significantly. This was the first project used the immersive technology.

Mixed reality affords the capability of keeping one foot in real world and the other in the virtual world. Without removing the headset, people can immerse themselves in the artificial environment created by mixed reality which allows people to interact with the virtual world using their hands. By means of next-generation imaging and sensing technologies, the user can manipulate real world as well as the virtual world objects and the environment proposed by MR. It brings two different worlds together and offers a rich experience that could change the way of user's daily activities.

Mixed reality is sometimes called as "enhanced AR" as it blends both augmented reality and virtual reality, but more similar to AR with higher physical interaction.

Mixed reality is the combination of augmented and virtual reality. Hence, the sensors used in MR are the mixture of sensors employed in AR and VR technologies. Sensors in MR head-mounted display are Spatial mapping sensors (stereo cameras, ToF sensor, structure-light sensor), Head trackers, Six degrees-of-freedom sensors, Spatial anchors, SLAM (simultaneous localization and mapping), Eye tracking sensors, and hand-gesture sensors. A brief description about most of the given sensors was explained in previous sections.

While coming to the MR in healthcare, Patient's previously taken CT scan reports can be overlapped with 3D digital prototype by using the prodigious technology called as mixed reality which allows surgeons to place the 3D model onto the patient's affected area during surgery. This is one of the extraordinary applications that helps surgeons to a great extent during surgeries and assists them to find the blood vessels accurately and move the respective blood vessels from one place to other part of the body in order to make the open wound to heal rapidly.

Significant benefits can be derived by implementing the AR and MR technologies in the areas of education and surgical practices. Major difference between the AR and MR is the interaction between the objects by the users other than that there is no difference to mention. The same becomes as the important advantage for MR technology mainly in the field of medicine particularly to the surgeons during surgeries. With the help of MR, surgeons be able to handle each and every parts of the body virtually as like in the real world, this leads to remote surgery.

In healthcare, MR can be used in medical schools to make students to understand about the anatomy of human being safely. Even a MR library could be created for case studies and practices. Patients also able to access their medical report to study about the diseases and the approaches, treatments available for getting cure. Many MNCs are currently doing research on these projects and developing products and applications that make patients and doctors to come together from their remote area itself. When an expert advice is needed in a surgery, it is possible to connect with an expert remotely and can get the guidance of them immediately for surgical decision-making situations. Endless applications will be developed in future in MR technology particularly for medicine.

While comparing medical applications of augmented reality, virtual reality, and mixed reality, all three technologies own their distinctive advantages and limitations. In terms of upcoming growth of 3D visualization environment and augmented reality for surgical procedure, mixed reality with its additional interactive abilities, has the potential to make the transformation in both the real and virtual environments of medicine.

MR vs VR   The virtual reality endows an artificial/virtual environment created with full of digital objects. A person be able to experience the 3D environment with the help of head-mounted display or a specialized VR headset that consists of video as well as audio and other sensing elements too. VR head-mounted display comes with handheld modules and special gloves used by the person in the virtual environment to make interaction with different objects there and the VR headset display remains black once the power turned off. Though, mixed reality mixes both real and virtual objects and produces an environment, where a person can interact with all the existing objects even without wearing any gloves or handheld sticks and another feature offered by mixed reality is, the MR headset which would become a see-through like a normal glass when the power for the headset is turned off.

MR vs AR   Augmented reality uses the real world objects and overlapping with virtual object on it. Yet, the person cannot be able to interact with the objects directly which are available on the 3D environment. For instance, consider a 3D object has been created using AR as well as using MR. A person be able to see the object with both AR and MR technology. But in AR, the person be able to only see the object whereas in MR, the person can see, sense, and touch the same 3D object. The AR technology requires hardware-like handheld sticks with cameras and screens while MR requires only a HMD (head-mounted display) that enables the person to interact with the objects in 3D environment directly by bare hands. HoloLens from Microsoft is a real time example for MR HDM.

Mixed Reality has quite a lot of applications, such as cybernetic (virtual) training for pilots, virtual education and training for surgeons, and remote guidance for engineers. The applications of augmented reality, virtual reality, and mixed reality are escalating from entertainment to medicine, to robotics. Some applications are,

- Entertainment – gaming, movies, and shows to offer a rich experience.
- Healthcare – Surgical simulations and training for fresher.
- Aerospace – Pilot training.

- Virtual tour – from home, travel to any place includes museum, colleges or another planet to explore.

5.8   Data Handling: AR, VR, and IoT

Massively a new trend is rising by encompassing three great pulsating and innovating technologies such as AR (augmented reality), VR (virtual reality), and IoT (internet of things).

In this era, the digitalization becomes the reason for this hottest trend in information technology and ICT (information and communication technology). Most of all the applications are transferring a very big volume of data over internet to one another. Due to this type of transactions, the network faces hassle in data handling and leads to security, privacy, and cyber threats. It consumes people and high processes to manage the data and it is hard to share the Big Data in a cost-effective, practical, and meaningful way. A framework has been developed by IBM to deal with the Data handling, based on four distinct 'V's [16]. They are Volume: convey a message that the excel sheet is not enough to hold the "big data"; Velocity: data visualization and handling takes place as soon as the data have been received; Variety: collect various types of data such as plain text, sensor data, rich document, etc., and analyze it accordingly; and Veracity: have to find out the reliability of the received data because trust is most important in data handling over the internet. Data Handling plays a vital role already in the field of data science, helps data scientists to realize the pattern and structure that the data holds, before causing serious issues over the network.

AR and big data have constantly gone together. In a real-time environment, to render the information virtually, a large data set is necessary for AR and the same is provided by Big data. Data visualization depends on type of information, techniques used for visualization and compatibility of data. Big Data needs to be transformed as human intellectual is inhibited [17]. AR meets Big data since AR and big data have a logical maturity that certainly makes both giant technique to be united in the visualization part. The pace of hitching AR and big data to raise new exciting applications is beginning to have a concrete existence [18]. In [19], the proposed is the increase of big data visualization in virtual reality environments to prevailing considerations of human insight and communication via a phenomenological lens and the concepts of personified interaction and perception. Hence, the fundamental perception of effective data visualization is to represent congested and complex data in a way that is more convenient for the user [20].

The graphical representation (Fig. 5.5) given below represents the approximate amount of data received and handled by AR/VR applications.

The arena of sensor technology is tremendously broad, and its future growth will encompass the interaction of every scientific and technical aspects. The

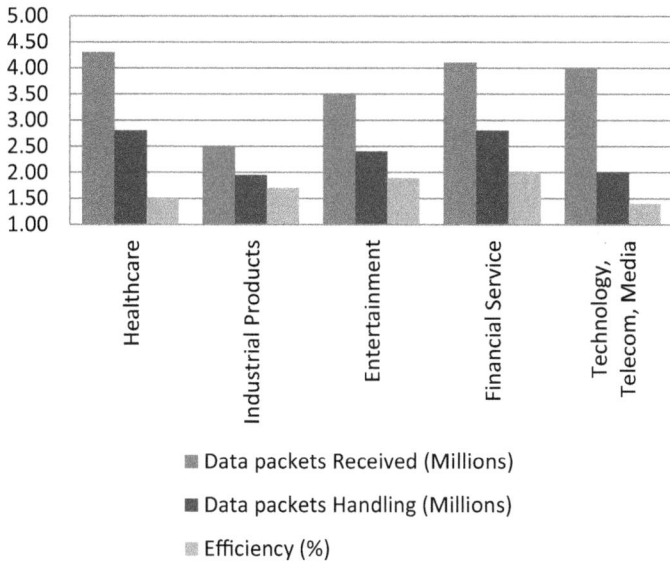

Fig. 5.5 Data Analytics in various applications of AR/VR

basic definitions of sensors and its terminology have been briefly presented, still considerable uncertainty exists in the sensor technologies, classifications, and its applications. Most of the modern sensors are integrating few types of signal processing in transmitting information as signals. The backend processes of sensors are well-hidden from the user end in modern sensors today. Novel materials are used to create more precise sensors to use in high-end technologies.

From internet of things (IoT), to augmented reality (AR), to virtual reality (VR), to mixed reality (MR), and now reaches AI (artificial intelligence) applications for each and every sector. By these advancements in emerging technologies, the universe is overfilled with numerous projects to make humanitarian aid as more effective. From 3D gaming headset, movies, virtual tour, and interior design experience to never-ending applications in elevating the human life better and ease. One of the best examples of AR technology is the game "pokemon Go", it reaches to every nook and corner in kids' world. Even adults get addicted over the game since it gives unique and different experience. Apart from the entertainment and other applications, the primary use of these emerging technologies is in the field of medicine. It saves life of many people. It cures so many traumas and pains of young and old people to a greater extent. The next upcoming technology is the Robotics. Robotics in medicine will be the pinnacle of technology in healthcare. These technologies play a vital role in terms of advancement in the medical field and the same is illustrated in the Fig. 5.6.

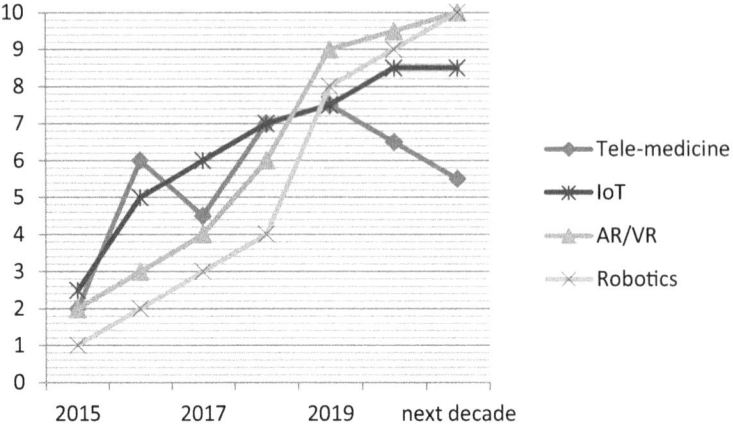

Fig. 5.6 Timeline of Technology in Health Care

5.9 Conclusion and Future Scope

By the above discussed applications, the AR and VR make their presence into the hearts of most of the users' globally. By collaborating these different technologies on a single network layer, IoT infrastructure, mobile devices, and applications be able to interact with each other and permit the advanced technology such as AR and VR along with IoT grow into globally accessible by all level of users and offer opportunities to companies to connect with various set of people around the world. Therefore, to make the virtual world to be a real one, sensor technology plays a vital role to invent newer applications with the help of emerging technologies in all walks of life.

Future work would be the optimization of sensors, precise data analytics to be done for improved accuracy. Security must be provided great for the confidential biomedical data exchanges between one another by using emerging technologies like blockchain.

References

1. M. Zheng, P.X. Liu, R. Gravina, G. Fortino, An emerging wearable world: New gadgetry produces a rising tide of changes and challenges. IEEE Syst. Man, Cybern. Mag. **4**(4), 6–14 (2018). https://doi.org/10.1109/msmc.2018.2806565
2. J. Priya, M. Gunasekaran, Security-aware and privacy-preserving communication in the internet of things: A review. 2019 5th Int. Conf. Adv. Comput. Commun. Syst., 225–230 (2019)
3. G. Fortino, A. Guerrieri, W. Russo, C. Savaglio, Internet of things based on smart objects. Fortino P. Trunfio, 49, 1–27 (2014) [Online]. Available: http://link.springer.com/content/pdf/10.1007/978-3-319-00491-4.pdf; http://link.springer.com/10.1007/978-3-319-00491-4

4. C. Chakraborty, B. Gupta, S. K. Ghosh, A review on telemedicine-based WBAN framework for patient monitoring, *Telemed. e-Health*, **19**(8), 619–626, (2013). https://doi.org/10.1089/tmj.2012.0215.
5. S.R. Khan, M. Sikandar, A. Almogren, I. Ud Din, A. Guerrieri, G. Fortino, IoMT-based computational approach for detecting brain tumor. Futur. Gener. Comput. Syst. **109**, 360–367 (2020). https://doi.org/10.1016/j.future.2020.03.054.
6. Q. An et al., Evaluation of wearable gyroscope and accelerometer sensor (PocketIMU2) during walking and sit-to-stand motions. Proc. – IEEE Int. Work. Robot Hum. Interact. Commun., 731–736 (2012). https://doi.org/10.1109/ROMAN.2012.6343838
7. W. Ying, W. Aimin, Augmented reality-based upper limb rehabilitation system. ICEMI 2017 – Proc. IEEE 13th Int. Conf. Electron. Meas. Instrum **2018**, 426–430 (2017). https://doi.org/10.1109/ICEMI.2017.8265843
8. J.A. Garcia, K.F. Navarro, The mobile RehApp™: An AR-based mobile game for ankle sprain rehabilitation. SeGAH 2014 – IEEE 3rd Int. Conf. Serious Games Appl. Heal. Books Proc. (2014), https://doi.org/10.1109/SeGAH.2014.7067087
9. Y. Zhang, R. Gravina, H. Lu, M. Villari, G. Fortino, PEA: Parallel electrocardiogram-based authentication for smart healthcare systems. J. Netw. Comput. Appl. **117**(June), 10–16 (2018). https://doi.org/10.1016/j.jnca.2018.05.007
10. F. Anderson, T. Grossman, J. Matejka, G. Fitzmaurice, YouMove: Enhancing movement training with an augmented reality mirror. UIST 2013 – Proc. 26th Annu. ACM Symp. User Interface Softw. Technol., 311–320 (2013), https://doi.org/10.1145/2501988.250204.
11. A. Borresen et al., Usability of an immersive augmented reality-based telerehabilitation system with haptics (Artesh) for synchronous remote musculoskeletal examination. Int. J. Telerehabilitation **11**(1), 23–32 (2019). https://doi.org/10.5195/ijt.2019.6275
12. Y. Shelke, C. Chakraborty, Augmented reality and virtual reality transforming spinal imaging landscape: A feasibility study. IEEE Comput. Graph. Appl. **1716**, 1 (2020). https://doi.org/10.1109/MCG.2020.3000359
13. Y. Jin, J. Monge, O. Postolache, W. Niu, Augmented reality with application in physical rehabilitation. 2019 Int. Conf. Sens. Instrum. IoT Era, ISSI 2019, 17–22 (2019), https://doi.org/10.1109/ISSI47111.2019.9043665.
14. J. Liu, J. Mei, X. Zhang, X. Lu, J. Huang, Augmented reality-based training system for hand rehabilitation. Multimed. Tools Appl. **76**(13), 14847–14867 (2017). https://doi.org/10.1007/s11042-016-4067-x.
15. N. Butti et al., Virtual Reality Social Prediction Improvement and Rehabilitation Intensive Training (VR-SPIRIT) for paediatric patients with congenital cerebellar diseases: Study protocol of a randomised controlled trial. Trials **21**(1), 1–12 (2020). https://doi.org/10.1186/s13063-019-4001-4.
16. https://www.bigdataframework.org/four-vs-of-big-data/
17. A.N. Ramaseri Chandra, F. El Jamiy, H. Reza, Augmented reality for big data visualization: A review. Proc. – 6th Annu. Conf. Comput. Sci. Comput. Intell. CSCI 2019, 2020, 1269–1274 (2019), https://doi.org/10.1109/CSCI49370.2019.00238.
18. C. Bermejo, Z. Huang, T. Braud, P. Hui, When augmented reality meets big data. Proc. – IEEE 37th Int. Conf. Distrib. Comput. Syst. Work. ICDCSW 2017, no. October, 169–174 (2017), https://doi.org/10.1109/ICDCSW.2017.62
19. M. Teras, S. Raghunathan, Big data visualisation in immersive virtual reality environments: Embodied phenomenological perspectives to interaction. ICTACT J. Soft Comput. **05**(04), 1009–1015 (2015). https://doi.org/10.21917/ijsc.2015.0141.
20. A. Moran, V. Gadepally, M. H. – … (HPEC), 2015 IEEE, and U. 2015, Bachelor thesis – improving big data visual analytics with interactive virtual reality, Ieeexplore.Ieee.Org, no. 2014 (2016) [Online]. Available: https://dspace.mit.edu/handle/1721.1/105972%; http://ieeexplore.ieee.org/abstract/document/7322473/

Chapter 6
Body Sensor Networks as Emerging Trends of Technology in Health Care System: Challenges and Future

N. Jaya Lakshmi and Neetu Jabalia

6.1 Introduction

In today's express, digital world Information Technology is dominating every field including healthcare industry [1]. The information technologies have the potential to impact various fields such as genome analysis, medical science, and public health. The emerging field of health informatics and its associated practices offers new opportunities and it is very promising approach [2]. Storing patient's records in an electronic format has significant advantages and offers improved and affordable health care facilities [3]. The current technological developments in the healthcare can be attributed to creation of Artificial intelligence (AI), Bigdata, Internet of things (IoT), Blockchain, and Cloud-based Technology [4].

Healthcare is such a vast ecosystem and digital transformations start from personal healthcare, pharma industry, medical insurances to real-time healthcare monitoring, and healthcare building amenities. Applications of IoT in use of robotics, biosensors, smart beds, smart pills, and the various healthcare specialties are never-ending. As, the emerging healthcare sectors are producing hefty volumes of data on patient history, pathological reports, treatment planning, bills and insurance coverage, demographics – drawing the attention of clinicians and researchers towards progressive information technology.

Therefore, this chapter discusses the overview of health informatics approaches which are entwined with techniques such as AI, block chain, cloud computing, big data, and Internet of things (IoT). The next section will focus on significant role of these technologies in healthcare. It will also highlight the implementation of technologies in current pandemic outbreak, i.e., COVID-19. Further, this chapter will

N. Jaya Lakshmi · N. Jabalia (✉)
Amity Institute of Biotechnology, Amity University, Noida, Uttar Pradesh, India
e-mail: njabalia@amity.edu

© The Author(s), under exclusive license to Springer Nature Switzerland AG 2021
C. Chakraborty et al. (eds.), *Efficient Data Handling for Massive Internet of Medical Things*, Internet of Things,
https://doi.org/10.1007/978-3-030-66633-0_6

present the emerging role of bioinformatics in healthcare system. A major hurdle in adopting healthcare informatics is the hesitation associated with patient's data privacy and security. Hence, the last section emphasizes the need to recognize the advantages and challenges of implementing health informatics globally.

6.2   Technologies in Healthcare

The emerging information technologies shaping-up future of healthcare by implementing technologies such as AI, big data, block chain, IoT, machine learning, and deep learning (Fig. 6.1). Artificial Intelligence is an approach of enabling a computer system or software to think like an intelligent human being. Intelligence is defined as the capability of a system to perform tasks such as calculations, reasoning, perceiving relationships and analogies, learn from experiences, storing and retrieving data based on memory, solving problems, comprehending complex ideologies, employing natural language processes fluently and classifying, generalizing, and adapting to new states [5]. Due to its diverse nature, AI is exploited by biologists across the globe to solve complex biological problems by applying algorithms to massive biological data obtained after experimental studies [6]. From bio-imaging, signal detection, sequencing analysis, protein structure folding to molecular modeling for drug discovery artificial intelligence improve the practices of computational biology to yield cheaper yet accurate solutions [7]. This chapter mainly discusses the basic aspects of the data science in public health sector. Further, it will provide an insight into the various dimensions, recent developments, and the future prospects. Machine learning (ML) is a part of AI whereas deep learning is a particular technique in machine learning. ML is considered a sub-set of Artificial Intelligence (AI), in other words it is an implementation of AI.

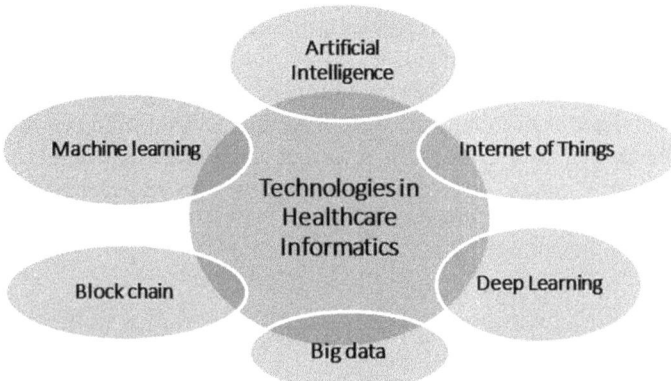

Fig. 6.1 Schematic Representation of Health informatics Components

Learning basically refers to the process of acquiring a specific skill or knowledge during a study or experience. Machine learning is an application of computer sciences, which allows a computer system to learn a specific piece of data and develop itself from this study without the need of explicit programming [8]. One can infer from this process that machine learning operates in two steps namely the training phase and testing phase [9]. A model is defined with some parameters present in a data pool where the system learns the parameters based on their relationships and inherent properties in the training phase. This model is tested on a new dataset to predict the learnt outcomes [10]. The ultimate goal of the model is to make generalized yet accurate predictions in the future, or descriptive to gain knowledge from new and large datasets, or both [11, 12].

Deep Learning is a branch of machine learning that takes inspiration from the structure and functioning of the human brain called artificial neural networks. Neural networks mimic the neuronal circuit in human brain; therefore, deep learning is a type of imitation of human brain [13]. It learns high-level abstractions and transformations in datasets by exploiting hierarchical architectures of input data thereby reducing the need for preprocessing [14]. Deep learning can be applied to modeling complex linear and nonlinear applications, moreover, they have multiple implementations especially in the field of pattern recognition for bioinformatics, medical image analysis, maintenance of healthcare data, and for drug discovery (Table 6.1) [22].

Major applications of Deep Learning in clinical imaging analyses are divided into six main groups (Fig. 6.2):

(i) Classification which involves the identification of specific features in an image;
(ii) Detection, involves locating these picked features;
(iii) Segmentation process in other words is to fragment an image into multiple chunks;
(iv) Reconstruction is the process of rebuilding the features into their original conditions;
(v) Registration is the procedure of integrating two different images into one;
(vi) Dose estimation, which is the process of estimating the right dose quantity of a substance [23].

Deep Learning classification models have been extensively exploited in oncology research and clinical studies for detecting tumor type (Benign, malignant or equivocal), tumor stratification, and grading. The abstraction and exploration of quantitative features from medical imaging datasets can help in developing a better understanding of tumor characteristics, including lesion grade and staging, potentially may allow avoiding biopsies. Lesion segmentation is an important ML application in medical imaging for automatic tumor segmentation that supports planning for radiotherapy treatments. Convolutional Neural Networks (CNNs) have proved to be the most effective neural networks in image segmentation in case of gliomas, breast cancers, prostate cancer, and lung cancers [24, 25]. According to the WHO, Cardiovascular diseases are the number 1 cause of the mortality globally therefore placing paramount focus on early detection of cardiovascular diseases. Deep learn-

Table 6.1 Tools based on Deep learning for Biological Analysis

Name of Application	Description
DeepBind	DeepBind specificities can be visualized in the form of weight-based position matrices or mutation maps which specify how variations alter binding with sequence of interest [15].
CellProfiler	Identifies and measures different biological entities in images. The applications demonstrated in the study referred are counting yeast colonies and their classification, annotating cell microarrays, yeast patch assay, tumor quantification in mice, and measuring tissue topology dimensions [16].
TITER	Translation Initiation siTE detectoR is a deep learning tool aimed at predicting translation initiation sites using sequencing data. TITER identifies vital sequence signatures [17].
DeepCpG	A DNN-based computing tool that determines methylation states in single cells and detects variable sites for DNA methylation. It takes advantage of the relationship between sequence pattern and their state of DNA methylation along with the nearby CpG regions, taking into account both inter and intra cellular sites [18].
Deep-CRISPR	Deep-CRISPR is based on a hybrid deep neural network. It can be used in different Cas9 Species for single-guide RNA on-target identification and efficacy prediction and also overcomes off-target binding [19].
DeepLOC	DeepLOC uses RNN framework to process the query protein sequence and identify sites using attention mechanisms for the subcellular localization [20].
LncADeep	LncADeep is markov model-based tool for identifying and functional annotation of long noncoding RNA which uses KEGG and Reactome databases for enriching the model. For functional annotation, lncRNA's interacting proteins are predicted using deep learning networks based on sequence and structure information [21].

ing algorithms play a crucial role in rapid and efficient in analyzing images produced by diagnostic procedures such as cardiac ultrasound, angiography, and magnetic resonance imaging, and computed tomography. The analysis includes detecting edges, texture features, morphological sieving, along with the construction of shape models and template matching algorithms. Several Classification studies on angiography images and echocardiography videos to predict the onset of coronary artery disease, plaque formation, and valve calcification using Multilayer Perceptrons, Convolutional neural network or Fusion neural networks that combine the spatial and temporal data obtained by echocardiography signals. A major limitation of existing Deep Learning techniques is the use of single sets of medical imaging data, those crucial parameters like genetic factors other relevant clinical constraints. Therefore, Radiologists initially refer to nonimaging information, such as clinical history, to help diagnose the disease in people. For radiologists, it is time consuming to identify sub-anatomic structures within medical images and perform measurements in order to attain quantification for the image-based diagnosis. However, advancement in deep learning allows accurate segmentation of 3D aCNNimages (Left Ventricle, Right Ventricle, and myocardium) to estimate cardiac parameters such as cardiac ejection fraction, volume, and mass by segmentation methods [26].

Fig. 6.2 Tasks in Deep
Learning

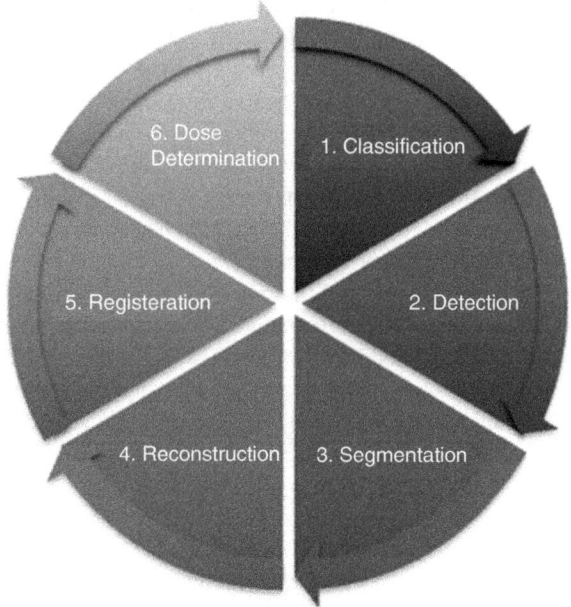

Next to cardiology, Neurology is perhaps one of the medical fields in which clinical images are extensively used both for research purposes in relation to the brain development, monitoring, and for diagnostic procedures linked to neurological disorders. CNN-based neurological models have achieved a high level of accuracy in relation to the prevention of Alzheimer's disease. In multiple sclerosis imaging, both the white and gray matter are affected, so normalization methods that depend on the brain tissue may introduce bias or remove biological changes of interest [27].

Big Data is used to define data with colossal volume or complications which cannot be handled by traditional data processing techniques. First and foremost is the volume of data that is growing rapidly in the biomedical informatics fields. The second feature is the diversity in data types and structures. The third distinctive feature of big data is velocity, refers to generating and handling data [28]. Big Data setup is a framework, which entails significant components including Hadoop (hadoop.apache.org), massively parallel processing, NoSQL databases that are used for Big Data storage, processing, and analysis [29]. Hadoop is a big data analysis platform that is highly effective for processing biologically pertinent data sizes, when we consider computing hours for both split and un-split datasets. Apache Hadoop has Packages like Cloudburst, MapReduce, Eoulsan, Crossbow, Contrail, Myrna, DistMap, and Seal that can accomplish several NGS applications, such as quality checking, de novo assembly, adapter trimming, read mapping, quantification, variant analysis, expression analysis, and annotation [30]. While debate is still on for the actual definition and limitations of Big Data and its advantages of healthcare, Big Data has been proven itself in three key aspects of healthcare- first prevention of diseases, identifying amendable risk factors in disease, and drug discovery for changing health behaviors [31].

Blockchain technology is being posited as the next frontier in healthcare sector. It is a distributed network containing public ledgers, recording transactions, and asset monitoring [32]. This technology is believed to bring significant progress in medical records management and insurance claims, aid clinical investigations and biomedical researches and progress biomedical and health care data ledgers [33]. This approach facilitates the switch from institution driven interoperability to patient-centered interoperability [34].

The basic idea behind Internet of Things is the linking of smart objects or things to Internet in a transparent manner. This allows exchanging information between all components, and conveys it to the user securely [35]. IoT-supported gadgets assist remote monitoring in the healthcare industry and enhanced patient involvement and gratification due to easy and effective communication with physicians and are commonly called as Internet of Healthcare Things (IoHT) or Internet of Medical Things (IoMT) [36].

Earlier in traditional healthcare systems, information management was paper based and later it was substituted by the Healthcare Information System (HIS). However, the HIS also seemed ineffective because of numerous concerns such as data storage volume, system integration, high expenses of operating, and system maintenance [37]. Cloud computing is a progressive and affordable approach that enables real-time data collection, data storage, and give-and-take amongst healthcare organizations. Cloud network is equipped with high-throughput and high-volume storage capacity. While conducting data computing on high population of patient's data, privacy and security are the aspects to be considered. Both are major concerns for adopting cloud-based healthcare facilities. Therefore, healthcare organizations must have electronic medical records in order to utilize the cloud networks [38].

6.3 Significant Role of Technologies in Health Care

The innovations of the digital world have revolutionized the healthcare system to attain sustainability goals by balancing the link healthcare experts and patients thereby yielding rapid, affordable, and efficacious treatments for all diseases. In healthcare, technology is progressively playing a significant part in practically all the procedures, from patient registration to record keeping, from pathology reports to personal care policies [39].

6.3.1 Artificial Intelligence (AI)

The advent of Artificial intelligence is at par with healthcare professionals and aids them to make accurate medical choices or even substitute human decisions in active zones of healthcare such as radiology. It has also shown significant potential in the healthcare marketing. AI utilization in the healthcare business is estimated to boom by 40% annually reaching a target of $6.6 Billion by 2021. Artificial Intelligence algorithms process various types of clinical data that include Diagnostic Imaging, Sequencing, Microarray, Electrodiagnosis, Monitoring, Mass screening, and Disability Evaluation [40]. AI has various applications in health informatics such as automate reminders, identifying people at high risk, and delivering personalized dosage recommendations. Google's DeepMind created an AI-based application for breast cancer analysis. The algorithm outperformed all human radiologists on pre-selected data sets to identify breast cancer, on average by 11.5% [41].

6.3.2 Blockchain and Data Security

Blockchain claims to redefine the fundamental operational strategies of colossal sectors – including digital healthcare marketing. Blockchain provides a safe yet branched database which operates without a dominant authority or proprietor. To promote legitimacy and transparency of healthcare information based on pre-existing data, from monitoring authorizations in electronic health records (EHR) to rationalizing claim and complaint processes. Data Security and privacy is one of the top priorities in the Blockchain developers [42]. A successful example of this is MedRec, a collaborative blockchain project of MIT Media Labs and Beth Israel Deaconess Medical Center. This system provides a decentralized style to manage consents, authorization, and data sharing amongst healthcare organizations. This project enables patients to monitor who can access their personal healthcare records. A key feature is that patient consents, data storage location, and audit logs are pooled on a blockchain to generate an automated method to share data for clinical and research practice, without actually storing the data in the blockchain. The healthcare information stays within EHR systems and requires additional softwares to allow interoperability [43].

6.3.3 Voice Search

Voice is the most recent target of healthcare market promotion strategies that has been on the ascent since the release of android phones and smart-speakers (with Amazon's Echo and Google Home). About 46% of adults in US households use voice assistants at home and the number is only anticipated to increase in the coming years. It is arguably one of the most compelling devices in the market today. Voice assistants are improving patient care by growing efficacy and offering a novel experience by providing a plethora of benefits. Patients can access medical records, check and deliberate healthcare-related issues, and communicate using this service. This is especially helpful for the elderly patients [44]. Hossain et al. proposed a cloud-based smart healthcare nursing system called Voice pathology detection (VPD) method which takes input as voices and an electroglottograph signal. This input instrument is linked to the Internet so that caught signals are transferred to the cloud which are further processed and categorized as normal or pathological with a confidence score. The outcome is then sent to Physicians who make the final decision and take suitable action [45].

6.3.4   Healthcare Trackers

Fitbit and jawbone have become our new fitness trainers. For people looking to improve their health, wearable fitness tracking gadgets provide an easy and real-time approach monitors one's health and to motivate them towards leading a healthy disease-free lifestyle that is driven by personal data-based understanding which is offered by such devices [46]. However multiple factors including interpersonal effect, personal creativity, individual's efficacy, attitude towards a wearable fitness tracker, well-being, and assumed cost of the device affect an individual's acceptance towards these trackers [47].

6.3.5   Chatbots

A chatbot offers users with a text-based conversation like the ones usually used on messaging applications, including SMS, social network systems, and web-based applications. Compared to the communicability of traditional interfaces, chatbots in healthcare provide a plethora of advantages and the prospect for improving patient medical record management, clinical management, aid in emergency situations, or with first aid. A major aspect of User experience is the interface that links a user and the service. In an effort to improve the human-computer interaction, engineers constantly come up with new technologies. Conversational interfaces are aimed to let users to communicate or to chat with bots by means of voice (voicebot) or text (chatbot) [48]. HOLMeS stands for Health On-Line Medical Suggestions, a medical recommendation system developed to autonomously contact with the user by understanding natural language in a chat and substituting a human physician. It is made of diverse components to deliver numerous innovative eHealth services through an instinctive chat service [49].

6.3.6   Virtual Reality (VR)

Virtual reality (VR) is improving the lives of patients and physicians alike. In the next few decades, we might watch surgeries as if we used the surgical blade on an organ or one could visit the picture-perfect Swiss Alps simply lying on their hospital bed. VR is a great tool with unrivalled engagement. VR also provides an immersive view where patients can get a virtual tour of the hospital and often helps them to cope with pain. VR is being used to train future doctors for actually carrying out surgeries. Such softwares are developed and provided by companies like Osso VR and ImmersiveTouch and are in active use with promising results. Women are being equipped with VR headsets to visualize soothing landscapes so as to help them get through labor pain. VR has been in use to reduce pain associated with surgeries, cardiac, neurological, and gastric problems in patients by distracting them from the stimulus of pain [50, 51].

6.3.7   Augmented Reality (AR)

Augmented reality varies from VR in two aspects: Here the users are in touch with reality throughout the experience and it adds information to the eyesight rapidly. These unique features have made augmented reality powerful component of future medicine; both on the healthcare experts and the patient's perspective. Using this method, medical students have access to detail and accurate, albeit virtual, and depictions of the human anatomy to study the subject without the need of real bodies [47]. Luo et al. describe the head-mounted display visualization which helps visually impaired patients instead of physicians. They utilized an optically transparent system to superimpose contour images from a camera connected for normal vision. The system was developed to assist patients with tunnel vision, mending their visual search practice [52, 53].

6.3.8   Internet of Medical Things (IoMT)

Internet of Medical Things (IoMT) plays a significant part in healthcare market to improve the accuracy, dependability, and efficiency of electronic instruments used for providing medical support to patients. Researchers from different parts of the world are coming together to develop a digitized healthcare system which links the accessible medical assets and healthcare facilities [54]. Georges Matar et al. offered a method to check patient posture by utilizing their body weight which applies pressure on specifically designed mattress; he used this measured pressure for monitoring patient posture. He validated this study using Cohen's Coefficient, where the value of the coefficient was 0.866 indicating high accuracy of prediction. According to him, the aim of this project was to cut down storage requirements along with computational costs [55].

6.3.9 Digitization of Healthcare Records

Electronic medical records or Electronic health records (HER) have created immense strides in the concentration and effectiveness of patient clinical data, it also finds use in population studies bringing in a huge cultural swing in the upcoming decades of data-driven medicine. Multiple data elements are collected in Electronic health records: daily charts, medical administration, physical assessments, on-admission nursing notes, healthcare plan, referrals, existing conditions or symptoms, medical history, life style, physical examinations, diagnosis, tests, medical procedures, treatments, medications, discharge, journals, findings, and immunization [56]. Raj Kumar et al. designed a representation of patients' complete raw EHR records on the basis of Fast Healthcare Interoperability Resources (FHIR) format. Further, this data is used with deep learning models for effectively forecasting multiple medical events from many centers without the need of integrating site-specific data [58]. Successful management of EHRs will offer key advantages just not only for patient's safety and quality of health care services but also make healthcare amenities more affordable [57].

6.3.10 Telemedicine/Telehealth

Studies reliably show the advantages of telehealth, particularly in rural areas whose access to resource are limited compared to main cities. Additionally, telemedicine centers will likewise lessen organization maintenance expenses by disposing the requirement of leaving work to go to a primary healthcare facility. Several medical labs use android devices connected to affordable telehealth equipment's, such as blood glucose monitors and electrocardiogram device [58]. Telemedicine offers clinical services linked to information technology, video imaging, and telecommunication connections to allow doctors to deliver healthcare services at a distance [59]. Teleradiology and telepsychiatry were among the earliest telemedicine applications [60]. Compared to telemedicine, which is specifically defined as the provision of medical services at a distance by a physician, telehealth is a canopy that encompasses telemedicine and a variety of nonphysician facilities, including telenursing and telepharmacy [61]. The main aim of telehealth application is to ease the burden on health care system and providing good healthcare facilities based on long-term follow-up for diagnostics and mediation strategies [62]. A few concerning clinical demerits of telehealth are poor standards of patient- physician relationships, physical examinations, and healthcare with remote appointments than physical meetings and abuse complaints [63, 64].

6.3.11   mHealth/Mobile Health

M-health provides an easy solution for an issue commonly overlooked in the clinical field: how to get to the correct data when and where it is required in highly dynamic and branched heath care systems [65]. M-health is liberating medical gadgets of wires and cords and permitting doctors and patients alike to check on medical practices on the go. Androids phones enable healthcare experts to easily access and send information. Doctors and healthcare providers can use mHealth applications for orders, documentation and just to gather adequate information when with patients. Huang et al. present WE-Care, a smart tele-1cardiological system that provides mhealth facilities in the form of wearables and mobile 7-lead ECG equipment. This application reduces the feedback time by distributing the detection process between mobile phone and the linked server so that diagnostic ability of ECG device can be utilized. The algorithm is designed to identify the aberrations in the ECG records and produces warnings if required; doctors get access to the alerts and ECG data further utilized conduct detailed analysis at the application end [64]. A randomized clinical study of a mHealth application aimed for weight loss and HbA1c reduction in Type 2 Diabetes Mellitus patients showed promising results [65]. This way mHealth changes the manner in which healthcare systems were perceived.

6.3.12   Portal Technology

Patients are gradually becoming dynamic players in their own healthcare; definition has almost shifted to personal care, and portal technology is a powerful tool in achieving these goals. Additionally, medical information accessibility is also increasing. The US portable healthcare recording systems employ a database which stores the details of the patients that can be accessed by the physicians and patients. Each patient is allotted a card with unique id and password to access this information. A doctor who is handling a particular patient's case can review and update their clinical data [66]. A different kind of application of portable technology is the use of portal UV disinfectants that prevent patients against infections acquired in the hospital environment that can be caused by pathogenic microbes such as *Clostridium difficile,* vancomycin-resistant *Enterococcus,* and methicillin-resistant *Staphylococcus aureus* [67].

6.3.13   Self-Service Kiosks

The self-service kiosk is an explicit type of Self Service Technology employed in healthcare facilities. They are generally installed on large touch screen panels or small monitors and keypad combos. (GG) Self-service kiosks can accelerate procedures like hospital registration. Patients can effectively do all procedures linked to registration in a hassle-free manner without the need to communicate with whole lot of administration. This allows cost cutting on staffs. Automated kiosks can help patients with payments, id verification, documentation, and other registration requirements [68]. Yet, Healthcare systems should be thoughtful while integrating it to make sure human to human communication is not entirely eradicated. If a person needs to communicate to the authorities, they should be able to allow such provisions. Lyu et al. designed self-service physiology-based kiosk that combines multiple biosensors and medical devices to take up user's physiological parameters such as plasma glucose, heart pulsing rate, blood oxygen, height, and weight. These measurements are vital to understand user's health condition. This system was designed with the aim to improve Human Machine Interactions and to calculate measurements accurately [69].

6.3.14   Remote Monitoring Tools

Monitoring patients' health at home can decrease costs and needless appointments to clinics. For heart patients, a cardiac cast with a pacemaker regularly transmits data to a monitoring center. So in case of emergencies, the physicians can be immediately informed and reached out for help. This technology is very helpful for people suffering with chronic disorders. Several studies have shown that remote monitoring tools have been successful in reducing emergency department or urgent hospital visits especially for patients suffering from cardiovascular diseases with implantable [70, 71].

6.3.15   Nanotechnology

Nanoparticles and nanodevices function as mini surgeons employing specialized drug delivery systems for complex diseases like cancer, Alzheimer's as a treatment tool. In 2014, researchers from the Max Planck Institute designed scallop-like microbot designed to literally swim through bodily fluids. Small, smart pills like the PillCam are already in use for colon exams in a noninvasive, patient-friendly way. In 2018, MIT researchers created an electronic pill that can be controlled wirelessly and transmit diagnostic data or drug release mediated by android phone instructions. At CES 2020, France-based Company called Grapheal demonstrated its smart patch that allows continuous monitoring of wounds and its graphene core can even stimulate wound healing. Nanotechnology has numerous applications in the field of medical science that include bioimaging, sensing, synthetic grafts, and target-specific delivery of genes, drugs, and bioactives [72].

6.3.16 Robotics

Robotics is one of the rapidly emerging and sensational technologies in healthcare. The innovations in this field are cutting-edge from robotic carts that moves equipment's at hospital to super-smart surgeon robots, pharmabots. The year 2019 was a great year for exoskeletons. It saw Europe's first exoskeleton-aided surgery and a tetraplegic man capable of controlling an exoskeleton with his brain. There are loads of other applications for these sci-fi suits from aiding nurses through lift elderly patients to helping patients with spinal cord injury. Robot companions also have their place in healthcare to help alleviate loneliness, treat mental health issues, or even help children with chronic illness. The Jibo, da Vinci Pepper, Xenex Germ-Zapping Robot, Paro, and Buddy robots are successful instances of robotics in healthcare and personal care. These robots have cameras, special sensors, and mics to communicate with its owner. For instance, ikki from an Australian startup is helping children with chronic illnesses monitor their medications, temperature, and breathing rate while keeping them company with music and stories. Another example is Cyberknife, a robotic surgery system developed in 1990s that carries out radiation therapy on tumors with supreme precision and is now being used in hospitals to treat patients with surgically complicated cancers [73].

6.3.17 3D-Printing

AI is a game changer in healthcare because when AI combined with three-dimensional (3D) printing technologies, it could increase the performance by reducing the risk of error and facilitating automated production. Nowadays, 3D printing has become an essential and potentially transformative approach to revolutionize health care rapidly. 3D-printing can bring wonders in all aspects of healthcare such as biotissues, artificial limbs, pills, and blood vessels. In November 2019, scientists at the Rensselaer Polytechnic Institute in New York developed a method to 3-Dimensional print living skin along with blood vessels. This development proves crucial for skin grafts for burn victims. Also, helping patients in need are NGOs like Refugee Open Ware and Not Impossible which 3D-print prosthetics for refugees from war-torn areas. The pharmaceutical industry is also benefiting from this technology. FDA-approved 3D-printed drugs have been a reality since 2015 and researchers are now working on 3D-printing polypills. These contain several layers of drugs so as to help patients adhere to their therapeutic plan [74].

6.3.18   Sensors and Wearable Technology

Wearable medical instruments and biosensors are efficient tools for collecting patient health information. Wearable electronic technologies integrate an electronic device into clothing, accessories, human skin, or implanted in vivo and detect biological components which are further used for body sensing, data storing, and mobile computing [75]. The advent of microelectromechanical systems has led to the development of miniaturized wearables that can be used for a range of applications [76]. A sensor can be as simple as device that sends alert to healthcare providers when the patient falls from the bed or pH bandages that can measure the skin pH and identify whether the cut or wound is infected. A wearable technology developed by Roy et al. assists in carrying out sweat analysis by measuring Na+ ion concentration using a polyvinyl chloride doped with ionophore and ion exchanger on Carbon Nanotube electrodes. Sweat Analysis is essential as its contents are biomarkers for a various disease like osteoporosis, hyponatremia, drug abuse, and cystic fibrosis [77]. One of the most developed biosensors are glucometers that have evolved from finger-prick-based blood glucose sensors to noninvasive glucometer that simply require a press of the finger on the sensing device (example: DiaMonTech, Cnoga), employs a nonperceptible electric current across the skin to extract a small quantity of analyte-glucose into a blotch positioned on the skin. These biosensors are being designed to provide astonishing features like voice readout for visually impaired patients, glucose pens that can be easily carried in the patient's pockets, and glucose sensors linked to mobile applications such as DiabetesPal, Dlife, and MyGlucoseBuddy. Table 6.2 shows the other types of sensors and their properties.

6.3.19   Wireless Communication

It is only recent that instant messaging system is being employed in hospitals instead of pagers and beeping devices. Vocera Messaging offers users to send posts like lab tests and alert signals to others using smartphones, web-based servers, or third-party clinical networks. These messaging systems can speed up the communication processes while still tracing and sorting information in a secure approach. Wireless-equipped healthcare systems can distantly and constantly observe the patients' health condition in both domestic and outdoor settings, so that the patient does not feel constricted to stay at a place. Timely finding of patients' emergency states based on wireless communications enables provision of timely first-aid and access to patients' health data in a ubiquitous method, thus refining both systems dependability and productivity [78]. CareNet is an Integrated Wireless Sensor Networking Environment for Remote Healthcare that provides dependable and secure information transfer between patients' homes and the healthcare providers [79]. Several healthcare companies such as TactioHealth sync with the modern fitness trackers like Bodymedia

Table 6.2 Common sensors used in healthcare

Type of sensor	Measurable Quantity	Functionality of sensor	Market products
Thermometer	Body temperature (°C, °F, or °K)	Measures patient's temperature at different body parts including oral, temporal, tympanic, and rectal	Pipercare, leelvis infrared, Clinitemp plastic strip thermometer
Glucometer	Plasma glucose Levels (mg/dL)	Glucometers are extensively used by diabetic patients to monitor glycemic variability.	Accu-Check lancing device, One touch Select Strips, Dr. Morepengluco One
Blood Pressure Sensor	Systolic, diastolic, and mean arterial pressure (mmHg)	Blood pressure sensors are used by patients with cardiovascular conditions	Omron Blood Pressure Monitor, BMP barometric pressure sensor, Vernier sensor
Pacemaker	Atrial, ventricular electrical pulses (bpm)	Real-time embedded sensor systems which maintain synchronized heart rates	Medtronic, Boston Scientific, Biotronik heart pacemaker
Oximeter	Blood oxygen saturation (SpO2) (%)	Measures the saturation of oxygen carried in RBCs	Accu-sure finger pulse oximeter, Newnik Pulse oximeter
Electro encephalography sensor	Voltage fluctuations (mV/s)	EEG signals evaluate the intracranial activity with electrodes placed on scalp.	Neurosky, Olimex, and sky technology neurosensor
Airflow sensors	Volumetric air flow rate is measured in "standard cubic centimeters per minute" (SCCM)	Silicon-based sensors that operate on differential air pressure and heat transfer commonly used in anesthesia delivery systems and heart pump	MQ135, Omron D6F, and Sensirion AG flow sensor

Fit, Fitbit, and Withings Pulse. It also stocks patient's glucose levels, A1c, and other important data and lets them print out detailed reports for your doctor.

6.3.20   Medical Tricorder

The Viatom CheckMe Pro is one such palm-sized gadget which can measure ECG, heart rate, oxygen saturation, temperature, blood pressure, and more. A smartphone application known as "Medical Tricorder" exploits android phone's inertial electro sensors when located on the human's chest, it proficiently captures the motion patterns produced by heart pumping. Through the obtained ballistocardiograph signal, the system effectively computes the heart rate in real time comparing it to the values of standard clinical grade electrocardiographs. These signals can be made readily available to clinicians for detection of heart defects at primary stage itself without involving healthcare staff [80].

6.3.21 Real-Time Locating Services

While GPS systems are successful in locating assets but they fail in indoor setting. Therefore, real-time location systems have become an essential service to solve tracking problems. Real-time locating services are of prime importance in effectively detecting emergency conditions in healthcare setting. The tracking facility can be installed in wide range of subjects-medical instruments, patients to healthcare staff. A real-time tracking system essentially consists of location sensors known as receivers or readers that receive wireless signals from the subject of interest (person/object) installed with a tag. Surveillance also has some boundaries, mainly in dynamic places like emergency units but tracing movements with real-time locating services highlight possible concerns in productivity and operations. At a fundamental level, these services make sure that equipment's and supplies are not stolen, as they are fairly expensive, also allow verification of its proper use. The same principle also applies to safeguarding of patient records as the healthcare is responsible for its security. However, the functionality of these devices must not be misinterpreted. Real-time locating system does not constantly track speed, direction, or spatial positioning of tracked assets and persons [81].

Hence, this is revolutionary time for healthcare due to development of digital health.

6.4 Potential Role of Technologies in COVID-19

The beginning of 2020 has seen the emergence of coronavirus outbreak caused by a novel virus called SARS-CoV-The sudden explosion and uncontrolled worldwide spread of COVID-19 show the limitations of existing healthcare systems to timely handle public health emergencies. In such contexts, inno-vative technologies such as blockchain and Artificial Intelligence (AI) have emerged as promising solutions for fighting coronavirus epidemic. On the one hand, blockchain can combat pandemics by enabling early detection of outbreaks, protecting user privacy, and ensuring reliable medical supply chain during the outbreak tracking. On the other hand, AI provides intelligent solutions for identifying symptoms caused by coronavirus for treatments and supporting drug manufacturing.

Today our world is trapped under an evasive pandemic called COVID 19 which has claimed upto 661k lives and still counting. COVID 19 is a highly communicable disease caused by a subfamily of a coronavirinae specifically known as SARS CoV-2 of beta coronavirus family. COVID19 has severely impacted economies, academics, transport, and politics but the worst hit is on healthcare systems [82].

The extent of clinical manifestations in this respiratory disease may be acute, moderate, or chronic depending upon the pre-existing comorbidities. So it can be treated with effective measures taken at the right time. But the sudden outburst and hysterical spread of COVID-19 globally show the overall flaws and limits of our existing healthcare facilities indicated by the inefficient handling of this public health emergency [83].

In this pandemic, nonmedical technologies such as artificial intelligence and blockchain arose to provide innovative solutions to tackle new problems emerging every day. Blockchain helps fighting the pandemic by aiding early detection of plague, guarding patient's record privacy, and warranting dependable medical services during the disease outbreak. AI offers intelligent solutions for detecting symptoms produced by the virus for effectively treating patients and aiding drug discovery and manufacture [84].

AI is a potent tool to combat the COVID19 pandemic. For example, Beck and his coworkers (2020) designed a deep learning algorithm to detect effective drugs for the drug-repurposing, i.e., identifying a swift drug using present drugs in market that can cure infected patients. This approach helps just not only in saving the expenses of drug discovery but also reduces the timeline [85].

In the situation of COVID-19, big data refers to the patient's information including admission-notes, X-Ray report, patient disease history, list of doctors, and nurses, and close contacts [82, 86]. Big data potentially provides a number of promising solutions to help combat COVID-19 epidemic. By combining with AI analytics, big data helps us to understand the COVID-19 in terms of outbreak tracking, virus structure, disease treatment, and vaccine manufacturing [87].

In USA, the George Washington University Hospital has utilized various telemedicine approaches, which include video consultation and live informative webinars to give remote medical advices to numerous people [88]. The Rush University Medical Center (USA) has adopted telemedicine platforms to assist on-demand video consultations. However, these health professionals were using such consultations not only to provide medical advices to patients but also to test them for the COVID-19 [89].

During outbreak, Infervision Company launched a coronavirus AI solution that assists front-line healthcare workers to screen and monitor the disease effectively. Similarly, during COVID-19, Ant Financial, a blockchain platform, helps to quicken the claim processes to reduce the incidences of physical meeting between patients and healthcare workers [90].

As the overall incidences of COVID-19 are rapidly increasing Machine Learning and Cloud Computing can be employed efficiently to trace the disease, hypothesize spread of the epidemic and design policies and guidelines to prevent its spread. Tuli and et al. (2020) develop Generalized Inverse Weibull distribution, a prediction framework for the growth and trends of COVID-19 pandemic using machine learning and cloud computing [91].

Andhra Pradesh and Assam (India), have executed telemedicine services to facilitate remote communication of probable COVID-19 patients with health experts [92, 93]. The Sheba Medical Center (Israel's largest hospital), several telehealth technologies were used to screen 12 Israeli passengers who were on board in the cruise quarantined in Japan for some weeks. However, the Sheba Medical Center deployed telemedicine services not only to treat these travelers remotely but also to make sure that least human contact was made while handling them within the hospital premises [94, 95]. A study compared the effectiveness of real- time location services in contact tracing for covid19 in healthcare workers of Singapore of preventing the spread of this infectious disease [96].

Wearable sensors aid in the real-time monitoring of heart rate, heart rate variability, resting heart rate, body temperature, arterial oxygen saturation (SPO2) respiration rate, and blood glucose levels for asymptomatic and mild-symptom home-based COVID-19 patients, along with specific parameters for patients with comorbidities like diabetes or chronic obstructive pulmonary disease and patients with severe symptoms in hospital intensive care units (ICU). Conventional sensors that measure heart rate and respiration rate can serve as potential markers of COVID-19 infection and are already measured by wearable devices such as the Apple Watch, Fitbit, Zephyr BioHarness, or VivaLNK Vital Scout [97, 98]. To enhance accuracy of detection of COVID-19, RT-PCR is aided by imaging informatics employed to analyze routine CT scans or X-ray images for detection and monitoring disease progression. In healthcare settings, multimodal dataset is intricately analyzed to support healthcare providers to develop better and efficacious treatments plans when managing for severe stage COVID-19 patients [99, 100]. Behavioral informatics is also being exploited to study human behavior data in the situation of self-quarantine, or community-quarantine in different countries to drive execution of better policies and laws [101]. These studies also help in providing a better grasp of human behavior by assessing patterns in the mental, emotional, and physical data so as to provide ample support to help people cope with self-quarantine, and any other potential agoraphobia post self-quarantine [102]. In rehabilitation informatics, medical data are being analyzed to comprehend the effect of the disease on affected organs like lung and heart functions post recovery in patients with varying stages of COVID-19 [103, 104]. In infectious disease modeling, epidemiological models have been built with field data to predict the rate of COVID-19 spread so as to assist policy makers in taking proper actions. The outbreak figures are analyzed for population health management and COVID-19 care resources supply chain management [105, 106].

6.5   Impact of Bioinformatics in Health Care

Bioinformatics is the integration of biology, mathematics, and computer science. It utilizes various in silico approaches and tools to predict biological information (Table 6.3). The computational tools are beneficial in analyzing metabolic disorders and genetic defects. Healthcare information includes physiological characteristics based on affected organs, cost reports, claim bills, and assessments linked to patient contentment [107].

Table 6.3 Bioinformatics Techniques and Approaches used in Health Informatics

S. No.	Bioinformatics Techniques	Approach (Tool/Database/Software)
1	Microarray analysis	GEO
2	Next gene sequencing	Strand NGS, DESeq (R package) EdgeR, TopHat/Cufflinks
3	Pathway analysis	KEGG, Reactome, BioGRID, STRING
4	Protein modeling and docking analysis	Sequence Databases: Uniprot
		Structure Databases: PDB
		Modeling Database: SWISS-MODEL, I-TASSER, Phyre2 Server
		Structure Refinement: SAVS, RAMPAGE
		Protein-Ligand Docking: SWISSDOCK, GLIDE (Shrodinger)
		PPI-Docking: HADDOCK, CLUSPRO
5	Genetic Variation	TOOLS: NovoAlign, SAMToolsGenome Analysis ToolKit
		Variant Annotation Databases: dbSNP
6	Sequence analysis	Alignment tools: BLAST, L-Align, CLUSTALW, MUSCLE, T-COFFEE
		Sequence Databases: NCBI Entrez, Ensemble, Uniprot

The identification of biomarkers is based on omics studies, which is generally done to predict consequences in a precision medicine such as patient disease vulnerability, analysis, diagnosis, prognosis, and response to therapeutics. Hence biomarker discovery tool has been developed, i.e., BioDiscM, which is a stand-alone program based on machine learning [108]. To classify the microarray cancer data, AI techniques has been utilized in gene selection tool [109]. Other application, AI in bioinformatics is drug repurposing and classification based on imaging data [110].

6.5.1 Genome Sequencing

Biological data science is an emerging area that has complemented computational techniques and the usage of contemporary high-performance structures that include CPU clusters, clouds, GPUs, and field programmable gate arrays. Next Gen Sequencing analysis needs computing all pairwise read alignments or all pairwise read-genome mapping software's like BLAST are computationally infeasible either due to the large size of query data or the software's are not designed for that specific task [111]. This is where big data comes into play. Cloudburst is a parallel-computing model that allows sequenced genomes to be mapped by utilizing short read mapping that enhances the scalability of sequencing data [112]. Biological databases play a noteworthy role in storing big data. Biological Databases such as the virulence factor database http://www.mgc.ac.cn/VFs/ that offers comprehensive information about virulence factors of bacteria that are medically proven to be pathogenic [113].

The Big Data has revolutionized several sectors of technology; the healthcare market has however been slow and has finally reached the period where big data can fully renovate the business for the better [114]. Big Data can increase operational efficiency, aid prediction and planning response to treatment, optimize the quality of monitoring of clinical trials, and reduce healthcare expenditure at multiple levels from patients to hospitals to governments. Combining the efforts interdisciplinary fields such as genomics and big data empowered by machine learning algorithms that can identify disease biomarkers, predict disease diagnosis, progression stage and prognosis in critical life-threatening diseases like cancer, neurological disorders like Parkinson, Schizophrenia, and Alzheimer. Reconstructing regulatory pathways from gene expression data is another well-developed field that uses a high-throughput genome scale data. Network reading approaches can be divided into five groups based on the primary model in each instance: regression, mutual information, correlation, Boolean regulatory networks, and other methods [115]. Figure 6.3 shows major applications of big data are genomics which is expected to be the future of healthcare [116].

The other side of genomics data is the multifaceted phenotypic data with which the sequence information is being correlated. Phenotypic data come from a variety of sources such as simple and unorganized textual data from electronic health records, biological function measurements from laboratories, sensors, and electronic trackers, and bioimaging data [117].

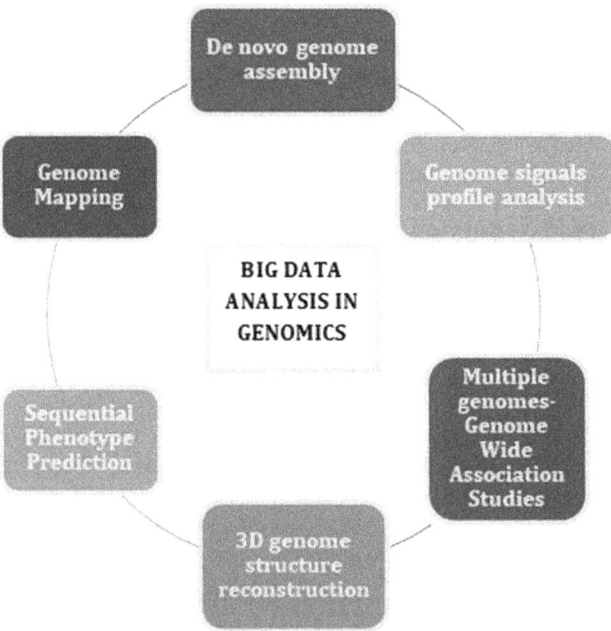

Fig. 6.3 Applications of Big DATA in genomics

6.5.2 Revolutionizing Drug Development

Drug discovery plays a key role in the pharma and biotech industries. The major objective of drug development is to create novel drugs in less time utilizing bioinformatics techniques. The drug discovery process has been reformed with the use of high-throughput technologies in biosciences that include – genomics, proteomics, metabolomics, and microbiomics. Novel trends and fast progress in drug discovery have led to success of the bioinformatics tools [118]. Cutting-edge in silico methodologies have given a remarkable opportunity to pharmaceutical corporations to identify novel drug targets which in turn quicken the success and time for conducting clinical trials for drug discovering [119]. The traditional drug discovery process was more serendipitous rather than a planned process. But today, drug discovery involves a streamlined progression from identification to optimization. Recently, companies such as Innoplexus are making it possible for pharma industries to revolutionize their drug discovery processes by harnessing AI-powered solutions. AI can help experts at various stages of drug discovery, expanding options for researchers involved in laboratory and computation-based research (in vitro, ex vivo, in silico), and facilitating translational medicine and bioinformatics.

Current drug discovery requires significantly time-consuming efforts in order to search literature such as publications and presentations to identify connections between genes, molecular targets, pathways, and drugs. Such efforts require searching through disparate databases and using search engines with inadequate understanding of the language of life sciences, leaving researchers with an incomplete picture of the connections and interactions between biological entities. This limitation makes it challenging to identify and test new methods (new targets, molecules, pathways, patient stratification, genomic sequencing, etc.) and find new indications to target. Highly advanced technology developed by Innoplexus enables researchers to have nearly all online published life science data at their fingertips and easily see connections between closely and distantly related entities [120].

6.6 Challenges and Future in Health Informatics

Healthcare modernization is led by a number of trends including increasing healthcare costs, an elderly population, and the rising occurrence of chronic disorders that necessitates long-term personal care. As technology advances and the productivity of the healthcare business have also risen, so are the number of people profiting from the healthcare industry. Moreover, the uses of devices that collect huge volumes of data are crucial for the shift to evidence based and prevention-based medications that the industry has adopted. These approaches lead to a more successful treatment for patients [121].

There are several challenges when it comes to wide scale implementation health informatics. The first and foremost challenge is providing data security and privacy during confidential transmissions of patient information that must comply with bio-ethical and legal agreements [122]. These guidelines are being constructed for med-ical websites; however, doctors and healthcare professional are yet to be trained efficiently enabling them to accurately guide and interpret the content to patients [123, 124]. Health informatics approaches are aimed to attain an ideal balance between cost efficiency and quality of service but they are often limited by the poor return investments in information management and technology [125]. AI- powered Clinical decisions support system that uses historical and current data to provide treatment plans, maximizes resource utilization, and cost procedures. Their adapt-ability has been fairly low due to the negligence of medical professionals, limita-tions in software systems and algorithms, and partly because of the effort in capturing expert knowledge. It also raises questions on the allocation of responsibil-ity when a machine-based decision system fails to provide the correct solutions. Technologies such as robotic surgery and implantable controller devices based on artificial intelligence are yet to seek approval in several countries as their efficacy and safety in regards to human life are yet to be proved [126, 127]. To address these issues, information must be operationalized, adjusted according to clinical work-flow along with generating ethical guidelines for responsibility of the data, integrat-ing standard data models, and provision of supportive infrastructure to make sense of the collected data for patients themselves.

The future of healthcare will rest upon three sectors: a digitalization, data sci-ence, and a patient-centric approach. Information technology will be the heart of this revolution, helping in cost reduction, improving productivity, and discovering new economies of scales for better efficiency and good patient care. IT can also mess up today's organizations and fundamentally alter healthcare delivery through personalized medicine and connected care. Predictive Analytics and IoT will form the future of many businesses, including healthcare. However, before these new technologies can truly deliver value to patients such as improving survivability and life expectancy or giving predictive and prescriptive indicators for ailments, health-care associations must first figure out their data strategies. This includes recording of data, storage of raw data, and ensuring security of data and utilizing it for greater patient insights [128].

Medical informatics is currently in the early stages of budding. Today, as an interdisciplinary field, it forms one of the bases for medicine and health care. As a consequence, considerable responsibility rests on medical informatics for refining the health of people, through its contributions to high quality, well-organized health care provisions, and to ground-breaking research in biomedicine and related health and computer sciences. Future research fields might range from seamless interactiv-ity with automatic data capture and storage, via informatics diagnostics and thera-peutics, to living labs with data analysis procedures, involving sensor-enhanced ambient environments [129].

The development in healthcare system is progressing by implementing informa-tion technology. Hence, today, health informatics is a combination with rapidly evolving technologies such as AI, big data, block chain, cloud technology, and inter-net of medical things which improves efficiencies and offers multiple avenues of streamlining healthcare delivery. It accelerates resource availability, boosts interoperability while lowering the costs but still there is need of better protocols, web services, and electronic medical record with better clinical decision support systems because there are few barriers in digitalized healthcare system such as security concern, system downtimes, and lack of patient data privacy. Programmers are still working on the drawbacks of these techniques and hence, the future is bright for the modern junctures between technology and healthcare.

References

1. G.N. Reddy, G.J. Reddy, Study of cloud computing in healthcare industry. arXiv preprint arXiv:1402.1841 (2014)
2. H. Thimbleby, Technology and the future of healthcare. J. Public Health Res. **2**(3), e28 (2013)
3. R. S. Dick, E. B. Steen, D. E. Detmer (eds.), *The Computer-Based Patient Record: An Essential Technology for Health Care* (National Academies Press, Washington, 1997)
4. S.S. Gill, S. Tuli, M. Xu, I. Singh, K.V. Singh, D. Lindsay, S. Tuli, D. Smirnova, M. Singh, U. Jain, H. Pervaiz, Transformative effects of IoT, Blockchain and Artificial Intelligence on cloud computing: Evolution, vision, trends and open challenges. Internet Things **8**, 100118 (2019)
5. S. Russell, P. Norvig, *Artificial Intelligence: A Modern Approach* (Pearson, Hoboken, 2002)
6. A. Narayanan, E.C. Keedwell, B. Olsson, Artificial intelligence techniques for bioinformatics. Appl. Bioinforma. **1**, 191–222 (2002)
7. G. Nápoles, I. Grau, R. Bello, R. Grau, Two-steps learning of Fuzzy Cognitive Maps for prediction and knowledge discovery on the HIV-1 drug resistance. Expert Syst. Appl. **41**(3), 821–830 (2014)
8. A. Burkov, M. Lutz, *The Hundred-Page Machine Learning Book* (Creative Commons, USA, 2019)
9. C.M. Bishop, *Pattern Recognition and Machine Learning* (Springer, New York, 2006)
10. T. Hastie, R. Tibshirani, J. Friedman, *The Elements of Statistical Learning: Data Mining, Inference, and Prediction* (Springer, New York, 2009)
11. E. Alpaydin, *Introduction to Machine Learning* (MIT press, Cambridge, 2020)
12. A. Frolova, M. Obolenska, Integrative approaches for data analysis in systems biology: Current advances, in *2016 II International Young Scientists Forum on Applied Physics and Engineering (YSF)*, (IEEE, Piscataway, 2016), pp. 194–198
13. I. Arel, D.C. Rose, T.P. Karnowski, Deep machine learning-a new frontier in artificial intelligence research. IEEE Comput. Intell. Mag. **5**(4), 13–18 (2010)
14. Y. Guo, Y. Liu, A. Oerlemans, S. Lao, S. Wu, M.S. Lew, Deep learning for visual understanding: A review. Neurocomputing **187**, 27–48 (2016)
15. B. Alipanahi, A. Delong, M.T. Weirauch, B.J. Frey, Predicting the sequence specificities of DNA- and RNA-binding proteins by deep learning. Nat. Biotechnol. **33**(8), 831–838 (2015)
16. M.R. Lamprecht, D.M. Sabatini, A.E. Carpenter, CellProfiler™: Free, versatile software for automated biological image analysis. BioTechniques **42**(1), 71–75 (2007)
17. S. Zhang, H. Hu, T. Jiang, L. Zhang, J. Zeng, TITER: Predicting translation initiation sites by deep learning. Bioinformatics **33**(14), i234–i242 (2017)
18. C. Angermueller, H.J. Lee, W. Reik, O. Stegle, DeepCpG: Accurate prediction of single-cell DNA methylation states using deep learning. Genome Biol. **18**(1), 1–3 (2017)
19. G. Chuai, H. Ma, J. Yan, M. Chen, N. Hong, D. Xue, C. Zhou, C. Zhu, K. Chen, B. Duan, F. Gu, DeepCRISPR: optimized CRISPR guide RNA design by deep learning. Genome biology, **19**(1), 1–18 (2018)

20. J.J. Almagro Armenteros, C.K. Sønderby, S.K. Sønderby, H. Nielsen, O. Winther, DeepLoc: Prediction of protein subcellular localization using deep learning. Bioinformatics **33**(21), 3387–3395 (2017)
21. C. Yang, L. Yang, M. Zhou, H. Xie, C. Zhang, M.D. Wang, H. Zhu, LncADeep: an ab initio lncRNA identification and functional annotation tool based on deep learning. Bioinformatics, **33**(22), 3825–3834 (2018)
22. Y. LeCun, Y. Bengio, G. Hinton, Deep learning. Nature **521**(7553), 436–444 (2015)
23. F. Piccialli, V. Di Somma, F. Giampaolo, S. Cuomo, G. Fortino, A survey on deep learning in medicine: Why, how and when? Inf. Fusion **66**, 111–137
24. R. Cuocolo, M. Caruso, T. Perillo, L. Ugga, M. Petretta, Machine Learning in oncology: A clinical appraisal. Cancer Lett. **481**, 55–62 (2020)
25. A.R. Ali, Deep Learning in Oncology–Applications in Fighting Cancer (2017)
26. K.K. Wong, G. Fortino, D. Abbott, Deep learning-based cardiovascular image diagnosis: A promising challenge. Futur. Gener. Comput. Syst. **110**, 802–811 (2020)
27. A.A.A. Valliani, D. Ranti, E.K. Oermann, Deep learning and neurology: A systematic review. Neurol. Ther. **8**(2), 351–365 (2019)
28. J. Luo, M. Wu, D. Gopukumar, Y. Zhao, Big data application in biomedical research and health care: A literature review. Biomed Inf Insights **8**, BII–S31559 (2016)
29. T.R. Rao, P. Mitra, R. Bhatt, A. Goswami, The big data system, components, tools, and technologies: A survey. Knowl. Inf. Syst. **60**(3), 1–81 (2019)
30. R. Tripathi, P. Sharma, P. Chakraborty, P.K. Varadwaj, Next-generation sequencing revolution through big data analytics. Front. Life Sci. **9**(2), 119–149 (2016)
31. R. Pastorino, C. De Vito, G. Migliara, K. Glocker, I. Binenbaum, W. Ricciardi, S. Boccia, Benefits and challenges of Big Data in healthcare: An overview of the European initiatives. Eur. J. Pub. Health **29**(Supplement_3), 23–27 (2019)
32. H.J. Yoon, Blockchain technology and healthcare. Healthcare Inf. Res. **25**(2), 59–60 (2019)
33. T.T. Kuo, H.E. Kim, L. Ohno-Machado, Blockchain-distributed ledger technologies for biomedical and health care applications. J. Am. Med. Inform. Assoc. **24**(6), 1211–1220 (2017)
34. W.J. Gordon, C. Catalini, Blockchain technology for healthcare: Facilitating the transition to patient-driven interoperability. Comput. Struct. Biotechnol. J. **16**, 224–230 (2018)
35. Y.I.N. Yuehong, Y. Zeng, X. Chen, Y. Fan, The internet of things in healthcare: An overview. J. Ind. Inf. Integr. **1**, 3–13 (2016)
36. R. Karjagi, M. Jindal, IoT applications in healthcare (2020), https://www.wipro.com/en-IN/business-process/what-can-iot-do-for-healthcare. Accessed 30 July 2020
37. M. Masrom, A. Rahimli, A review of cloud computing technology solution for healthcare system. Res. J. Appl. Sci. Eng. Technol. **8**(20), 2150–2153 (2014)
38. H.A. Aziz, A. Guled, *Cloud Computing and Healthcare Services* (CRC Press, Boca Raton, 2016)
39. B. Mesko, Future of healthcare: 10 ways technology is changing healthcare (2020), https://medicalfuturist.com/ten-ways-technology-changing-healthcare. Accessed 25 July 2020
40. F. Jiang, Y. Jiang, H. Zhi, Y. Dong, H. Li, S. Ma, Y. Wang, Q. Dong, H. Shen, Y. Wang, Artificial intelligence in healthcare: Past, present and future. Stroke Vasc. Neurol. **2**(4), 230–243 (2017)
41. S.M. McKinney, M. Sieniek, V. Godbole, J. Godwin, N. Antropova, H. Ashrafian, T. Back, M. Chesus, G.C. Corrado, A. Darzi, M. Etemadi, International evaluation of an AI system for breast cancer screening. Nature **577**(7788), 89–94 (2020)
42. S. Angraal, H.M. Krumholz, W.L. Schulz, Blockchain technology: Applications in health care. Circ. Cardiovasc. Qual. Outcomes **10**(9) (2017)
43. A. Azaria, A. Ekblaw, T. Vieira, A. Lippman, Medrec: Using blockchain for medical data access and permission management, in *2016 2nd International Conference on Open and Big Data (OBD)*, (IEEE, Piscataway, 2016), pp. 25–30
44. D. Dojchinovski, A. Ilievski, M. Gusev, Interactive home healthcare system with integrated voice assistant, in *2019 42nd International Convention on Information and Communication*

Technology, Electronics and Microelectronics (MIPRO), (IEEE, Piscataway, 2019), pp. 284–288

45. M.S. Hossain, G. Muhammad, A. Alamri, Smart healthcare monitoring: A voice pathology detection paradigm for smart cities. Multimedia Syst. **25**(5), 565–575 (2019)

46. S. Asimakopoulos, G. Asimakopoulos, F. Spillers, Motivation and user engagement in fitness tracking: Heuristics for mobile healthcare wearables, in *Informatics*, vol. 4, (Multidisciplinary Digital Publishing Institute, Basel, 2017), p. 5

47. S.Y. Lee, K. Lee, Factors that influence an individual's intention to adopt a wearable healthcare device: The case of a wearable fitness tracker. Technol. Forecast. Soc. Chang. **129**, 154–163 (2018)

48. S. Valtolina, B.R. Barricelli, S. Di Gaetano, Communicability of traditional interfaces VS chatbots in healthcare and smart home domains. Behav. Inform. Technol. **39**(1), 108–132 (2020)

49. F. Amato, S. Marrone, V. Moscato, G. Piantadosi, A. Picariello, C. Sansone, HOLMeS: EHealth in the big data and deep learning era. Information **10**(2), 34 (2019)

50. L.R. Valmaggia, L. Latif, M.J. Kempton, M. Rus-Calafell, Virtual reality in the psychological treatment for mental health problems: A systematic review of recent evidence. Psychiatry Res. **236**, 189–195 (2016)

51. C.S. Lányi, Virtual reality in healthcare, in *Intelligent Paradigms for Assistive and Preventive Healthcare*, (Springer, Berlin, Heidelberg, 2006), pp. 87–116

52. W. M. Carroll (ed.), *Emerging Technologies for Nurses: Implications for Practice* (Springer Publishing Company, New York, 2020)

53. M. Danciu, M. Gordan, A. Vlaicu, A. Antone, A survey of augmented reality in health care. Acta Technica Napocensis **52**(1), 13 (2011)

54. G.J. Joyia, R.M. Liaqat, A. Farooq, S. Rehman, Internet of Medical Things (IOMT): Applications, benefits and future challenges in healthcare domain. J. Commun. **12**(4), 240–247 (2017)

55. G. Matar, J.M. Lina, J. Carrier, A. Riley, G. Kaddoum, Internet of things in sleep monitoring: An application for posture recognition using supervised learning, in *2016 IEEE 18th International Conference on e-Health Networking, Applications and Services (Healthcom)*, (IEEE, Piscataway, 2016), pp. 1–6

56. K. Häyrinen, K. Saranto, P. Nykänen, Definition, structure, content, use and impacts of electronic health records: A review of the research literature. Int. J. Med. Inform. **77**(5), 291–304 (2008)

57. H.M. Krumholz, Big data and new knowledge in medicine: The thinking, training, and tools needed for a learning health system. Health Aff. **33**(7), 1163–1170 (2014)

58. C. Chakraborty, B. Gupta, S. K. Ghosh, A Review on Telemedicine-Based WBAN Framework for Patient Monitoring, Int. Journal of Telemedicine and e-Health, Mary Ann Libert inc., **19**(8), 619-626 (2013)

59. E.R. Dorsey, E.J. Topol, State of telehealth. N. Engl. J. Med. **375**(2), 154–161 (2016)

60. R.S. Weinstein, E.A. Krupinski, C.R. Doarn, Clinical examination component of telemedicine, telehealth, mhealth, and connected health medical practices. Med. Clin. **102**(3), 533–544 (2018)

61. R.S. Weinstein, A.M. Lopez, B.A. Joseph, K.A. Erps, M. Holcomb, G.P. Barker, E.A. Krupinski, Telemedicine, telehealth, and mobile health applications that work: Opportunities and barriers. Am. J. Med. **127**(3), 183–187 (2014)

62. B.G. Celler, N.H. Lovell, D.K. Chan, The potential impact of home telecare on clinical practice. Med. J. Aust. **171**(10), 518–521 (1999)

63. C. Chakraborty, B. Gupta, S. K. Ghosh, D. Das, C. Chakraborty, Telemedicine Supported Chronic Wound Tissue Prediction Using Different Classification Approach, Journal of Medical Systems, **40**(3), 1–12 (2016)

64. A. Huang, C. Chen, K. Bian, X. Duan, M. Chen, H. Gao, C. Meng, Q. Zheng, Y. Zhang, B. Jiao, L. Xie, WE-CARE: An intelligent mobile telecardiology system to enable mHealth applications. IEEE J. Biomed. Health Inform. **18**(2), 693–702 (2013)
65. C.L. Bentley, O. Otesile, R. Bacigalupo, J. Elliott, H. Noble, M.S. Hawley, E.A. Williams, P. Cudd, Feasibility study of portable technology for weight loss and HbA1c control in type 2 diabetes. BMC Med. Inform. Decis. Mak. **16**(1), 92 (2016)
66. C. Logan, Portable health care history information system. U.S. Patent 7,039,628 (2006)
67. Health Quality Ontario, Portable ultraviolet light surface-disinfecting devices for prevention of hospital-acquired infections: A health technology assessment. Ont Health Technol Assess Ser **18**(1), 1 (2018)
68. H. Takyi, V. Watzlaf, J.T. Matthews, L. Zhou, D. DeAlmeida, Privacy and security in multi-user health kiosks. Int. J. Telerehabilitation **9**(1), 3 (2017)
69. Y. Lyu, C.J. Vincent, Y. Chen, Y. Shi, Y. Tang, W. Wang, W. Liu, S. Zhang, K. Fang, J. Ding, Designing and optimizing a healthcare kiosk for the community. Appl. Ergon. **47**, 157–169 (2015)
70. G. Boriani, A. Da Costa, A. Quesada, R.P. Ricci, S. Favale, G. Boscolo, N. Clementy, V. Amori, S. Mangoni, L. Stefano, H. Burri, MORE-CARE Study Investigators, Effects of remote monitoring on clinical outcomes and use of healthcare resources in heart failure patients with biventricular defibrillators: Results of the MORE-CARE multicentre randomized controlled trial. Eur. J. Heart Fail. **19**(3), 416–425 (2017)
71. M. Landolina, G.B. Perego, M. Lunati, A. Curnis, G. Guenzati, A. Vicentini, G. Parati, G. Borghi, P. Zanaboni, S. Valsecchi, M. Marzegalli, Remote monitoring reduces healthcare use and improves quality of care in heart failure patients with implantable defibrillators: The evolution of management strategies of heart failure patients with implantable defibrillators (EVOLVO) study. Circulation **125**(24), 2985–2992 (2012)
72. M. Singh, S. Singh, S. Prasad, I.S. Gambhir, Nanotechnology in medicine and antibacterial effect of silver nanoparticles. Dig. J. Nanomater. Biostruct. **3**(3), 115–122 (2008)
73. J.R. Adler Jr., S.D. Chang, M.J. Murphy, J. Doty, P. Geis, S.L. Hancock, The Cyberknife: A frameless robotic system for radiosurgery. Stereotact. Funct. Neurosurg. **69**(1–4), 124–128 (1997)
74. H. Dodziuk, Applications of 3D printing in healthcare. Pol. J. Cardiothorac. Surg. **13**(3), 283 (2016)
75. J. Chen, J. Zheng, Q. Gao, J. Zhang, J. Zhang, O.M. Omisore, L. Wang, H. Li, Polydimethylsiloxane (PDMS)-based flexible resistive strain sensors for wearable applications. Appl. Sci. **8**(3), 345 (2018)
76. T. Shany, S.J. Redmond, M.R. Narayanan, N.H. Lovell, Sensors-based wearable systems for monitoring of human movement and falls. IEEE Sensors J. **12**(3), 658–670 (2011)
77. S. Roy, M. David-Pur, Y. Hanein, Carbon nanotube-based ion selective sensors for wearable applications. ACS Appl. Mater. Interfaces **9**(40), 35169–35177 (2017)
78. X. Shen, J. Misic, N. Kato, P. Langenörfer, X. Lin, Emerging technologies and applications of wireless communication in healthcare. J. Commun. Networks **13**(2), 81–85 (2011)
79. S. Jiang, Y. Cao, S. Iyengar, P. Kuryloski, R. Jafari, Y. Xue, R. Bajcsy, S.B. Wicker, CareNet: An integrated wireless sensor networking environment for remote healthcare, in *BODYNETS*, (2008), p. 9
80. C. Gavriel, K.H. Parker, A.A. Faisal, Smartphone as an ultra-low-cost medical tricorder for real-time cardiological measurements via ballistocardiography, in *2015 IEEE 12th International Conference on Wearable and Implantable Body Sensor Networks (BSN)*, (IEEE, Piscataway, 2015), pp. 1–6
81. M.B. Kamel, G. Berry, Real-time locating systems (RTLS) in healthcare: A condensed primer. Int. J. Health Geogr. **11**, 25–25 (2012)
82. Q.V. Pham, D.C. Nguyen, W.J. Hwang, P.N. Pathirana, Artificial intelligence (AI) and big data for coronavirus (COVID-19) pandemic: A survey on the state-of-the-arts. IEEE Access **8**, 130820–130839 (2020)

83. G. Lalit, C. Emeka, N. Nasser, C. Chinmay, G. Garg, Anonymity preserving IoT-based COVID-19 and other infectious disease contact tracing model. IEEE Access **8**, 159402–159414 (2020). https://doi.org/10.1109/ACCESS.2020.3020513, ISSN: 2169-3536

84. D. Nguyen, M. Ding, P.N. Pathirana, A. Seneviratne, Blockchain and AI-based solutions to combat coronavirus (COVID-19)-like epidemics: A survey (2020)

85. B.R. Beck, B. Shin, Y. Choi, S. Park, K. Kang, Predicting commercially available antiviral drugs that may act on the novel coronavirus (SARS-CoV-2) through a drug-target interaction deep learning model. Comput. Struct. Biotechnol. J. **18**, 784–790 (2020)

86. S. Chae, S. Kwon, D. Lee, Predicting infectious disease using deep learning and big data. Int. J. Environ. Res. Public Health **15**(8), 1596 (2018)

87. M. Eisenstein, Infection forecasts powered by big data. Nature **555**(7695), S2–S4 (2018)

88. S. Gilgore "GWU hospital tackles COVID-19 with new testing site, telemedicine and outreach on D.C.'s east side" (2020), https://www.bizjournals.com/washington/news/2020/04/08/gwu-hospital-tac%kles-covid-19-withnew-testing.html. Accessed 28 July 2020

89. M. Shah, A. Tosto, "Industry voices-how rush University medical center's virtual investments became central to its COVID19 response" (2020), https://www.fiercehealthcare.com/hospitals-health-systems/industryvoic%es-how-rush-university-system-for-health-s-virtual. Accessed 28 July 2020

90. B. Marr, Coronavirus: How artificial intelligence, data science and technology is used to fight the pandemic (2020). Retrieved 30th March.

91. S. Tuli, S. Tuli, R. Tuli, S.S. Gill, Predicting the growth and trend of COVID-19 pandemic using machine learning and cloud computing. Internet Things, 100222 (2020)

92. The Hindu BusinessLine, Covid-19: AP launches telemedicine facility [Online] (2020). Available: https://www.thehindubusinessline.com/news/national/covid-19-ap-launches%-telemedicine-facility/article31332943.ece

93. A. Chakraborty, "Assam: Telemedicine, video monitoring for COVID19 home-quarantined people in Dhemaji" (2020), https://nenow.in/health/assam-telemedicine-videomonitoring-for-covid-1%9-home-quarantined-people-in-dhemaji.html Accessed 28 July 2020

94. V. Chauhan, S. Galwankar, B. Arquilla, M. Garg, S. Di Somma, A. El-Menyar, V. Krishnan, J. Gerber, R. Holland, S.P. Stawicki, Novel coronavirus (COVID-19): Leveraging telemedicine to optimize care while minimizing exposures and viral transmission. J. Emerg. Trauma Shock **13**(1), 20 (2020)

95. J. Comstock, "Israel's Sheba hospital turns to telehealth to treat incoming coronavirus-exposed patients" (2020), https://www.mobihealthnews.com/news/europe/israels-sheba-hospital-turns%-telehealth-treat-incoming-coronavirus-exposed-patients. Accessed 28 July 2020

96. H.J. Ho, Z.X. Zhang, Z. Huang, A.H. Aung, W.Y. Lim, A. Chow, Use of a real-time locating system for contact tracing of health care workers during the COVID-19 pandemic at an infectious disease center in Singapore: Validation study. J. Med. Internet Res. **22**(5), e19437 (2020)

97. D.R. Seshadri, E.V. Davies, E.R. Harlow, J.J. Hsu, S.C. Knighton, T.A. Walker, J.E. Voos, C.K. Drummond, Wearable sensors for COVID-19: A call to action to harness our digital infrastructure for remote patient monitoring and virtual assessments. Front. Digital Health **2**, 8–16 (2020)

98. J.P. Navis, L. Leelarathna, W. Mubita, A. Urwin, M.K. Rutter, J. Schofield, H. Thabit, Impact of COVID-19 lockdown on flash and real-time glucose sensor users with type 1 diabetes in England. Acta Diabetol., 1–7 (2020)

99. A. Haghanifar, M.M. Majdabadi, S. Ko, Covid-cxnet: Detecting covid-19 in frontal chest x-ray images using deep learning. arXiv preprint arXiv:2006.13807 (2020)

100. S. Lalmuanawma, J. Hussain, L. Chhakchhuak, *Applications of Machine Learning and Artificial Intelligence for Covid-19 (SARS-CoV-2) Pandemic: A Review* (Chaos, Solitons & Fractals, 2020), pp. 110059–110065

101. C.J.C. Nicomedes, R.M.A. Avila, An analysis on the panic during COVID-19 pandemic through an online form. J. Affect. Disord. **276**, 14–22 (2020)
102. H. Wang, T. Li, S. Gauthier, E. Yu, Y. Tang, P. Barbarino, X. Yu, Coronavirus epidemic and geriatric mental healthcare in China: How a coordinated response by professional organizations helped older adults during an unprecedented crisis. Int. Psychogeriatr. **32**(10), 1117–1120 (2020)
103. V. Balachandar, I. Mahalaxmi, S.M. Devi, J. Kaavya, N.S. Kumar, G. Laldinmawii, N. Arul, S.J.K. Reddy, P. Sivaprakash, S. Kanchana, G. Vivekanandhan, Follow-up studies in COVID-19 recovered patients-is it mandatory? Sci. Total Environ. **729**, 139021–139030 (2020)
104. Y.M. Zhao, Y.M. Shang, W.B. Song, Q.Q. Li, H. Xie, Q.F. Xu, J.L. Jia, L.M. Li, H.L. Mao, X.M. Zhou, H. Luo, Follow-up study of the pulmonary function and related physiological characteristics of COVID-19 survivors three months after recovery. EClinicalMedicine **25**, 100463–100472 (2020)
105. K. Govindan, H. Mina, B. Alavi, A decision support system for demand management in healthcare supply chains considering the epidemic outbreaks: A case study of coronavirus disease 2019 (COVID-19). Transp. Res. Part E Logist. Transp. Rev. **138**, 101967–101981 (2020)
106. A. Amini, W. Chen, G. Fortino, Y. Li, Y. Pan, M.D. Wang, Editorial special issue on "AI-driven informatics, sensing, imaging and big data analytics for fighting the COVID-19 pandemic". IEEE J. Biomed. Health Inform. **24**(10), 2731–2732 (2020)
107. V. Majhi, S. Paul, R. Jain, Bioinformatics for healthcare applications, in *2019 Amity International Conference on Artificial Intelligence (AICAI)*, (IEEE, Piscataway, 2019), pp. 204–207
108. Executive office of the president and council of economic advisers, economic report of the president (2008)
109. T.W. Shi, W.S. Kah, M.S. Mohamad, K. Moorthy, S. Deris, M.F. Sjaugi, S. Omatu, J.M. Corchado, S. Kasim, A review of gene selection tools in classifying cancer microarray data. Curr. Bioinforma. **12**(3), 202–212 (2017)
110. A. Serra, P. Galdi, R. Tagliaferri, Machine learning for bioinformatics and neuroimaging. WIREs Data Min. Knowl. Discovery **8**(5), e1248 (2018)
111. Z. Yin, H. Lan, G. Tan, M. Lu, A.V. Vasilakos, W. Liu, Computing platforms for big biological data analytics: Perspectives and challenges. Comput. Struct. Biotechnol. J. **15**, 403–411 (2017)
112. M.C. Schatz, CloudBurst: Highly sensitive read mapping with MapReduce. Bioinformatics **25**(11), 1363–1369 (2009)
113. L. Chen, D. Zheng, B. Liu, J. Yang, Q. Jin, VFDB 2016: Hierarchical and refined dataset for big data analysis—10 years on. Nucleic Acids Res. **44**(D1), D694–D697 (2016)
114. M. Leclercq, B. Vittrant, M.L. Martin-Magniette, M.P. Scott Boyer, O. Perin, A. Bergeron, Y. Fradet, A. Droit, Large-scale automatic feature selection for biomarker discovery in high-dimensional OMICs data. Front. Genet. **10**, 452 (2019)
115. R. Nambiar, R. Bhardwaj, A. Sethi, R. Vargheese, A look at challenges and opportunities of big data analytics in healthcare, in *2013 IEEE International Conference on Big Data*, (IEEE, Piscataway, 2013), pp. 17–22
116. H. Fröhlich, R. Balling, N. Beerenwinkel, O. Kohlbacher, S. Kumar, T. Lengauer, M.H. Maathuis, Y. Moreau, S.A. Murphy, T.M. Przytycka, M. Rebhan, From hype to reality: Data science enabling personalized medicine. BMC Med. **16**(1), 150 (2018)
117. R. Bhardwaj, A. Sethi, R. Nambiar, Big data in genomics: An overview, in *2014 IEEE International Conference on Big Data (Big Data)*, (IEEE, Piscataway, 2014), pp. 45–49
118. F.C. Navarro, H. Mohsen, C. Yan, S. Li, M. Gu, W. Meyerson, M. Gerstein, Genomics and data science: An application within an umbrella. Genome Biol. **20**(1), 109 (2019)
119. S.S. Ortega, L.C.L. Cara, M.K. Salvador, In silico pharmacology for a multidisciplinary drug discovery process. Drug Metab. Pers. Ther. **27**(4), 199–207 (2012)

120. V.S. Rao, K. Srinivas, Modern drug discovery process: An in silico approach. J. Bioinf. Sequence Anal. **3**(5), 89–94 (2011)
121. M.K. Hassan, A.I. El Desouky, S.M. Elghamrawy, A.M. Sarhan, Big data challenges and opportunities in healthcare informatics and smart hospitals, in *Security in Smart Cities: Models, Applications, and Challenges*, (Springer, Cham, 2019), pp. 3–26
122. H. Liyanage, S.T. Liaw, J. Jonnagaddala, R. Schreiber, C. Kuziemsky, A.L. Terry, S. de Lusignan, Artificial intelligence in primary health care: Perceptions, issues, and challenges: Primary health care informatics working group contribution to the yearbook of medical informatics 2019. Yearb. Med. Inform. **28**(1), 41 (2019)
123. M.A. Winker, A. Flanagin, B. Chi-Lum, J. White, K. Andrews, R.L. Kennett, C.D. DeAngelis, R.A. Musacchio, Guidelines for medical and health information sites on the internet: Principles governing AMA web sites. JAMA **283**(12), 1600–1606 (2000)
124. R.A. Meinhardt, New "E-sign" law enables electronic prescriptions. Drug Benefit Trends **12**(9), 23–49 (2000)
125. A.C. Norris, J.M. Brittain, Education, training and the development of healthcare informatics. Health Informatics J. **6**(4), 189–195 (2000)
126. K.W. Goodman, *Ethics, Computing, and Medicine: Informatics and the Transformation of Health Care* (Cambridge University Press, Cambridge, 1998)
127. S. Johnson, Pathways of care: What and how? J. Managed Care **1**(1), 15–17 (1997)
128. H. Heathfield, D. Pitty, R. Hanka, Evaluating information technology in health care: Barriers and challenges. BMJ **316**(7149), 1959 (1998)
129. R. Haux, Medical informatics: Past, present, future. Int. J. Med. Inform. **79**(9), 599–610 (2010)

Chapter 7
Smart Sensor Technologies for Healthcare Systems

Avinash Sharma, Rasmeet Kaur, and Dharminder Yadav

7.1 Introduction

The internet of things can be characterized as a combination of two terms: one is the internet, which is characterized as systems that can interface billions of clients using a standard web convention. A few gadgets such as a cell phone, as well as personal systems and business associations, are associated with the internet. The subsequent term is things; this fundamentally means these gadgets or items that transform into smart objects. Also, it is likewise a piece of all objects of this real world. The digital media communicate with the physical world utilizing plenty of sensors and actuators. The IoT can likewise be characterized as "An open and complete framework of insightful articles that can auto-sort out, exchange information and assets, acknowledging, and portraying in contempt of situations and changes in the surrounding". The evolution of the IoT has been fundamentally deduced by the stipulation of prodigious partnerships that residue to worth exceptionally from the presentiment and stability supervised through the ability to follow all objects through the item chains in which they are engrafted. The ability to code and trace entities has allowed companies to be increasingly productive, accelerate forms, decrease errors, prevent burglary, and fuse complex and versatile authoritative arrangement through the IoT. The IoT is a mechanical upset that speaks to the future of registering and interchanges and its advancement depends on zestfully dedicated development in several significant areas through isolated sensors to nanotechnology.

A. Sharma (✉)
Deemed to be University, Mullana, Ambala, Haryana, India
e-mail: asharma@mmumullana.org

R. Kaur · D. Yadav
Department of Computer Science, and Application, Glocal University, Saharanpur, UP, India

© The Author(s), under exclusive license to Springer Nature Switzerland AG 2021
C. Chakraborty et al. (eds.), *Efficient Data Handling for Massive Internet of Medical Things*, Internet of Things,
https://doi.org/10.1007/978-3-030-66633-0_7

They are going to label each item for identifying, robotizing, checking, and controlling.

As per the existing scenario, more than 100 countries are involved in the business of information, headlines, and evaluations by way of the internet, whereas talking about things that possibly any object or individual which can be identifiable by this current actuality. These entities assimilate other electronic items we experience and utilize gradually and items that move automatically, for example, equipment and items; however "things" that we do not typically regard as electronic, for instance, food, clothes, components, and concentrated things; milestones, and masterpieces, and all sorts of occupations, ways of life, and modernity. Hence, it is clearly stated that things, possibly living beings, such as humans, animals, trees, as well as non-living things such as objects, machines, etc.; hence, things are actual entities in this world. There is no special definition available for the IoT; certainly, there is a group of scholars, analysts, white-collar workers, innovators, and technicians who have defined the term. What all the definitions share to all intents and purposes is the possibility that the basic description of the web concerned the facts assembled by solitary. On the other hand, the following variant considers facts and figures made by entities. The appropriate description for the IoT would be:

The IoT space prompts the universe of innovation, and correspondence to another period where items can convey, process, and change the data according to the prerequisites. The label Internet of Things was coined in 1999 by Kevin Auston, the Executive Director of Auto-ID Labs and the idea of the IoT became popular in 2003. At the point when the idea of such correspondence appeared, organizations concentrated on it, attempted to appraise its noteworthiness, and started to acknowledge its roles and the connected future viewpoints. During that time these organizations started putting resources into the IoT space. The present web is changing step by step as its application getting increments and new improvements in its engineering. The Web of Things is another transformation of the internet. The Web of Things can be said to be the development of internet providers. It gives a platform for correspondence between objects where articles can arrange and oversee themselves. It makes objects themselves conspicuous. The Web of Things permits everybody to be connected whenever and wherever.

The IoT had a pre-eminent effect on society; there are further connected objects, in contrast to individuals, across the earth. The frameworks and facts that stream from them will bolster a remarkable scope of applications, and chances of financial gain. As with any revolution, there is an equal chance for critical difficulties as well; given the IoT, threats to protection and security challenges have the best potential to cause damage.

In straightforward words, when the articles or things associated with one another utilize standard conventions and standard foundation they can communicate with one another, and every one of these items/things can be observed and constrained by anyplace, and whenever utilizing the web then it tends to be called the IoT. In the design of the framework all things such as objects in keen homes, vehicles, electronic devices, and so on, are associated with the web, the IoT is developing, continuing the recent and most advertised plan in the technology world. During the past decade, the IoT has stood out by expecting the perception of a worldwide infrastructure of grouped tangible entities, certifying anytime, anywhere network for anything, and not just for anyone. The IoT can also be recognized as a planetary system that allows the correlation of human-to-human, human-to-objects, and objects-to-objects, which is anything on earth, by giving a special personality to each item. The IoT depicts a scene where anything can be connected and conveyed in an insightful manner. The greater part of us considers "being connected" as far as electronic devices go, for instance, servers, computers, tablets, and cell phones. The IoT is regarded among the most remarkable territories of upcoming transformation and is increasing huge contemplation across an immense range of livelihoods. The official appraisal of the IoT can be completely acknowledged when interconnected objects can interact with each other, and, united with the seller, oversaw stock framework, client support structure, livelihood insight implementations, and business investigation. Gartner (2014) conjectured that by 2020, the IoT would arrive at 26 billion units, a rise from 0.9 billion in 2009, and will affect the facts accessible to gracefully chain accomplices, and how the flexible chain works. From the production line, transport from stockpiling to merchandise, and reserving, the IoT is evolving forms of livelihood by giving increasingly precise and ongoing clarity into the progression of materials and items. Companies will put assets into the IoT to overhaul industrial facility work processes, revamp the following of materials, and streamline transport costs. For instance, John Deere, as well as UPS, are using IoT-sanctioned armada following advancements to reduce expenses and upgrade productivity flexibly.

As there is a continuation in the revolution, we are moving in the direction of a general public, where everything and everybody will be interconnected. The IoT is examined as the upcoming estimation of the internet that confers machine-to-machine (M2M) learning. The essential idea of the IoT is to allow the independent and assured interrelation and trade of figures between real-world gadgets and applications. Most cell phones include various sensors and actuators that can detect, perform calculations, make insightful choices, and transmit helpful data across the internet. Using a framework of these sorts of gadgets with multiple sensors can bring forth enormous astonishing applications, and administrations that can bring huge individual, proficient, and financial advantages. The IoT comprises items, sensor gadgets, correspondence foundation, a computational, and a handling unit that might be put on the cloud, a dynamic and activity-conjuring framework. These tangible objects are equipped with radio-frequency identification (RFID) labels or other standardized tags that can be detected by the smart sensor devices. The sensors convey object-explicit data over the internet to the computational and handling unit. A blend of multiple sensors can be utilized for the planning of excellent administrations. The after-effect of handling is then passed to the dynamic and activity summoning framework that decides a mechanized activity to be conjured up. The IoT is a hot exploration theme that is attracting increased notoriety for the researcher's community in industry just as in government. Numerous European and American associations, as well as multinational organizations are engaged with the plan and improvement of IoT to obtain distinctive kinds of supportive and incredible robotized administrations.

The internet has extensively developed over the last few years, connecting billions of things all around. These things have distinct sizes, proportions, preparations, and computational force, and reinforce a distinctive variety of applications. Hence, the traditional internet converges into a technology-friendly future internet, called the IoT. The IoT interfaces genuine entities, and inserts the insight into the system to adroitly process the article-explicit data, and make co-operative self-sufficient choices. With the headway in transformation, these devices are preparing energy, and storage capabilities that are fundamentally inflated whereas their size has diminished.

The sensors impart object-explicit data over the internet to the computational and preparing unit. An amalgamation of numerous sensors can be utilized for the structure of savvy administrations. The consequence of preparing is then passed to the dynamic and activity-summoning framework that decides a mechanized activity to be conjured up. The IoT is made up of the four components mentioned below:

- *Sensors/devices:* These devices accumulate facts from their surroundings, and negotiate them into worthwhile data.
- *Connectivity:* the data collected by sensors pass to a cloud infrastructure. To transport data a medium is required. Various mediums such as Bluetooth, WiFi, Cellular Network, and satellite networks are used to connect the sensors with the Cloud.
- *Data processing:* the software performs data processing when they move to the Cloud.
- *User interface:* later, the information is made available to the end-user. A user has an interface on which they can check their IoT system.

7.1.1   Introduction to Smart Sensor Technology

In a sensor, an electrical yield is created when joined with some associating equipment and this is named a smart sensor. Intelligent sensors are likewise called smart sensors, which is a progressively valuable phrase in the current age (see Figs. 7.1 and 7.2).

Sensors obtain data from preferred environments and convert their physical attributes into measurable electrical signals. These attributes include temperature, mass, speed, pressure, or presence of warm bodies such as humans. The microprocessor processes these electrical signals to produce outputs that correspond to a set of actions. The system finally communicates the output with receivers in the intended devices for favorable functioning. To achieve the understanding of smart sensors in a different class first, think about the meaning of a standard sensor. As a rule, a sensor is a gadget that is intended to gain data from an object, and change it into an electrical signal. A conventional amalgamated sensor can be separated into three sections:

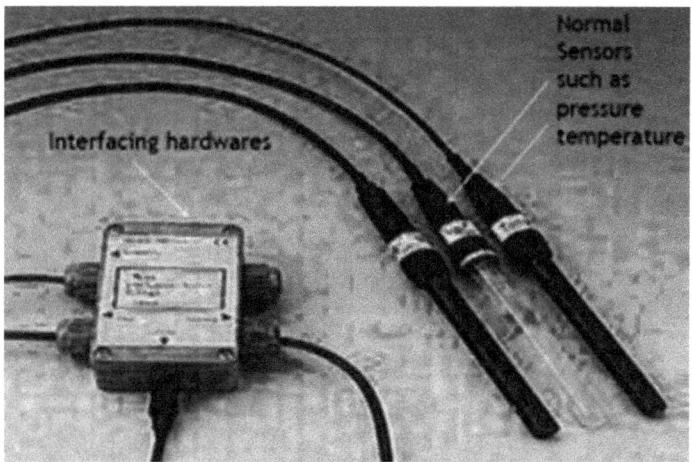

Fig. 7.1 Example of a smart sensor

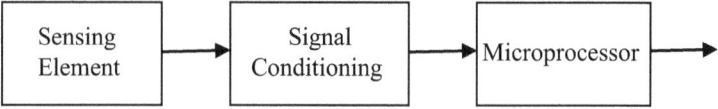

Fig. 7.2 Smart Sensor

(I)   the detecting component
(II) signal molding and handling
(III) a sensor interface

The fundamental contrast between an intelligent sensor and a standard incorporated sensor is its knowledge abilities, for example, the onboard chip (As shown in Fig. 7.2). The microchip is regularly utilized for computerized handling, analog to digital, or frequency to code conversions, which can encourage self-identification, or self-adjustment (dynamic) capacities. It can likewise choose when to dump/store information, and control when, and to what extent it will be completely alert to limit power utilization [1].

7.1.2   The Architecture of a Smart Sensor

In Fig. 7.3, A1, A2…An are amplifiers, and S/H1, S/H2…S/Hn is the sample that holds circuits corresponding to various sensing elements consequently. The analog signal is periodically sampled to receive a digital conversion of an analog signal, and that persistent value is held and is transformed into digital words. Every sort of

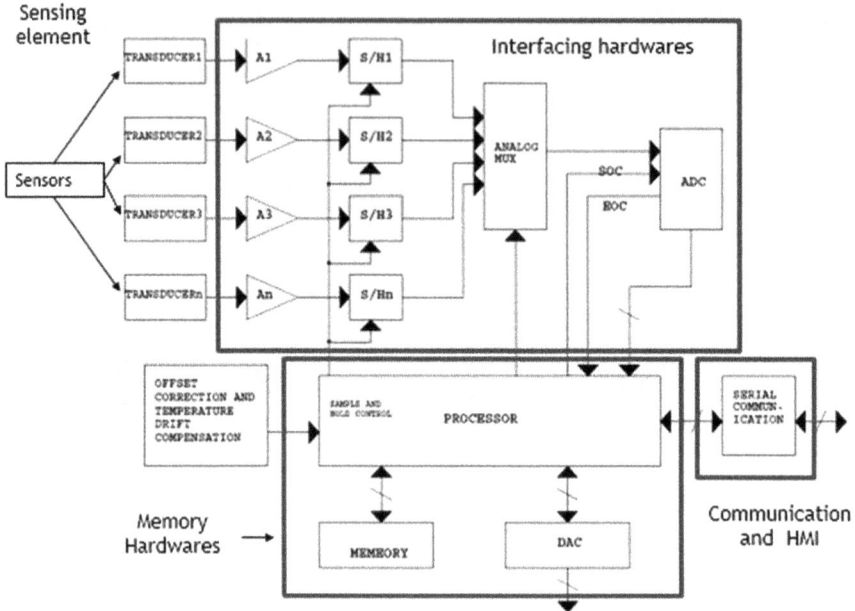

Fig. 7.3 Architecture of smart sensors. *HMI* human–machine interface

analog-to-digital converter (ADC) should hold or proceed by a circuit. This circuit holds onto the voltage at the input to the ADC converter persistently throughout the whole transformation time. Transformation times fluctuate extensively, from nanoseconds to microseconds to hundreds of microseconds.

The ADC initiates transformation as it gets the start of the conversion signal from the processor and it sends the end of the transformation signal to the processor when the transformation is over. Outputs of every sample and hold circuits are multiplexed collectively to use a single ADC, which will diminish the cost of the chip. Offset compensation and correction consist of one ADC for computing a reference voltage and another for the zero. Obligating two channels of the multiplexer and using a single ADC for the entire system can circumvent the addition of an ADC for this. It helps in offset correction and zero compensation of gain because of temperature drifts of the acquisition chain. Moreover, a smart sensor also incorporates internal memory so that we can store the required data and program [3].

Intelligent sensors with an installed chip and remote correspondence can essentially change how common frameworks are checked, controlled, and maintained. A 2002 National Research Council report noted that the utilization of network frameworks of embedded computers, and sensors all through society could overshadow every single past achievement in data transformation. In any case, no system yet exists that can permit the dispersed figuring worldview offered by smart sensors to be utilized for auxiliary wellbeing checking, and control frameworks; current algorithms accept that all information is gathered and handled centrally. Such a methodology does not scale to frameworks with thickly instrumented varieties of sensors that will be required for the up and coming age of auxiliary wellbeing checking and control frameworks.

Over time there has been a decrease in the size of smart sensors. The utilization of microelectromechanical systems (MEMS) has made the fantasy about having omnipresent detecting, and specifically little "brilliant" detecting, conceivable. MEMS gadgets are made utilizing very large-scale integration technology (VLSI) and can epitomize both mechanical and electrical capacities. MEMS can be utilized in a domain to both detect and incite. Detecting necessitates a physical or substance marvel being changed over to an electrical sign for showing, preparing, transmitting, or potentially recording. Incitation inverts this stream and changes via an electrical sign to a physical or concoction change in nature. The principle advantage to applications of this innovation and its structured worldview is scaling down. MEMS highlights are regularly of micrometric size. MEMS gadgets can be found in a wide range of uses, from accelerometers for airbag arrangement to an electronic molecule detector that aids in atomic, organic, and synthetic assessment. In addition, the cost of the smart sensors is diminishing. Large-scale manufacturing of MEMS and microchips for an assortment of uses has decreased their price to a number of dollars, and with their expanding prevalence, they could be reduced to portions of a dollar. Improvement in the advancements for other significant parts, for example, memory, radio transmitters, and batteries, will permit increasingly competent and durable gadgets, lessening the cost of maintenance.

At long last, all smart sensors are now wireless, with the information passing dependent on radiofrequency (RF) correspondence. There are a few conventions for dispatching the information. One of the most mainstream is Bluetooth, a short-go radio innovation planned for rearranging correspondence between internet gadgets, just as between gadgets and the web. Most of these sensors are imagined to utilize the low transmitted capacity to avoid substantial expenses related to registering the sensor with the Federal Communications Commission. In this way, a smart sensor as characterized in this way has four significant highlights:

(I) On-board focal handling unit (CPU)
(II) Small size
(III) Wireless
(IV) The guarantee of being inexpensive

To put things in their appropriate specialized perspective, the following section sums up past exploration of remote sensors and describes the brilliant sensors produced for a structural building framework.

7.1.3   Technologies Entailed in Making the Sensor "Intelligent"

Micro-Electromechanical System

This framework encourages the sensor to work distinctly by permitting it to keep up with the huge volume of information in only a blink of an eye. The run of the mill information that is gathered by the sensor is prepared with the chip, which, by a propelled computation, eradicates or stores the information. The significant favorable circumstances of MEMS technology amalgamates limiting vitality and materials, revised repeatability, enhanced precision just as dilated affectability, and decision-making.

Very Large-Scale Integration Technology

Very large-scale integration technology is the procedure of scaling down PC chips and embedding an enormous number of transistor gates on an isolated silicon semiconductor wafer. VLSI has numerous points of interest, for instance, reducing the dimension of circuits, and the cost of the objects, accelerating the circuit, with low power utilization while inhabiting a moderately confined space.

7.2   Sensors, Healthcare, and the IoT

The IoT is a popular expression today, and this modern innovation has teamed up with the clinical and medical service applications to convey case results [5]. As per expectation, the IoT-based healthcare showcase is soaring and will reach about $136.8 billion by 2021. There is no uncertainty that the IoT will smooth out the whole procedure. This driving innovation has improved the assignment of human services experts. They have the chance to obtain all data and information on their smart gadgets the same number of the propelled clinical types of gear is associated with the patient's body to screen the indispensable boundaries. Aside from that, the IoT, consolidating with medical services, has started a much better approach to dealing with the assets. The clinical staff can check their huge load of products effectively, and maintain it. Additionally, it has become simpler to adhere to the directions from the specialist, and this assists with reducing the expense of treatment for the patients. The IoT applications, regardless of whether for city foundations, manufacturing plants, or wearable gadgets, utilize huge varieties of sensors gathering information for transmission over the internet to a central, cloud-based asset management system [14]. Investigation programming running on the cloud computers reduces the immense volumes of created information to significant data for clients, and orders to actuators pull out in the field.

Sensors are the vital elements in IoT achievement; however, these are not traditional sorts that essentially convert physical factors into electrical signs. They are expected to advance into something increasingly complex to play out an actual and financially suitable job inside the IoT condition.

Sensors need to add a few attributes to go forward as IoT segments:

- Low cost, so that a huge number of sensors can be deployed
- Physically small, to "vanish" subtly into any condition
- Wireless, because wired linking regularly is unrealistic
- Self-recognizable proof and self-approval
- Very low energy, so that it is easy for it to get by for long periods without changing the battery
- Self-indicative and self-mending
- Self-aligning, or acknowledges adjustment orders through remote connection
- Data pre-preparation, to decrease the load on passages, programmable logic controllers, and cloud assets

Data from numerous sensors can be consolidated, and related to construed decisions about dormant issues, for example, temperature sensor and vibration sensor information can be used to recognize the beginning of mechanical malfunction.

Smart sensors are worked as IoT segments that transform the current reality variable that they're estimating into a computerized information stream for transfiguring to an entryway. The application calculations are performed by an implicit chip unit (MPU). These can run sifting, pay, and some other procedure-specific sign molding roles. The MPU's knowledge, which can be used for various capabilities, can also lessen the burden on the IoT's increasingly central assets such as adjustment facts can be sent to the MPU so that the sensor is naturally set up for any creative modifications. The MPU can discover any creative boundaries that begin to float previous adequate standards, and produce alerts as needed; administrators would then be able to take precautions before a disaster occurs.

The sensor could work in a "report by special case" mode if suitable, where it certainly conveys information. This diminishes both the burden on the core computing asset and the smart sensor's energy requirements, normally a basic primacy, as the sensor must rely upon a battery or energy source without equated power.

With the condition that the smart sensor remembers two components for the investigation, the sensor's self-diagnostics can be indigenous. Any emerging drift in one of the sensor's component yields can be identified right away. Also, if a sensor collapses completely, for instance, because of a short circuit, the procedure can proceed with the second estimating component. On the other hand, a test can contain two sensors that cooperate for improved observation of criticism.

The word "smart" has been used many times for different sensors. The significance has also been holding forth by the in-tune appearance of as good as ever plans in the revolution. The rapid advancements in the technology, imparting conservativeness, and propelled microchip coordination, make the use of sensors practically limitless.

The smart sensor has clever capacities, for example, remote interaction, and being an on-board microcontroller. It can be used to convert analog data to the digital form, digital processing, decision making, and two-way transmission. Smart sensors have varying points of interest, in contrast with ordinary sensors, for example, compact size, negligible energy utilization, and high throughput.

A smart sensor can be viewed as an analog or digital transducer with added detecting and processing capacities. It comprises a transduction segment, signal molding gadgets, and a processor that underpins some knowledge in a solitary bundle. This coordinated gadget sensor, which has the hardware and the transduction component together on one Si wafer, is known as framework on-chip.

7.2.1 Focal Points of IoT in Healthcare

Lower Cost many devices can follow wellbeing condition. Subsequently, clinical representatives can screen patients' wellbeing continuously. Thus, individuals do not need to visit specialists consistently. It involves fewer costs. Besides, individuals can be at home, on the off chance that they are not truly sick, and specialists will see each change using telemedicine.

Improved Treatment Outcome Advancessuch as cloud computing, and the availability of clinical gadgets permit specialists to see constant information about patients using the IoT-based wellbeing observation framework. Therefore, specialists can investigate symptoms more quickly and give the appropriate therapy. This prompts better considered outcomes.

Better Illness Control there is relentless control because of current advancements. Along these lines, accepting new information consistently, specialists can recognize disease early and start treatment quicker.

Fewer Mistakes mechanized procedures such as division of information, obtaining information, and information-driven choices can decrease analysis errors. The IoT and important gadgets can help with flexible control, and taking medicine; thus, there will be fewer costs. Also, the control procedure will turn out to be increasingly precise.

Remote Patient Care there are a few countries in which telemedicine is utilized effectively, for example, Singapore. Specialists can see their patients at any time using a wellbeing observation framework that is dependent on the IoT.

Maintenance of Clinical Gadgets clinical gadgets are costly, and any hardware requires appropriate maintenance methodology to work properly. The IoT can help with this because this innovation will ascertain every conceivable issue with any gadget.

More Trust Towards Doctors the IoT in medical clinics offers patients a chance to speak with their primary care physicians without any problems. In addition, specialists can help patients at any time. This builds the patients' trust.

7.2.2 Burdens of the IoT in Healthcare

Secrecy of Patients secrecy has consistently been a significant problem. Taking into account that a specialist's work with individual data of their patients, people ought to be sure that these are kept private. Tragically, there is a chance of hacking this information and gaining admittance to the social insurance IoT environment [13].

Accidental Failures one little mistake in the IoT-enabled patient wellbeing checking framework can have a genuine effect. No innovation can forestall disappointment. Thus, it is imperative to think about everything concerning application advancement and equipment manufacture.

Malware the internet is loaded with viruses these days and can taint any working frameworks, for example, IoT applications in the medical services field. Be that as it may, introducing effective antivirus programs and firewalls can offer security.

Lack of Encryption one more security choice is modifying the encryption framework. It is ready to shield the framework from unapproved access. Tragically, only a few frameworks have extraordinary encryption; thus, every individual can gain admittance to it.

7.2.3 Existing Solutions on the Market

Apple Watch App to Fight Depression
The research structure Cambridge Cognition and a pharmaceutical organization chose to make an Apple Watch application that offers specialists a chance to examine the working of psychological elements of patients who experience the ill effects of depression.

This issue is very far-reaching these days; thus, this application can bring plenty of benefits. It can accumulate inactively and dynamically high-recurrence information about the mental state of the individual; specialists receive these data routinely. Consequently, medical professionals make more precise decisions and administer improved therapy.

Intel Health Application Platform
The Intel Health Application Platform (IHAP) is another IoT framework that can consider patients remotely. It is agreeable because there is no need to have a cell

phone or tablet. IHAP includes equipment, a gadget that provides a chance to interface with a client using programming from Intel. All information is stored in the cloud and any approved individual can access these data.

Mobile Health

Mobile health is also known as mHealth, a versatile strategy for observing and dealing with one's wellbeing can be a genuine lifeline for present-day patients, to all intents and purposes everyone who uses cell phones consistently. Adaptable wellbeing is a developing sector that serves intensely basic clinical situations as well as standard therapy cases. Such applications can be utilized as your out, and out medicinal services center where you can get access to significant clinical information, dissect your living behavioral patterns, look after other body-imparted IoT sensors, and consult your doctor with a single tap.

Healthcare frameworks pioneer attempts to benefit from these patterns, making new applications intended to connect with clients in the setting they are generally comfortable with. The HealthWorks Collective recently distributed a few insights into the utilization of versatile human services applications. They expressed:

- There are over 97,000 wellbeing and wellness applications accessible for download to versatile or tablet gadgets.
- 52% of cell phone clients gather wellbeing-related data on their gadgets.
- 15% of 18- to 29-year-olds have wellbeing applications previously installed on their personal digital assistants.
- 8% of cell phone clients between the ages of 30 and 49 have downloaded clinical applications.
- 40% of specialists believe that these portable apparatuses can reduce the quantity of on-site clinical visits.
- More than 25% of American doctors are utilizing, in any event, one mHealth application.
- 93% of specialists state that portable applications can improve the nature of a patient's wellbeing.
- Portable healthcare applications can be utilized in an assortment of approaches to improve wellbeing.

TempTraq is a small wearable gadget that fits easily under the arm. The gadget tracks the temperature of the wearer, sending it through the Cloud to a portable application. Parents can screen their children's temperature while they are sleeping without waking them. TempTraq is accessible at CVS pharmacy, Target, and on the web.

Spok Mobile is an application intended to improve the continuity of care by connecting the center point and talked human services supplier model to a safe dashboard that encourages correspondence between a consideration group. The application is interoperable with electronic health records and emergency clinic planning.

Abilify MyCite was recently approved by the FDA. Abilify MyCite is an aripiprazole tablet with a little ingestible sensor inserted into the pill. At the point when the pill hits the stomach lining of the patient, a little ping goes out to a cell phone application. This mHealth application has been endorsed for the treatment of psychological illness, where the consistency of medications is famously troublesome.

Although these three creative models are intriguing, they are, actually, the tip of the mHealth iceberg. With all forecasts demonstrating boundless increments in client appropriation by patients and specialists, portable applications are sure to venture into the work processes of each training program, regardless of how large or small.

Advanced Authority Partners
Telehealth is unalterably attached to the portable application range of medical services. Telemedicine carries the specialist to the patient's preferred advanced gadget, regardless of whether a cell phone, tablet, or work area. With a cell phone, patients can connect with their doctor of choice with the bit of a catch. This makes telehealth a kind of unique virtual house call that is as cozy and patient-engaged as it is proficient.

In 2017, there were more than 30 million telehealth visits. That number increased by 8 million experiences from the previous year. Patients of any age are becoming increasingly comfortable with a telehealth application on their cell phone. The Harvard Business Review proposed that 97% of patients are happy with their first utilization of the innovation and state that the apparatus improved their relationship with their doctors.

Concerning mHealth applications, telehealth is one of the most well-known. These instruments have overcome any barriers to the connection between doctor and patient, bringing social insurance into homes, schools, and workplaces, improving access for a large number of Americans.

OrthoLive offers an mHealth arrangement that is a protected, reasonable choice for orthopedic practices. Get in touch with us to discuss our imaginative social insurance application and how it could change your supplier's persistent connections.

7.3 Smart Sensor Technology in Healthcare

Sensors have consistently spoken to a basic part in many frameworks that need to ensure trustworthiness and huge accomplishments. The industrial world provides an ideal model. During the most recent years, such instruments have expanded their capacities, on account of the mixture of functionalities that only certain gadgets had before, arriving at a degree of brilliance that has permitted them to grow their range of applications. The utilization of smart sensors in wearables has been seen to be expanding generally. Smart sensors are discovered in application in a few wearable clinical gadgets, and are utilized in blood glucose observation, smart biomedical detecting, etc. Innovative advancements in sensors have made new inroads into clinical wearables. Wearable clinical gadgets with installed brilliant sensors send data about patient wellbeing to medical services experts and custodians, in this way speeding the way toward regulating clinical guides. The appropriation of brilliant sensors for medical services applications is relied upon to flood in the coming years, thus boosting the income development of the worldwide smart sensor showcase.

In numerous ventures, sensors have assumed a crucial role in distinguishing synthetic, natural, physical signs, etc. In healthcare, to convey care legitimately to a patient's sensors gives the mechanical vision of perusing, tallying, arranging and automated direction.

These days, the IoT being a distinct advantage in the human services field as it joins sensors, microcontrollers, doors, and a microchip to investigate, and sends sensor information to the Cloud and afterward onto custodians. Smart sensors transform healthcare. Technology ends up being an advantage for every human. The following highlights of smart or clinical sensors are:

Caution Ahead of Schedule for Clinical Issues according to necessity, various kinds of sensors are available on the market that produce analytics to notify physicians. These sensors could show symptoms of a cardiovascular breakdown, kidney failure, stroke, etc., before the attack happens, For instance, injectable biosensors are effectively used to identify cancer during the beginning phase.

Enable Neural Technologies smart sensors or smart neural gadgets end up being an advantage for patients in looking after problems, for example, rheumatoid joint inflammation or Parkinson disease, or neural detour innovations especially for the paralyzed sufferer.

Intelligent Clinical Gadgets with expanding requests, sensors are utilized to mechanize clever clinical gadgets. To satisfy the constant patient needs different smart gadgets are made that join information investigation and sensor information, and change drug conveyance.

Oversee Ceaseless States of Patients various minuscule's, high-goals sensors permit patients and medical professionals to deal with an ongoing patient interminable condition, such as coronary illness, diabetes, different sclerosis, and so forth. To give ongoing suggestions to patients' different progressed explanatory motors could screen signals from numerous sensor types.

7.3.1 Benefit of Using Smart Sensor Technology in Healthcare

7.3.1.1 Reducing Waiting Times in Emergency Room

Barely anything is as exhausting as going to the emergency room. Aside from the subsequent clinical costs, emergency room visits take a long time to complete. Owing to some ongoing resourcefulness, and the IoT, at any rate, one medical clinic, Mt. Sinai Medical Center in New York City — adequately cut waiting times for half of their emergency room patients who need inpatient care. It is their collaboration with GE Healthcare, and new, IoT-based programming, called AutoBed, that keeps an eye on occupancy among 1200 units and components in 15 unique measurements to survey the requirements of individual patients. It is a profoundly viable framework that features some of the more creative and energizing uses of the IoT.

7.3.1.2 Remote Health Monitoring

Every now and again, the sufferer does not need to go to an emergency room or medical clinic. The clearest and main uses of human services and the IoT is for remote wellbeing checking, some of the time called telehealth. Besides the fact that it reduces expenditure and removes the need for specific appearances, it improves the patient's quality of life by saving them the bother of movement. On the off-chance that a patient has restricted mobility or relies upon open transportation, something as basic as this can improve things significantly.

7.3.1.3 Ensuring the Convenience and Attainability of Critical Hardware

Present-day medical clinics need cutting edge programming and tools to work. Like every single electronic entity, this is also prone to multiple threats such as power failure or system failure. An innovative IoT-based arrangement, called an e-Alert by Phillips, is expected to settle that issue. Instead of trusting that a gadget will fail, Philips' new framework adopts a proactive strategy by essentially observing clinical equipment, and alerting emergency clinic staff when there is any problem.

7.3.1.4 Tracking Staff, Patients, and Inventory

Safety is the most important challenge of any emergency clinic or clinical office. It is quite tough to maintain the greatest security measures without the ability to follow resources, individual members of staff, patients, and tools throughout the building. This is an assignment that is effortlessly accomplished in smaller establishments, so why shouldn't bigger institutions that include different structures and grounds, as well as a huge number of patients and staff do this? Many are going to the IoT and constant area frameworks to encourage following of resources. In addition, it is a cheap technique for observing everyday activities in a medical clinic setting; however, it is an inconspicuous, powerful front line.

7.3.1.5 Enhanced Drug Management

One of the main empowering forward leaps concerning medical services and the IoT comes in the form of new types of physician-recommended medication. It appears to be a work of science fiction; however, pills containing infinitesimally tiny sensors can impart a sign to an external gadget, typically fixed to the body, to guarantee appropriate measurement and usage. Such data could be priceless with regard to ensuring that patients take their medicines, and endorse future medications. In addition, patients additionally approach the data using a helpful cell phone application, to follow their exhibition, and to improve their propensities.

7.3.1.6 Tending to Chronic Disease

Repeated medical obstacles are rarely energizing, yet enormous forward leaps are being made in the nursing of such problems, and much of it is an immediate after-effect of the IoT. There is no single advancement or gadget that is helping to treat the chronic ailments in the twenty-first century; it is the blend of wearable technology, latest investigation, and versatile relativity. Resources such as Fitbit utilize the IoT to screen individual wellbeing, possibly imparting these data to a specialist to prevent having to explain repeated events. An organization called Health Net Connect has recently settled on a popular diabetic administration program to improve clinical treatment and reduce clinical expenses for patients, and they have just delivered some energizing outcomes.

Starting a Constant Change in Healthcare IT
The IoT can affect each individual across the globe at one time or another in their lifetimes. It has gone from the advanced processing plant floor to technology-based emergency clinics and clinical offices in an extremely short period of time, and it is an improvement that is now changing the business of social insurance IT. Let us examine a few different means of actualizing the IoT in human services.

- *Remote patient monitoring*: there are a considerable number of individuals who experience the ill effects of ceaseless illness and need to go to specialists normally [19]. Remote patient monitoring is a framework that is beneficial for individuals who have issues with the heart or for diabetics. Along these lines, the sufferer simply needs to carry the remote patient monitoring gadget that naturally alerts the specialist if the sufferer collapses.
- *Wearables*: these days, there are plenty of gadgets that patients can wear each day, for example, wellness groups, circulatory strain, pulse-measuring sleeves, etc. These mainstream devices screen the client's day-to-day activities, as well as gathering information about steps taken, calories consumed, etc. These gadgets change the patients' carries on with, particularly older individuals, as they permit continuous following of their wellbeing condition. Wearables can send warnings to the relatives about modifications in the normal exercises or some other variation in the condition of the client [11].

- *Better drug management*: to create and oversee medications, individuals spend a great deal of money. IoT gadgets can provide the chance of adhering to all security principles of the pharmaceutical market. Perhaps the best model is the smart vaccine fridge. It can keep vaccines from being ruined, and their conditions can be screened every minute of every day.
- *Hospital management*: all things considered, there are plenty of approaches to utilizing the IoT to upgrade ordinary emergency clinic activities and decrease costs. Lost and stolen hardware cost a lot of money. The issue can be settled by incorporating sensors to gear, for example, RFID or Bluetooth. This arrangement permits following the areas at any time.

7.3.2   Sorts of Sensors in the Clinical Field

In the clinical field, these days quiet take effectively part in the gathering and evaluating their reports. In the digitized scenario, different remote correspondence norms have permitted the sensor to create standard forms, for example, requiring dynamic patient cooperation to aloof shape, for example, with no need for persistent support [6].

The present enormous number of passive sensors are utilized that continually screen the patient's vital signs exclusively, and store that information or offer it remotely to medical services experts. By consolidating investigation and sensor information, analysis is made that depicts the early wellbeing state of the patient. Contingent upon the prerequisite, different kinds of sensors are being used. Wearables such as computerized watches, Fitbit, etc., are installed or worn on garments.

In healthcare, various sorts of detecting gadgets are utilized relying on the attributes, ease of use, and productivity. The benefits of smart sensors are that they are simple to design, have high trustability, are adaptable versatile systems, have the fewest inter-dependent links, and high performance. The preferences and detriments of brilliant sensors are clarified below.

The Disadvantages of Smart Sensors
For wired intelligent sensors, the multifaceted nature of the IoT is soaring; consequentially, the cost is likewise sky-high. They require making use of already defined built-in functions all along with the plan of the smart sensor. It demands actuators and sensors. Sensor alignment must be overseen by an external processor.

The sensors are used to analyze, screen, or serve illnesses in the clinical areas defined as clinical sensors. Clinical gadgets are arranged into various classes dependent on their hazard profile, namely, class I (lowest expected hazard), class IV (highest likely hazard), etc. The highlights and elements of clinical sensors of various sorts are described below.

Features of Clinical Sensors
- They should comply with the IEC 60601-1 wellbeing standard.
- They should agree to legal determinations including other requirements and principles for quality control, hazard the executives, convenience, and utilitarian wellbeing to guarantee that given gadget works accurately with reaction to given data sources.
- It has to convey exact estimation with great accuracy.
- The estimation should be exceptionally steady, and have a quick reaction time.
- They should provide digital results, for example, I2C to associate with microcontrollers/microchips.

With the ever-developing and maturing population, patient self-observation frameworks are becoming increasingly well known. Their notoriety comes from being both reliable and repeatable, notwithstanding being cost-effective. Sensor-studded observation instruments in this classification are likewise adaptable, as they can be utilized in clinics as well as at home. Choosing a sensor can be basic if the application and the boundaries that should be checked are unmistakably perceived. Implantable sensors are the most complex, followed by sensors used in catheters and body cavities, sensors that are on the outside but that communicate with body fluids, as well as sensors for external applications.

7.3.2.1 Implantable Sensors

Implantable sensors should be small, light, and capable of working with very little power consumption. They must not, above all, rot.

Being from class III clinical gadgets, such sensors naturally require FDA endorsement. It is normally expected for it to take 2–4 years for the advancement and execution of these sensors before proceeding to production. In general, these sensors are costly and need a professional to precisely implant them. The significant difficulty with such sensors is the energy requirement. Those that can work without power are ideal, but this type of sensor is fewer in number and also uncommon.

7.3.2.2 Piezoelectric Polymer Sensors

These are appropriate for vibration recognition owing to some features such as small size, being solid, sturdy, and requiring no power. These can be utilized in pacemakers to screen the activities of the patient. This sensor looks like a little cantilever beam with weight connected toward one side that flops with body development. The sensor produces a signal whenever the patient moves. When utilizing a pacemaker, for instance, the pacemaker at that point receives this sign and makes the heart beat at the ideal pace. Such sensors can discriminate between different exercises, for example, running and other physical exercises.

7.3.2.3 Sensors in Catheters and Body Cavities

The prerequisites for sensors that can be embedded through an entry point – commonly at the tip of a catheter – are less basic than implantable sensors. Contingent upon the surgery, such sensors must work for a couple of moments up to several hours and can be powered by using outside sources. A pair of coordinated thermistors at the tip of a catheter can be guided to various areas of the heart to gauge the flow of blood. To measure bloodstream concentrations, they can be warmed through the curl or flushed with cold liquid. As the bloodstream heats the fluid that arrives at the second sensor, the primary sensor is cooled more than the second when flushed with cold fluid. Because the temperature and volume of the fluid are regulated by a known distance between these two temperature sensors, the blood flow can be calculated by comparing the opposition estimations of the two sensors. No external force is needed for these thermistors.

7.3.2.4 Catheter Ablation Sensors

Catheter ablation sensors are embedded temporarily via an incision. The catheter tip holds a space for RF energy and a power load cell sensor. RF energy, similar to that utilized with implantable sensors to convey information, is frequently utilized in the removal cycle to wear out dead tissue. The power applied by the catheter tip to the objective tissue must not exceed the greatest qualities to avoid any chance of penetrating the objective tissue. TE's detecting innovation holds the guarantee of giving a triaxial power detecting framework ready to gauge tissue contact powers in every one of the three measurements at the same time.

7.3.2.5 Silicon MEMS-Based Disposable Pressure Sensors

Intrauterine pressure (IUP) sensors are used to measure constriction pressure and frequency during labor. The technique is more reliable than ordinary belts and is used in everyday situations. Extra features, such as amnion liquid mixture and extraction, can be added to these sensors, which are implanted in the amniotic sac after passing via the uterus. Once the child is ready to be delivered the sensor is removed.

7.3.2.6 Body Cavity Sensors

Body cavity sensors incorporate oral and rectal tests that gauge internal heat levels. These temperature sensors are intended to be very small and tough and are secured with a delicate covering material to ensure that the inner layer of the organs of the patient are not further harmed because of contact.

7.3.2.7 Micro-Thermocouple Sensors

The two metals emit a low specific voltage that can be calculated and analyzed using a thermocouple thermometer. Various individually insulated metals are used, and an overcoat is used to retain the bifilar configuration. Micro-thermocouples from TE are made entirely of biocompatible materials, making them ideal for use in clinical applications.

These sensors are utilized whenever exact temperature measurements are needed. The thermocouple comprises two different metals, combined on one side. A low voltage is delivered by the two metals that can be estimated and interpreted by a thermocouple thermometer. The disparate metals are independently protected, and a jacket is available to maintain a close bifilar setup.

7.3.2.8 External Sensors Exposed to Fluids

There seem to be just a few dispensable sensors that are placed outside of the body but that interact with bodily fluids. The dispensed pulse sensor (DPS) is an example of this). Such sensors are used in surgeries and intensive care units (ICUs) to continuously monitor the patient's circulatory strain. When undergoing medical procedures or in the ICU, this is the most reliable way of determining the pulse. The patient's information profile is then documented by plugging the disposable pulse sensor into a display. In order to avoid contamination, these sensors must be replaced every 24 h. The sensor used in the inflation of angioplasty inflatables is a particular form of sensor that makes contact with bodily fluids. There are elements of various kinds of clinical sensors for various applications as described below.

- Temperature tests: are used for internal heat level estimation. These aid in giving better prescriptions and treatment; they are termed thermometers.
- Force sensors: are used in dialysis machines.
- Airflow sensors: are used in sedation conveyance frameworks, laparoscopy, heart siphons, etc.
- Pressure sensors: are mainly used in infusion pumps, and sleep apnea machines. Most of these sensors are coordinated with implanted frameworks and are utilized for clinical determination, pulse observation, imbuement siphons, etc.
- Implantable pacemaker: a continuously inserted sensor framework that conveys a synchronized cadenced electronic improvement to the heart muscle to maintain a viable cardiovascular-pace.
- Oximeter: quantifies the division of oxygen-saturated hemoglobin relative to the complete hemoglobin level in the blood.
- Glucometer: estimates the assumed level of glucose fixation.
- Magnetometer: this determines the heading of a client by inspecting the adjustments in the earth's magnetic field around the client.
- Electrocardiogram (ECG) sensor: quantifies the electrical activity of the heart.
- Heart rate sensor: tallies how many times the heart contracts every minute.

- Electroencephalogram sensor: quantifies the electrical movement of thebrain.
- Electromyogram sensor: records electrical movement delivered by the skeletal muscles.
- Respiration rate sensor: tallies how frequently the chest rises in a minute.

7.4 Conclusion

Nowadays, it is hard to cherish the place of the IoT in human services. Smart objects, wearables, and the general degree of availability and developments in present-day clinical hardware have changed the business. M-Health being a standard, normal concept has decreased the number of physical visits to medical clinics. This is just a rough image of the accomplishments of Internet of Medical Things. It is evaluated that before the end of 2020, the base number of IoT gadgets introduced into medical services will be over 161 million units. Sensors and wearables authorize constant physiological checking with reduced manual mediation, and at a low cost. Sensors and wearables can be incorporated into various articles such as articles of clothing, eyewear, accessories, and different entities, for instance, wristwatches, earpieces, and cell phones. Many wearable items utilize numerous advanced sensors that are regularly included in sensor structures involving other stick-on sensors, as well as surrounded sensors.

In this chapter, we explore smart sensor technology and its utilization in healthcare. Section 7.1 is an introduction to the IoT and smart sensors, architecture, and the working of smart sensors, as well as the technologies that make a sensor intelligent. In Sect. 7.2 we describe the role of the IoT and sensors in healthcare. Section 7.3 explains the usage of smart sensor technology in healthcare. This section also elaborates on the benefits of smart sensor technology for healthcare and the various kinds of clinical sensors used in healthcare.

References

1. B.F. Spencer, E. Manuel, Ruiz-Sandoval, R. Kurata, Smart sensing technology: Opportunities and challenges. Struct. Control. Health Monit. **11**, 349–368 (2004) Copyright # 2004 John Wiley & Sons, Ltd
2. L. Catarinucci, D. Donno, L. Mainetti, L. Palano, L. Patrono, M.L. Stefanizzi, L. Tarricone, An IoT-Aware Architecture for smart healthcare systems. IEEE Internet Things J. https://doi.org/10.1109/JIOT.2015.2417684 Copyright (c) 2015 IEEE
3. Griggs K. N., O. Ossipova, P. Kohlios C., N. Baccarini A., A. Howson E., T. Hayajneh, Healthcare blockchain system using smart contracts for secure automated remote patient monitoring. J. Med. Syst **42**, 130 (2018) © Springer Science+Business Media, LLC, part of Springer Nature 2018
4. G. Manogaran, R. Varatharajan, D. Lopez, P. Kumar, R. Sundarasekar, C. Thota, A new architecture of Internet of Things and big data ecosystem for secured smart healthcare monitoring

and alerting system. Futur. Gener. Comput. Syst.. https://doi.org/10.1016/j.future.2017.10.045 0167-739X/© Elsevier B.V (2017)

5. P. Sundaravadivel, E. Kougianos, S.P. Mohanty, M.K. Ganapathiraju, Everything you wanted to know about smart healthcare. IEEE Consum Electron. Mag (2018). https://doi.org/10.1109/MCE.2017.2755378

6. P. Gupta, D. Agrawal, J. Chhabra, P.K. Dhir, IoT based Smart HealthCare Kit. International conference on computational techniques in information and communication technologies (ICCTICT) (2016)

7. H. Maheshwari, D. Yadav, U. Chandra, D.S. Rai, Forecasting epidemic spread of COVID-19 in India using Arima model and effectiveness of lockdown. Adv. Math. Sci. J **9**(6), 3417–3430 (2020)

8. G.W. Hunter, J.R. Stetter, P J. Hesketh, C.-C. Liu, Smart sensor systems,. ecsdl.org/site/terms_use. © ECS 2018

9. M.G. Golzar, Asan Pardazan Co., H.R. Tajozzakerin, A new intelligent remote control system for home automation and reduce energy consumption. Mathematical/analytical modelling. and computer simulation (AMS), IEEE (2010)

10. S. Baker, W. Xiang, I. Atkinson, Internet of Things for smart healthcare: Technologies, challenges, and opportunities. IEEE Access (2017). https://doi.org/10.1109/ACCESS.2017.2775180

11. S.H. Chang, R.D. Chiang, S.J. Wu, W.T. Chang, A context-aware, interactive M-health system for diabetics. IT Prof **18**(3), 14–22 (2016)

12. C.F. Pasluosta, H. Gassner, J. Winkler, J. Klucken, B.M. Eskofier, An emerging era in the management of Parkinson's disease: Wearable technologies and the Internet of Things. IEEE J. Biomed. Health Inform. **19**(6), 1873–1881 (2015)

13. Y. Yin, Y. Zeng, X. Chen, Y. Fan, The Internet of Things in healthcare: An overview. J. Ind. Inf. Integr. **1**, 3–13 (2016)

14. S.M.R. Islam, D. Kwak, H. Kabir, M. Hossain, K.-S. Kwak, The Internet of Things for health care: A comprehensive survey. IEEE Access **3**, 678–708 (2015)

15. D.V. Dimitrov, Medical Internet of Things and big data in healthcare. Healthc. Inform. Res **22**(3), 156–163, 7 (2016)

16. R. Kaur, B.L. Raina, A. Sharma, Internet of Things: Architecture, applications, and security concerns. J. Comput. Theor. Nanosci. **17**, 2469–2475 (2020)

17. U. Chandra, G. Shukla, H. Maheshwari, R. Kaur, Internet of Things (IoT) in agriculture. Inform. Stud. **7**(2), 32–36 (2020)

18. D. Yadav, H. Maheshwari, U. Chandra, Outbreak prediction of COVID-19 in most susceptible countries. Glob. J. Environ. Sci. Manage **6**(4) (2020)

19. C. Chakraborty, B. Gupta, S.K. Ghosh, Mobile metadata assisted community database of chronic wound. Int. J. Wound Med **6**, 34–42 (2014). https://doi.org/10.1016/j.wndm.2014.09.002

Chapter 8
Cloud and IoMT-Based Big Data Analytics System During COVID-19 Pandemic

Joseph Bamidele Awotunde, Roseline Oluwaseun Ogundokun, and Sanjay Misra

8.1 Introduction

The occurrence of coronavirus (COVID-19) is greater than that of respiratory infections syndrome (SARS) that took place in 2003. As of 12 August 2020, the reported cases are more than 73,435 deaths and more than 2000 deaths worldwide, and both COVID-19 and SARS are distributed across regions, infecting living beings [1, 2]. By contrast, in 2003, SARS claimed 774 lives, but in the shortest time, COVID-19 claimed more than that. But the significant difference among them is that since 17 years of SARS, other new power tools have emerged, which could be used as an instrument in fighting this virus and keeping it within reasonable limits. Internet of Things (IoT), wearable body sensor (WBS), and Machine Learning (ML) are examples of such tools. Recently, these methods have caused a paradigm shift in the healthcare sector, and the applicability of these methods in the COVID-19 outbreak might yield profit especially in predicting, monitoring, and diagnosing and treatment of patients during the outbreak. Their application in COVID-19 pandemic can expedite the diagnoses and monitoring of COVID-19 and can minimize the burden of these processes.

J. B. Awotunde
Department of Computer Science, University of Ilorin, Ilorin, Nigeria
e-mail: awotunde.jb@unilorin.edu.ng

R. O. Ogundokun
Department of Computer Science, Landmark University, Omu-Aran, Nigeria
e mail: ogundokun.roseline@lmu.cdu.ng

S. Misra (✉)
Center of ICT/ICE Research, CUCRID, Covenant University, Ota, Nigeria
e-mail: sanjay.misra@covenantuniversity.edu.ng

The outbreak of Coronavirus (COVID-19) infection at Wuhan, China, in December 2019 is spreading widely across the world. Globally, as stated to the WHO as of 1 September 2020, there were 25,328,298 identified COVID-19 cases, with 850,926 global deaths at 10:50 am CEST in 213 countries/regions [3]. Since it is a new pandemic, real drug strategies were not anticipated to be ready for any time soon; meanwhile, community-based control methods such as stay home policy and lock-outs were effectively applied by pretentious nations to squash the pandemic curve affecting an estimated 3 billion people worldwide [4, 5].

COVID-19 is exceptionally infectious and can spread complications before and after the onset. Monitoring and lockdown have to encompass anyone with symptoms and properly isolate persons who have been infected from those who are not, to allow adequate containment. Patients carrying the virus could either be symptomless (e.g., fever, sore throat, and sneezing) or have severe clinical signs (e.g., pneumonia, respiratory failure, and eventually death) [6, 7]. The transmittable SARS-CoV-2 condition is called "coronavirus disease" (COVID-19) [1, 5]. Gratitude to the recent developments in analytical practices including information and communication technologies (ICTs), machine learning (ML), and big data will aid manage the immense, unparalleled volume of data generated from patient monitoring, real-time tracking of disease outbreaks, now-casting/predicting patterns, daily situation briefings, and public updates [8].

Health professionals are in desperate need of technology for decision-making to tackle this epidemic and allow them to get timely feedback in real time to prevent its transmission. AI works to simulate the human intellect thoughtfully. This may as well play a crucial responsible in interpreting and recommending the creation of a COVID-19 vaccine. This result-driven engineering is employed to scan better, evaluate, forecast, and monitor current clinicians and patients expected to be in future. The relevant technologies relate to the monitoring of verified, recovered, and death cases.

In remote detection, prediction, surveillance, recovery, and therapy, the Internet of Things (IoT)-based system is very useful and paramount part in which telemedicine has recently been broadly applied. With interest in designing smart technologies, such as healthcare tracking systems, medical diagnosis, prediction and treatment systems, and smart healthcare, IoT has recently been implemented in the medical sector. Data are obtained from remote medical devices, such as CT machines and MRI machines, wearable sensors, and then distributed and reconfigured locally in three dimensions during the telemedicine process. The Internet of Medical Stuff (IoMT) provides a forum for sensors and machines to connect inside a smart world and to exchange knowledge across medical channels easily.

This pandemic has activated anxiety on public health surveillance and has generated an extraordinary need for remote patient monitoring. Internet of Medical Things (IoMT) smart healthcare is gaining impact to manage COVID-19 in this era of innovative digital expertise. The popularity of wearable devices provides a new perspective for the precaution of infectious diseases. Wearable devices are one solution that provides a practical option for the omnipresent, reliable, and accessible tracking of patients in chronic, relieve environments. Hence, wearable and implantable body area network structures are handy for the unceasing intensive care of the patient during COVID-19.

By benefiting from the full possibilities provided by Internet technology, the latest adaptation to numerous wireless technology places IoMT-based system as the next innovative technology. There is an immense growth in the volume of data produced by sensors, smartphones, social media, healthcare apps, temperature sensors, and numerous other technological applications and interactive resources that regularly produce vast volumes of organized, unstructured, or semi-structured data. The methods of searching for a database, mining, and reviewing data devoted to optimizing market efficiency are used in big data analytics. Big data analytics is the method by which massive data sets representing several categories of data are analyzed. Voluminous volumes of data have been produced as the miniaturization of IoMT devices has increased over the last decade. However, without analytical capacity, such data are not useful. Numerous solutions for big data, IoMT, and analytics have allowed individuals to gain useful insights into the comprehensive data produced by IoMT devices. Ses ideas are still in their infancy, however, and the domain needs a detailed investigation.

The data science analysis using big data analytics is newly evolving, intending to empower healthcare systems to connect, harness information, and convert it to usable knowledge and preferably personalized clinical decision-making. Utilizing and application of IoT-WBS-based system in the field of infectious diseases have implemented a range of improvements in the modeling of knowledge generation. Big data can be interpreted, stored, and collected in healthcare through the continually emerging field of these models, thereby allowing the understanding, rationalization, and use of data for various reasons. Therefore, this chapter proposes a framework for Cloud-IoMT-based big data analytics to guaranteeing better expansion and research against COVID-19. The hope of using the framework in COVID-19 will have a significant impact on the quality of outbreak diagnosis, prediction, and treatment. It can deliver quality care to patients across socioeconomic and geographic boundaries.

The organization of this chapter is as follows: Section 8.2 discusses the importance of IoMT-based system during COVID-19 pandemic. Section 8.3 presents the applicability and the usefulness of wearable body sensor networks during COVID-19. Section 8.4 presents the CI-WBSN framework for monitoring the elderly patient during the COVID-19 outbreak. Section 8.5 offers a practical case of CI-WBSN for watching older people. Section 8.6 presents result, discussion, and future research direction. Finally, Section 8.7 concludes this chapter and looks at the future direction of using IoMT-based system for battling infectious diseases.

8.2   Application of the Internet of Medical During COVID-19 Pandemic

IoT-based systems have provided various types of sensors and devices such as blood glucose tracking system that can be used in smart healthcare system for monitoring of several health-rated diseases [9, 10]. During this period of COVID-19 outbreak, the used of hybrid sensors with actuators as well as mobile equipment will really provide real-time monitoring and diagnosis of patient effectively and accurately globally [7, 11]. The IoMT-based system is a version of IoT-based systems in the healthcare systems using smart devices to capture data from the patient, and consequently process by the inbuilt Machine Learning algorithms for proper decision-making by medical professionals. Thus, this system can be used for proper decision-making by the government agency and medical experts during infectious disease outbreak [12, 13]. There are over 3.7 million smart devices that are linked together by various wireless technologies that can be used for various purposes in smart healthcare systems [14].

There are various types of commercial cloud that can be used as cloud infrastructure such as Amazon Web Services and Google Cloud Computing among other custom web services for data storage. Furthermore, IoMT services can be used for remote monitoring of patient for short- or long-term illness both in urban or rural areas globally. The system can be used by an elderly patient to diagnose, and monitor their health status using wearable devices without necessarily visiting the clinic or hospital. The health records they have obtained can be submitted to their doctor.

This could be shown that the IoMT system operates with a massive deployment of resources for detecting and controlling. The IoMT is regarded to be the large-scale application of machine type communication (MTC) equipment which performs sensing actuation activities through nominal human intervention. The number of Internet-connected objects is estimated to surpass the number of persons in the society. That is because IoT is focused on the reasonableness of networking specific physical gadgets via the connected networks, for instance, the majority of health gadgets linked to the Internet is growing exponentially everyday [15]. Besides, healthcare services are considered the largest target market for IoMT, with the pulse rate tracking being identified as the most significant benefit [16]. Use essential devices such as glucose levels pulse rate tracking, the IoMT systems used to implement urgent warning systems, and remote medical surveillance systems accessing data into more advanced technologies.

Such specific instruments, as a typical example [17], can track particular devices used by Bpacemakers. It would be advantageous to build such a program mainly for the aged, and those with serious illness. Health records will be sent to the health service via smartphone for screening, assessment, and interpretation. These systems need to ensure current efficiency, to be effective and efficient operate efficiently, to track the condition of the patient automatically, and to respond appropriately safely [18]. Therefore, these programs must gain patient trust in the protection of their patients' personal information. The devices, mobile, smart-home network, public contact networks, and hospitals network were exposed to numerous security concerns most of the time; the critical explanation was the weaknesses derived from wireless technology.

In these difficult COVID-19 period, older patients face many severe and critical problems [19]. The goal of IoMT is to link individuals to healthcare facilities to track and regulate vital signs of the human body using connectivity infrastructure

[20]. Telemedicine is becoming common in remote locations where, due to multiple reasons, accessibility to a professional physician is minimal [21].

Heart rate, electrocardiography, diabetes, and vital physiological signs, for example, can all be tracked remotely without the intervention of clinicians. Sensors and actuators are examples of devices that can accept data from a patient and send it to the cloud through a local gateway. The doctor reviews the data using any smartphone or laptop device that has been given to them, and then informs the patient or medical staff who is caring for them about the study [22]. Figure 8.1 describes the various methods and techniques used by IoMT to support the patient during COVID-19.

IoMT also helps physicians and healthcare practitioners to offer medical services to patients by providing them with solutions in crucial and rural locations [23, 24]. This approach also decreases the overall type of discomfort and increases the productivity of, among others, the doctors, workers, and nurses. It reduces unnecessary hospital admissions and the overall burden on healthcare organizations by linking older patients directly with their physicians and thus enabling health information to be transferred via a protected site.

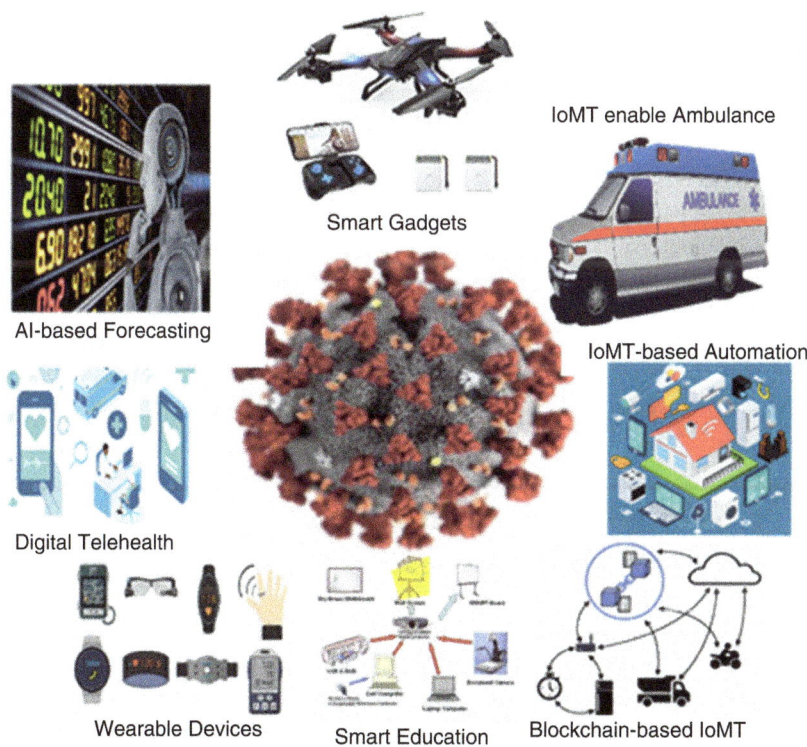

Fig. 8.1 Prospective applications of IoT to combat COVID-19

The IoMT is the expanded health-specific edition of the Internet of Things (IoT) [12]. Introduced to the present situation can be used to build a social forum to help individuals access appropriate treatment at home and to develop a robust repository on disease control for government and healthcare organizations by diagnosis and healthcare devices could be obtained for persons with minor symptoms (preventive disguises, thermometers, medicines, personalized COVID-19 infection diagnosis, and control kits). Patients were able to upload their overall health to the IoMT (clinical data storage) site online regularly and exchange their relevant data to area hospitals, the Center for Disease Control (CDC), and state and local health offices.

Now the global epidemic COVID-19 has become the primary hub of scientific research. The new digital technologies will act as a perfect solution to this worldwide crisis. IoMT can address the problem of detecting, surveillance, mapping contacts, and controlling this viral infection [5, 25].

Healthcare facilities could then provide electronic health evaluations regarding the health status of each individual. If appropriate, the administration (the CDC and state and municipal health offices) could assign resources and designate containment centers (guesthouses or regional quarantine establishments). Using the IoMT system, humans could supervise their disease activity automatically and receive appropriate healthcare needs without transmitting the disease to someone else. It will minimize global medical expenses, alleviate the pressures of the shortage of healthcare equipment, and provide a centralized database allowing the government to effectively track disease transmission, distribute supplies, and enforce emergency strategies.

The currently daunting COVID-19 disease outbreak circumstance is convincing for, among others, medical professionals, nurses, and medical employees. IoMT could be used to offer essential and relevant, positive, and motivating treatment services to its patients. This chapter provides the possibility of providing medical services to older patients via the IoMT program during the COVID-19 disease outbreak. During this epidemic, older patients also face many challenges, such as attending treatment facilities, buying medication, monitoring, and reporting. [26]. Through the IoMT strategy, these conflicts can be addressed more conveniently and easier. This also benefits the older patients who live or are trapped in some distant area where medical services cannot otherwise be given promptly and satisfactorily.

8.3 The Use of Wearable Body Sensors Network for Combating COVID-19 Outbreak

Technological advances of low-cost, insightful, compact, and insubstantial medical sensor networks have been accepted for positioning themselves ideally on the human body using wearable devices and sensors [27]. This helps in creating a system for long-term tracking of various major chronic physical diseases, delivering real-time input to users and medical workers, aiming to revolutionize health monitoring [27]. The WSN technologies are regarded as one of the leading scientific fields for enhancing the quality of care in the computer science and healthcare applications sectors [28].

Utilizing digital innovations such as wearable sensor networks and the IoMT movement are bringing improvement in COVID-19-guided surveillance of older patients [7]. Together with the IoMT-powered mobile devices, the processing strategies are supporting evolving and encouraging real-time healthcare systems in isolated areas. Meanwhile, electronic and wireless communication technologies have thoroughly changed the medical world by pressing smart and tiny sensors that can be used on or inside the human body.

The implementation of these sensing devices with evolving health technology is the fundamental change toward highly sustainable, intelligent, and omnipresent medical cities and homes for the elderly in isolated areas [29]. Body sensor networks (BSNs) is an improvisatory and prospective candidate for stepping up medical innovation and education to improve the healthcare platform further. Wearable sensor networks (WSNs) have revolutionized healthcare sectors with the introduction of various implantable and wearable sensors and devices, and has been used in several fields such as transportation, emergency services, healthcare, among others. The use of AI with wireless sensors with simulation has created an open research in the area of intelligent systems. This has resulted in the creation of interdisciplinary paradigm in ambient intelligence to resolve various healthcare challenges in our daily life [30].

The use of WSNs in smart healthcare system has created a wide range of applications and it can be used to solve various healthcare challenges. Thanks to the integration of single-chip sensors with mass production of WSN, the smart healthcare has really changed the healthcare industry with radio interfaces and computer chips [31]. The system can be used for various purposes like in emergency services, surveillances, agricultural practices, and in healthcare monitoring services. The most useful application of WSN during this pandemic is the tracking and monitoring of COVID-19 patients in real time globally [32–34].

The popular sensor nodes designed and placed in specified locations are limited when compared with the WSNs that can be installed with an ad hoc, thus making them robust, fault-tolerant, and cover larger area [35, 36]. This really helps in monitoring and tracking of patient in real time and remotely without any intervention of any kind. As a result, these strategies will alleviate burden and stress on healthcare personnel, resulting in the reduction of medical errors, reduce healthcare cost, and bring about patient satisfaction with an increase in medical professional effectiveness [37, 38].

The challenges and inaccuracies in the use of IoMT-based system are as a result of lack of reliable and detailed information at the right time because of the inaccurate diagnosis and prescription problems [38, 39]. The risk of death and inaccurate diagnosis would have been reduced if adequate precautions are offered to patients at the right time [40]. Medical experts need adequate information about any patient in order to ensure safety and thereby save lives at the right time and in real-time basis. As a result, patients with life-threatening diseases such as diabetes, heart disease, and high blood pressure need a healthy and low transmission latency. Sensor networks can be strategically placed on the human body to create a cluster WBAN, thus used to capture and collect disease signs and symptoms from patients [41, 42].

Also, as shown in Fig. 8.2, BSNs are made up of a large number of different biomedical sensors, and these sensing nodes wirelessly track and communicate abnormal changes in a patient's vital sign or physiological signals such as temperature, pulse, and blood pressure. Wearable sensors can collect and record data on one's diagnosable disorder and moving responses in real time.

This has really helped and changed the outlook of smart healthcare technology in recent years with introduction of various devices and sensors that can be embedded and implanted in human body. As applied to biomedical technology, this is known as biomedical sensor wireless networks (BWBSNs) [43, 44]. The WBSN allows for the embedding of low-power, remotely controlled smart ubiquitous sensor nodes to track body systems and their surroundings. Every node can detect, track, and send data to the Super Sensor. During the COVID-19 pandemic, selected sensors used in IoT for information collection and monitoring are depicted in Fig. 8.2.

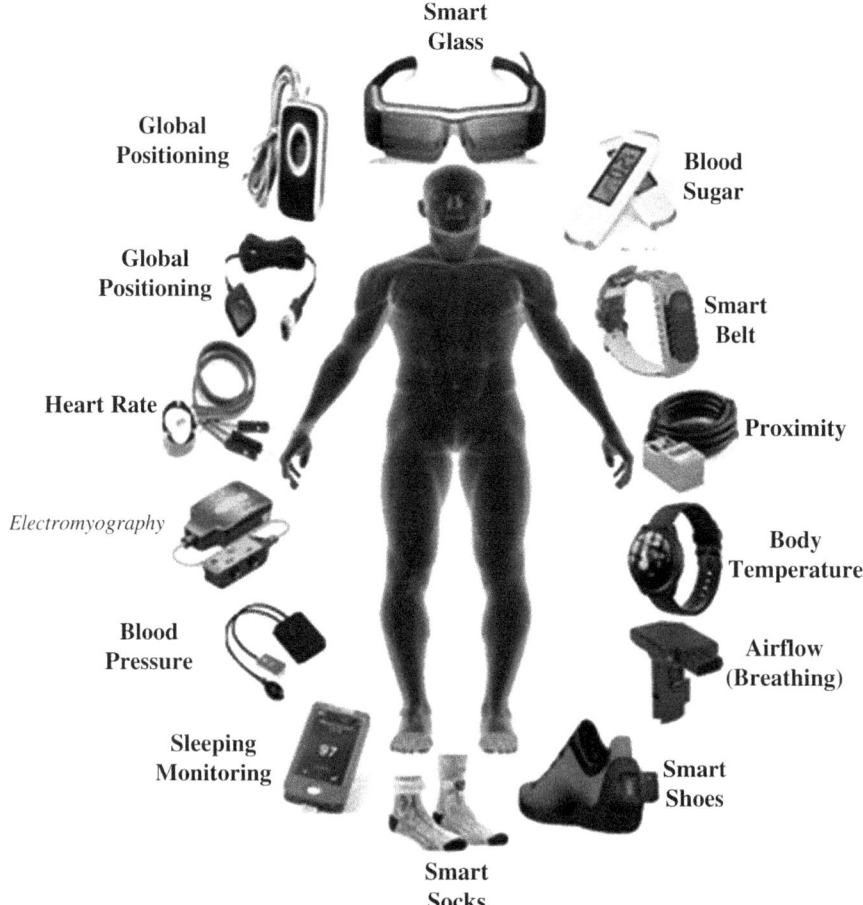

Fig. 8.2 Selected worthwhile sensor devices for collection data on IoT during COVID-19

8.4 Big Data Analytics Opportunities in IoMT-Based Platform

Big data analytics is quickly emerging as a crucial initiative for IoMT. One of the utmost influential characteristics of IoMT is its study of related stuff knowledge [45]. Big data analytics in IoMT requires the giving out of huge capacities of data and the storage of data in different storage technologies. Since big formless data are assembled unswervingly from web-aided possessions, broad data implementation will require lightning-fast analytics with extensive inquiries to enable establishments to access quick intuitions, make speedy verdicts, and relate with persons and other gadgets. Recognizing and motivating gadgets interconnect with the opportunity to exchange knowledge crosswise networks across a cohesive infrastructure and build a shared functioning image to allow creative applications [45].

In the healthcare industry, voluminous volumes of data were generated during the last few years. This rapid growth in data output has, however, produced difficulties in extracting useful knowledge from extensive medical data that can aid pandemic forecast and cure numerous sicknesses [46]. Data analytics can help healthcare professionals examine vast volumes of medical data and learn about a clinical history (with the understanding of private clinicians). Insurance firms might as well employ data mining for policymaking. Healthcare practitioners can also diagnose dangerous illnesses at an early stage and thereby avoid the loss of life [46]. The IoMT-based program created a smart healthcare framework contributing to the diagnosis of epidemics, treatments, and illness.

Smart health tracking apps have evolved exponentially in recent years. These devices generate massive quantities of data. Therefore, adding data processing to data obtained from baby monitoring, electrocardiograms, temperature sensors, or blood glucose level monitoring will assist medical professionals inaccurately determine patient clinical conditions. Data analytics allow healthcare practitioners to detect dangerous diseases at their first steps to aid rescue being. Data analytics increases the medical excellence of treatment, including ensuring patient health. Furthermore, the background of doctors can be checked by looking at the past of patient care, which can boost client loyalty, acquisition, and retention (Fig. 8.3).

Enhanced competency: The criteria for handling and storing data from progressive analytics utilization have hindered their implementation in numerous regions. Such obstacles are thus starting to collapse due to IoT [46]. Big data technology, for instance, Hadoop and cloud-based mining tools, provide substantial cost-cutting benefits relative to conventional mining techniques. Besides, traditional analytical methods involve data in a positive form, which is hard to do while employing IoMT-based data. Using existing big data solutions that develop around less-cost group infrastructure, though, will help boost the analytics capabilities and reduce computing costs.

Independence from data silos: The initiation of IoT, including empowering technology, for instance, cloud computing has enabled data storage towers to be

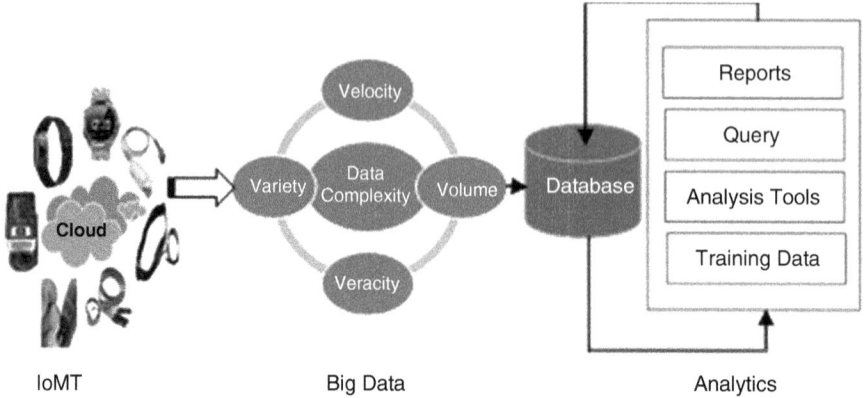

Fig. 8.3 The relationship between IoMT and big data

replaced in various realms [46]. Typically, each data type is deemed only usable for its context, but cross-domain data have arisen as powerful resolutions to various glitches [47]. Different data types, for instance, runtime data, system metadata, business data, retail data, and corporate data, can today be employed because of the numerous supporting technology that supports IoMT, including Big Data, Cloud, Semantic Web, and Data Storage.

Value-added applications: Deep learning [48], machine learning [49], and artificial intelligence are key innovations that offer value-added IoMT and big data applications. Before IoMT and cloud computing emerged, large volumes of data and processing resources remain inaccessible for many applications and hence prohibit them from employing such machinery. Various data analytics solutions [50], business intelligence systems [51], simulation frameworks [52], and analytics apps [53] have recently appeared. They have helped companies and enterprises change their processes, improve their profitability and diagnostics, and incrust them. This amount of specificity had not been available until IoMT appeared.

Decision-making: The explosion of IoMT-based apps, mobile phones, and social networks presents decision-makers with an ability to collect useful knowledge about their customers, forecast potential patterns, and identify fraud. By rendering knowledge accessible and available to enterprises, big data will create tremendous value, thus allowing them to reveal uncertainty and improve their performance. Considerable data engendered through IoMT and numerous analytical gadgets produce a wide range of healthcare system changes. These methods use statistical analysis, grouping, and clustering approaches to deliver diverse approaches to data mining [54–57]. Mining IoMT will also use big data to improve people's decision-making behaviors.

Big data analytics provides well-designed tools to analyze Big Data in IoMT in real time, generating accurate decision-making outcomes. Big data analytics focused on IoMT demonstrates complexity, growing scale, and capabilities of real-time data processing. Big data fusion with IoMT is introducing new possibilities for creating a smart healthcare environment. Big data analytics focused on IoMT has wide-ranging implementations in almost every industry. The key performance areas of healthcare analytics, however, are reduction in hospital backlog admissions, rating healthcare network, the accuracy of forecast and test tests, enhanced decision-making, efficiency, decreased risk assessment, and improved patient segmentation.

8.5 Framework for the Cloud and IoMT-Based Big Data Analytics System

The IoMT paradigm principle has many interpretations focused on the abstraction and description of IoMT domains [45]. It provides a reference model that distinguishes associations between different IoMT verticals [45]. The big data analytics architecture provides a data abstraction approach. The Cloud and IoMT-based architecture offer recognition for various sensors and devices, while the big data analytics provides an interpretation of the data gathered from these connected devices. Many current architectures provide a prototype that builds on the standard. For instance, [58], in a cloud-centric IoT environment, provided an IoT architecture with cloud computing at the core and a model of endwise engagement between different stakeholders.

However, for a closer comparison with the existing Cloud and IoMT-based big data analytics platform is an advantageous IoT–based big data analytics system focusing on IoT in communications [45]. The proposed framework is accomplished by seamless universal sensing, data processing, and information representation with MIoT as the unifying while also concentrating on interactions with MIoT. There has been no research in the recent literature on the proposed program to our knowledge that combines MIoT and big data analytics.

Figure 8.4 demonstrates the Cloud and IoMT-based big data analytics system. The framework comprises of perception layer with numerous radar gadgets and items which can be linked over a radio receiver link. This radio receiver link could be separate from Wi-Fi, ultra-wideband, RFID, ZigBee, and Bluetooth. The IoMT gateway tolerates the cyberspace and numerous networks to connect. The upper level is about big data analytics, where vast volumes of data obtained from radars are processed in the cloud and accessible by big data analytics apps. These frameworks provide API monitoring and a dashboard to aid in managing engine communication.

There are three layers in the proposed framework, namely, the first layer is called the perception, the second is the integrated Cloud and IoMT-based and big data analytics, and the third is the application layer. Figure 8.4 displays a thorough explanation of every layer, and its execution scenario is conversed.

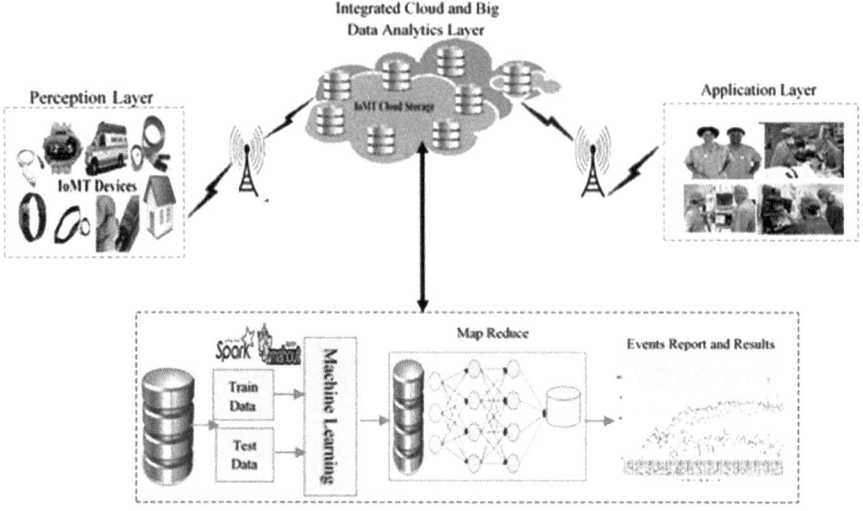

Fig. 8.4 The framework for COVID-19 pandemic using Cloud and IoMT-based and big data analytics

8.5.1 Perception Layer

The first layer was used to collect patient's information data from the built-in wearable sensor such as body temperature and heartbeat rate can be obtained by attaching it to the patient body. These sensors can also be positioned on the right wrist, left ankle, and chest to perceive and investigate the undertaking by innumerable parts of the body, posture sensing, and body position. For instance, the ePatch sensors placed on the chest is used to archive and tracks the ECG with physical efforts of a person. The obtained data from these wearable sensors are transferred and can be linked over a radio receiver link. This radio receiver link could be separate from Wi-Fi, ultra-wideband, RFID, ZigBee, and Bluetooth.

8.5.2 Integrated Cloud and IoMT-Based and Data Analytics Layer

The second layer collects the recorded and physical activities data from different IoMT devices and wearable sensors attached to the body of any person. The collected data will transmit through, and of Wi-Fi, ultra-wideband, RFID, ZigBee, and Bluetooth and the network gateways to the cloud platforms such as Amazon Web Service (AWS) or Cloud Google medium, where it is stored for real time of future analyzed at the big data analytics processor. The daily activities recorded can be processed and analyzed by select and extract features from multiple wearable sensors that are transferred to the HDFS big data processor and Cloudera virtual machine [59, 60]. Hadoop MapReduce can be used to execute the enormous amount of input data since it can process multiple cores in parallel.

Seventy percent to thirty percent of the input data is divided into rations, where 70% of the data is used for preparation purposes, and the remaining 30% of the information is used for research purposes and to estimate the physical movements of the data gathered under observation. Machine learning algorithms such as support vector machine, artificial neural network, deep learning, among others, can be used for the implementation of obtained data from these IoMT devices and wearable sensors using Mahout. The physical activities of the recorded actions over time can be calculated utilizing machine learning techniques. The attained outcomes from the big data processor after examination are communicated wirelessly to the application layer.

8.5.3 The Application Layer

The application layer is divided into data visualization and user interfaces. Data visualization techniques are divided into remote expert interface and monitoring interface, which are used to generate reports and sent to end-user interfaces.

Remote Expert Interface
The inaccessible experts use the interface to manage any allocated patients by generating results and documentations from the examination of the classifiers built on day-to-day events. Decisions are made, centered on patient data, body temperature, heartbeat diagnosis, and classification outcomes. In the case of emergencies such as high body temperature, high blood glucose falls detection and heart attacks, during the monitoring of a person during COVID-19 outbreak, warning notifications are sent to caregivers for more therapy advice to stratify hazards and initiate essential achievement strategies.

Monitoring Interface
The caregivers will be able to monitor the behavior of their close and precious ones in this interface. For instance, the patient is at risk or the heart rate is below 40 if the body temperature is too high >1800 °C, then all actions are null. The patient is at stake; in the event of an emergency, a warning notice via text message will be sent to the caregivers. These three layers are incredibly integrated and interoperable and move data effectively from wearable devices to sensors, gateways, server, storage, retrieval, research, and users.

The security of any IoT-based devices is very significant, thereby for efficient security requirements was considered in designing the system, such as security are access control, trust and privacy data authenticity and data should be regarded as in remote monitoring of the patient to combat COVID-19 pandemic. The DICOM and HIPPA international standard was also considered when the layers communication of clinical data and information and nonclinical [61].

8.6 The Practical Implementation Scenario of the Proposed Framework

The conceptual architecture consists of five main components of advanced technology: Big data processing software, cloud servers, IoMT gateway, network apps, and IoMT systems and sensors. Since IoMT devices and sensors produce an immense volume of data (Big Data), which is after that forwarded to a TCP (Transmission Control Protocol) port where an analytics platform is previously in succession and heeding to this channel. The tool mediator is set up with the actual data streams created by IoMT as the origin and the Apache as the sink so that after listening from the TCP port, the data are stored on Apache tools. The proposed analytics solutions are simplified (i.e., the big data analytics platform uses all of the Apache environment's virtual machines) to store the data. The IoMT-based instruments and monitors are single or multiple practical IoMT instruments such as blood pressure monitors, glucose sensors, temperature sensors, oxygen sensors, luminosity sensors, smoke/hazardous gas detectors, and others. Cloud storage is typically used to store the enormous amount of data produced by IoMT devices and sensors before submitting it to the computing software used by big data analytics.

The network tools are used to connect via any wireless network accessible among other components. The IoMT sensor data collection, optimization, and simulation can be conducted in the big data analytics software and even the building environment is managed based on the effects of the real-time data analysis. As mentioned previously, the data produced from the virtual sensors are ingested into the tools used by Apache. The data are processed in real time from the Apache application and will be saved in the cloud database for future use depending on the findings of the analytics.

For tracking purposes, the smartphone applications are empowered with IoMT-based devices providing real-time information using wireless network gateways, Wi-Fi network, RFID, etc. They have been used in different ways that are extensively useful to intensify the chance of monitoring and detecting infected people [7, 62]. The implementation of smartphone applications with IoMT-based platforms during COVID-19 outbreak might have the benefits of having a complete cloud database with COVID-19 outbreak data and information which government, physicians, and healthcare experts can use to monitor and allow the infected person receiving treatment from home. It is possible for the people to upload their health-related information to the cloud using an IoMT-based cloud database and get health advice from physicians' online without being physically present at the clinic. Treatment is being administered within this platform, and without expanding the contamination, the patient will be cured at home. The system is cost-effective when compared with the existing methods with direct contact and appointment with physicians, and the report can be used by the government to make better decisions and action in future pandemics. They will be able to manage the outbreak effectively [63].

The application of wearable smart glasses in IoMT-based devices has also proved useful in detecting the COVID-19 outbreak among people. This can also be replaced with thermometer guns with its characteristic of less human interaction. The smart glass empowered with thermal camera and with the functionality of optical imaging have been used to monitor people in a crowd [64]. The face recognition technology within the sensor captures the user's body temperature, and tracking of an infected person becomes more comfortable. The data from smart glasses become more reliable with the help of Google Location History, which can be used to track the infected patient contact within a given time. The report of the captured data can be handy from the IoMT-cloud database or sent to the physicians' smartphone for further actions [64]. For example, a Chinese company Rokid designed smart glasses with infrared devices to fight the COVID-19 outbreak and this can monitor up to 200 people [65]. The combination of Vuzix intelligent glasses with Onsight Cube camera thermal is another excellent example of these devices; in detecting high temperature the device is very helpful and provide a real-time report for medical centers.

Different IoMT smart thermometers that can be used to record constant measurement of body temperatures have been developed. They are created in various types such as radiometer, touch and patch; they are accurate devices and cost-effective [66]. The tools are beneficial in early diagnosis, treatment, and monitoring of COVID-19 patients and any suspicious cases that can arise from the outbreak. Also, infrared thermometers can spread the COVID-19 outbreak when used for taking body temperature because of the nearness of the infected person and the physician; thus, smart thermometers will be of help in such cases [67]. Different wearable thermometers can be used during this period such as IFiever, Isense, Ran's Night, Tempdrop, among others, which report the body temperature in real time on smartphones and can be used as sensors on IoMT-based devices. These touchable devices can be a stick or worn on the skin under clothing [66]. For example, In the USA, Kinsa's thermometers have been used to predict the most suspicious areas based on the recorded reports using temperature measurement to detect the highest of being infected with the COVID-19 virus [68–70]. This thereby helps the system to diagnose new COVID-19 patients without stress and increase people's daily lives.

Another acceptable sensor is the smart helmet with a thermal camera when compared with the infrared thermometer gun due to its lower human interactions [71]. The image and location of the user's face are taken when an optical camera detects the high temperature on the smart helmet and report it to the IoMT-cloud database. Experts can differentiate the infected person, and take necessary action immediately. The use of the devices allows physicians and other related officers have access in the crowd to personal information, dark spot visioning temperature, and facial recognition of the user.

The smart helmet has the storage capacity to keep all of the captured data within the helmet, and thus serve as a backup for the IoMT-cloud database [71]. Moreover, the smart helmet integrated Google Location, and the history of the infected person can be used to find the places after discovery [72]. This wearable device has been used successfully in countries such as Italy, the United Arab Emirates (UAE), and China to monitor crowds within two meters and has shown promising results [73, 74]. For instance, a Chinese company produced a smart helmet called KC N901 used for body temperature discovery with an accuracy of 96% and has been used by the countries as mentioned earlier [73–75].

Based on the specifications of popular therapeutic organizations and the physiognomies of entirely all forms of disease community, by offering primary diagnostic services for targeted remote health identification, experts can get the technical diagnostic facility at all periods and appropriately access their well-being information. At the same time, it is possible to monitor the development of all types of growing acute, chronic sickness inmates. Bettering care, antecedent detection, antecedent intervention, and early recovery will advance the value of the life of people with severe illness and decrease the risk of sickness. A delayed diagnosis will significantly reduce federal health benefits, revolving to prevent crucial disease.

Sustainable healthcare based on the IoMT-based sensor. Since IoMT-based system incorporates several physiological sensors into the body of patients, it could collect a range of critical physical markers and has the benefits of being relaxed, appropriate for the aging, progenies, and persons with physical and psychological sickness. Hence, utilizing these innovative wearable devices will create a modern medical infrastructure that incorporates less-power radio receiver networking, cloud computing, big data, and deep learning technologies to comprehend customized healthcare services based on simple physiological knowledge tracking. The core therapeutic services are primarily focused on a handful of huge sanitoria. IoMT-based expertise offers a way to exchange different sections of current medical services and is one of the critical steps for ensuring parity of health. Cloud and IoMT-based systems satisfy the demand of consumers in a timely way, consider the patient's current state of health, enhance contact between physicians and sick persons, and reduce the waiting period for therapeutic care, which will boost client loyalty and at the same time maximize hospital performance. Right telemedicine may achieve a standardized norm. Apart from smart healthcare, this theoretical system could be applied to other uses. Smart agriculture, intelligent vehicles, smart cities, and aircraft may be used to track and regulate sensors and equipment rates to ensure convenience, health, and protection.

8.7   Conclusion

The integration of computer and biomedical technologies in medical systems has supported healthcare events, for instance, real-time disease analysis, remote monitoring of patients, and real-time drug prescriptions, among others. The methods have significantly helped to store both patients' personal information and their symptoms on the cloud, which can help during the COVID-19 pandemic. This aids the quality of services provided by the physicians, thereby improve patients' satisfaction. IoMT and wearable sensors and devices can aid early diagnosis of COVID-19 pandemic and create ease of detection during response to the outbreak. These devices have a remarkable impact on the prompt detection of the COVID-19 outbreak. For instance, cloud and IoMT-wearable sensors have the capacity to show any part of them that is not functioning well when they are used to capture patient health status and thereby create big data. With the results from these devices, users can notice any change in their health condition frequently and book an appointment with a physician before it is generated to real disease or any symptoms appear. The implementation of cloud-IoMT-based wearable sensors will make the fight against COVID-19 pandemic easier and effective. Also, monitoring COVID-19 patients remotely would be more convenient and reduce the number of patients admitted into hospital or isolation centers.

In this chapter, the core principles of Cloud and IoMT-based big data analytics pieces of machinery in the medical sector were explored in depth. This chapter addressed the big data analytics focusing on IoMT, the possibilities, expectations, and threats in the healthcare sectors. We also proposed a Cloud and IoMT-driven integrated data analytics platform for the healthcare industry, focusing on a broad software application structure built on medical IoMT and big data applications. This chapter as well demonstrates the architecture of the extensive healthcare system based on IoMT, the technological problems, and some standard implementations relevant to comprehensive healthcare. Data safety and confidentiality will be looked at for future research with Cloud and IoMT-based big data analytics with healthcare systems. Machine learning approaches to solve the problem related to changing sensory inputs should be integrated. Developing countries, particularly African hospitals, should be thinking about how IoMT can be deployed in hospitals to reduce costs as it is feasible and economical. Government, medical, and research collaboration is relevant to improving IoMT implementation and deployment at our hospital. This chapter concluded that current big data analytics approaches based on IoMT were still in their initial development periods. Therefore, immediate analytics resolution that could offer speedy understanding would be necessary and helpful.

References

1. R.O. Ogundokun, J.B. Awotunde, Machine learning prediction for COVID-19 pandemic in India. medRxiv (2020)
2. M.É. Czeisler, M.E. Howard, R. Robbins, L.K. Barger, E.R. Facer-Childs, S.M. Rajaratnam, C.A. Czeisler, Early public adherence with and support for stay-at-home COVID-19 mitigation strategies despite adverse life impact: A transnational cross-sectional survey study in the United States and Australia. BMC Public Health **21**(1), 1–16 (2021)
3. COVID-19 Dashboard by the Center for Systems Science and Engineering (CSSE) at Johns Hopkins University (JHU) (2020), https://coronavirus.jhu.edu/map.html. Last accessed 1 Sept 2020

4. D. Dunford, B. Dale, N.L. Stylianou, M. Ahmed, I.d.l.T. Arenas, Coronavirus: The world in lockdown in maps and charts. BBC News (2020). Available at https://www.BBC.com/news/world-52103747

5. R.O. Ogundokun, A.F. Lukman, G.B. Kibria, J.B. Awotunde, B.B. Aladeitan, Predictive modelling of COVID-19 confirmed cases in Nigeria. Infect. Dis. Model. **5**, 543–548 (2020)

6. A. Perrella, N. Carannante, M. Berretta, M. Rinaldi, N. Maturo, L. Rinaldi, Editorial–novel coronavirus 2019 (Sars-CoV2): A global emergency that needs new approaches. Eur. Rev. Med. Pharmacol. **24**, 2162–2164 (2020)

7. X.V. Wang, L. Wang, A literature survey of the robotic technologies during the COVID-19 pandemic. J. Manuf. Syst. (2021). https://doi.org/10.1016/j.jmsy.2021.02.005

8. Z.S. Wong, J. Zhou, Q. Zhang, Artificial intelligence for infectious disease big data analytics. Infect. Dis. Health **24**(1), 44–48 (2019)

9. P.K.D. Pramanik, B.K. Upadhyaya, S. Pal, T. Pal, Internet of things, smart sensors, and pervasive systems: Enabling connected and pervasive healthcare, in *Healthcare Data Analytics and Management*, (Academic Press, London, 2019), pp. 1–58

10. E.A. Adeniyi, R.O. Ogundokun, J.B. Awotunde, IoMT-based wearable body sensors network healthcare monitoring system, in *IoT in Healthcare and Ambient Assisted Living*, (Springer, Singapore, 2021), pp. 103–121

11. A. Darwish, G. Ismail Sayed, A. Ella Hassanien, The impact of implantable sensors in biomedical technology on the future of healthcare systems, in *Intelligent Pervasive Computing Systems for Smarter Healthcare*, (Wiley, Hoboken, 2019), pp. 67–89

12. G.J. Joyia, R.M. Liaqat, A. Farooq, S. Rehman, Internet of Medical Things (IOMT): Applications, benefits, and future challenges in the healthcare domain. J. Commun. **12**(4), 240–247 (2017)

13. G. Manogaran, N. Chilamkurti, C.H. Hsu, Emerging trends, issues, and challenges on the Internet of Medical Things and wireless networks. Pers. Ubiquit. Comput. **22**(5–6), 879–882 (2018)

14. Y.A. Qadri, A. Nauman, Y.B. Zikria, A.V. Vasilakos, S.W. Kim, The future of healthcare Internet of Things: A survey of emerging technologies. IEEE Commun. Surv. Tutor. **22**(2), 1121–1167 (2020)

15. N. Alharthi, A. Gutub, Data visualization to explore improving decision-making within Hajj services. Sci. Model. Res. **2**(1), 9–18 (2017)

16. S.A. Parah, J.A. Sheikh, F. Ahad, N.A. Loan, G.M. Bhat, Information hiding in medical images: A robust medical image watermarking system for E-healthcare. Multimed. Tools Appl. **76**(8), 10599–10633 (2017)

17. A. Gutub, N. Al-Juaid, E. Khan, Counting-based secret sharing technique for multimedia applications. Multimed. Tools Appl. **78**(5), 5591–5619 (2019)

18. N. Alassaf, A. Gutub, S.A. Parah, M. Al Ghamdi, Enhancing the speed of SIMON: A light-weight-cryptographic algorithm for IoT applications. Multimed. Tools Appl. **78**(23), 32633–32657 (2019)

19. R.P. Singh, M. Javaid, A. Haleem, R. Vaishya, S. Al, Internet of Medical Things (IoMT) for orthopaedic in COVID-19 pandemic: Roles, challenges, and applications. J. Clin. Orthopaed. Trauma **11**, 713 (2020)

20. J.J. Rodrigues, D.B.D.R. Segundo, H.A. Junqueira, M.H. Sabino, R.M. Prince, J. Al-Muhtadi, V.H.C. De Albuquerque, Enabling technologies for the internet of health things. IEEE Access **6**, 13129–13141 (2018)

21. S.C.I. Chen, R. Hu, R. McAdam, Smart, remote, and targeted health care facilitation through connected health: Qualitative study. J. Med. Internet Res. **22**(4), e14201 (2020)

22. F. Ayeni, S. Misra, N. Omoregbe, Using big data technology to contain current and future occurrence of Ebola viral disease and other epidemic diseases in West Africa, in *International Conference in Swarm Intelligence*, (Springer, Cham, 2015), pp. 107–114

23. M.A. Jan, M. Usman, X. He, A.U. Rehman, SAMS: A seamless and authorized multimedia streaming framework for WMSN-based IoMT. IEEE Internet Things J. **6**(2), 1576–1583 (2018)

24. F. Qureshi, S. Krishnan, Wearable hardware design for the internet of medical things (IoMT). Sensors **18**(11), 3812 (2018)
25. S. Swayamsiddha, C. Mohanty, Application of cognitive Internet of Medical Things for COVID-19 pandemic. Diabetes Metab. Syndr. Clin. Res. Rev **14**, 911 (2020)
26. K. Liu, Y. Chen, R. Lin, K. Han, Clinical features of COVID-19 in elderly patients: A comparison with young and middle-aged patients. J. Infect. **80**, e14 (2020)
27. R. Gravina, P. Alinia, H. Ghasemzadeh, G. Fortino, Multi-sensor fusion in body sensor networks: State-of-the-art and research challenges. Inf. Fusion **35**, 68–80 (2017)
28. G. Fortino, R. Giannantonio, R. Gravina, P. Kuryloski, R. Jafari, Enabling effective programming and flexible management of efficient body sensor network applications. IEEE Trans. Hum. Mach. Syst. **43**(1), 115–133 (2012)
29. A.H. Sodhro, L. Zongwei, S. Pirbhulal, A.K. Sangaiah, S. Lohano, G.H. Sodhro, Power-management strategies for medical information transmission in wireless body sensor networks. IEEE Consum. Electron. Mag. **9**(2), 47–51 (2020)
30. S.I. Popoola, O.A. Popoola, A.I. Oluwaranti, A.A. Atayero, J.A. Badejo, S. Misra, A cloud-based intelligent toll collection system for smart cities, in *International Conference on Next Generation Computing Technologies*, (Springer, Singapore, 2017), pp. 653–663
31. P. Ajayi, N.A. Omoregbe, D. Adeloye, S. Misra, Development of a secured cloud based health information system for antenatal and postnatal clinic in an African Country, in *ICADIWT*, (2016), pp. 197–210
32. I. Elansary, A. Darwish, A.E. Hassanien, The future scope of internet of things for monitoring and prediction of COVID-19 patients, in *Digital Transformation and Emerging Technologies for Fighting COVID-19 Pandemic: Innovative Approaches*, (Springer, Cham, 2021), pp. 235–247
33. F. Li, M. Valero, H. Shahriar, R.A. Khan, S.I. Ahamed, Wi-COVID: A COVID-19 symptom detection and patient monitoring framework using WiFi. Smart Health **19**, 100147 (2021)
34. K.R. Venugopal, M. Kumaraswamy, An introduction to QoS in wireless sensor networks, in *QoS Routing Algorithms for Wireless Sensor Networks*, (Springer, Singapore, 2020), pp. 1–21
35. G. Fortino, S. Galzarano, R. Gravina, W. Li, A framework for collaborative computing and multi-sensor data fusion in body sensor networks. Inf. Fusion **22**, 50–70 (2015)
36. S. Iyengar, F.T. Bonda, R. Gravina, A. Guerrieri, G. Fortino, A. Sangiovanni-Vincentelli, A framework for creating healthcare monitoring applications using wireless body sensor networks, in *Proceedings of the ICST 3rd International Conference on Body Area Networks*, (2008), pp. 1–2
37. R. Kumar Behera, S. Kumar Rath, S. Misra, R. Damaševičius, R. Maskeliūnas, Distributed centrality analysis of social network data using MapReduce. Algorithms **12**(8), 161 (2019)
38. P. Ajayi, N. Omoregbe, S. Misra, D. Adeloye, Evaluation of a cloud based health information system, in *Innovation and Interdisciplinary Solutions for Underserved Areas*, (Springer, Cham, 2017), pp. 165–176
39. U. Varshney, Mobile health: Four emerging themes of research. Decis. Support. Syst. **66**, 20–35 (2014)
40. D.M. Benjamin, Reducing medication errors and increasing patient safety: Case studies in clinical pharmacology. J. Clin. Pharmacol. **43**(7), 768–783 (2003)
41. G. Fortino, A. Guerrieri, F.L. Bellifemine, R. Giannantonio, SPINE2: Developing BSN applications on heterogeneous sensor nodes, in *2009 IEEE International Symposium on Industrial Embedded Systems*, (IEEE, 2009), pp. 128–131
42. S. Vijendra, Efficient clustering for high dimensional data: Subspace based clustering and density-based clustering. Inf. Technol. J. **10**(6), 1092–1105 (2011)
43. S.K. Panigrahy, B.P. Dash, S.B. Korra, A.K. Turuk, S.K. Jena, Comparative study of ECG-based key agreement schemes in wireless body sensor networks, in *Recent Findings in Intelligent Computing Techniques*, (Springer, Singapore, 2019), pp. 151–161
44. F.J. Velez, R. Chávez-Santiago, L.M. Borges, N. Barroca, I. Balasingham, F. Derogarian, Scenarios and applications for wearable technologies and WBSNs with energy harvesting,

in *Wearable Technologies and Wireless Body Sensor Networks for Healthcare*, vol. 11, (The Institution of Engineering and Technology, London, 2019), p. 31

45. M. Marjani, F. Nasaruddin, A. Gani, A. Karim, I.A.T. Hashem, A. Siddiqa, I. Yaqoob, Big IoT data analytics: Architecture, opportunities, and open research challenges. IEEE Access **5**, 5247–5261 (2017)

46. A. Amini, W. Chen, G. Fortino, Y. Li, Y. Pan, M.D. Wang, Editorial special issue on "AI-driven informatics, sensing, imaging and big data analytics for fighting the COVID-19 pandemic". IEEE J. Biomed. Health Inform. **24**(10), 2731–2732 (2020)

47. A. Bröring, S. Schmid, C.K. Schindhelm, A. Khelil, S. Käbisch, D. Kramer, et al., Enabling IoT ecosystems through platform interoperability. IEEE Softw. **34**(1), 54–61 (2017)

48. X.W. Chen, X. Lin, Big data, deep learning: Challenges and perspectives. IEEE Access **2**, 514–525 (2014)

49. J. Qiu, Q. Wu, G. Ding, Y. Xu, S. Feng, A survey of machine learning for big data processing. EURASIP J. Adv. Signal Process. **2016**(1), 67 (2016)

50. V.O. Safonov, Example of a trustworthy cloud computing platform in detail: Microsoft azure, in *Trustworthy Cloud Computing*, (Wiley, Hoboken, 2016)

51. J. Vidal-García, M. Vidal, R.H. Barros, Computational business intelligence, big data, and their role in business decisions in the age of the internet of things, in *Web Services: Concepts, Methodologies, Tools, and Applications*, (IGI Global, Hershey, 2019), pp. 1048–1067

52. Y. Jeong, H. Joo, G. Hong, D. Shin, S. Lee, AVIoT: Web-based interactive authoring and visualization of indoor internet of things. IEEE Trans. Consum. Electron. **61**(3), 295–301 (2015)

53. M. Strohbach, H. Ziekow, V. Gazis, N. Akiva, Towards a big data analytics framework for IoT and smart city applications, in *Modelling and Processing for Next-Generation Big-Data Technologies*, (Springer, Cham, 2015), pp. 257–282

54. F.E. Ayo, R.O. Ogundokun, J.B. Awotunde, M.O. Adebiyi, A.E. Adeniyi, Severe acne skin disease: A fuzzy-based method for diagnosis, in *International Conference on Computational Science and Its Applications*, (Springer, Cham, 2020), pp. 320–334

55. T.O. Oladele, R.O. Ogundokun, J.B. Awotunde, M.O. Adebiyi, J.K. Adeniyi, Diagmal: A malaria coactive neuro-fuzzy expert system, in *Computational Science and Its Applications–ICCSA 2020: 20th International Conference, Cagliari, Italy, July 1–4, 2020, Proceedings, Part VI 20*, (Springer International Publishing, Cham, 2020), pp. 428–441

56. A.F. Jahwar, A.M. Abdulazeez, Meta-heuristic algorithms for K-means clustering: A review. PalArch's J. Archaeol. Egypt/Egyptol. **17**(7), 12002–12020 (2020)

57. F. Stephany, N. Stoehr, P. Darius, L. Neuhäuser, O. Teutloff, F. Braesemann, The CoRisk-index: A data-mining approach to identify industry-specific risk assessments related to COVID-19 in real-time. arXiv preprint arXiv:2003.12432 (2020)

58. J. Gubbi, R. Buyya, S. Marusic, M. Palaniswami, Internet of Things (IoT): A vision, architectural elements, and future directions. Futur. Gener. Comput. Syst. **29**(7), 1645–1660 (2013)

59. S. Kunnakorntammanop, N. Thepwuttisathaphon, S. Thaicharoen, An experience report on building a big data analytics framework using Cloudera CDH and RapidMiner Radoop with a cluster of commodity computers, in *International Conference on Soft Computing in Data Science*, (Springer, Singapore, 2019), pp. 208–222

60. R. Gravina, C. Ma, P. Pace, G. Aloi, W. Russo, W. Li, G. Fortino, Cloud-based activity-aaService cyber–physical framework for human activity monitoring in mobility. Futur. Gener. Comput. Syst. **75**, 158–171 (2017)

61. L. Syed, S. Jabeen, S. Manimala, Telemammography: A novel approach for early detection of breast cancer through wavelet-based image processing and machine learning techniques, in *Advances in Soft Computing and Machine Learning in Image Processing*, (Springer, Cham, 2018), pp. 149–183

62. M.A. El Khaddar, M. Boulmalf, Smartphone: The ultimate IoT and IoE device, in *Smartphones from an Applied Research Perspective*, (InTech, Rijeka, 2017), p. 137

63. T. Yang, M. Gentile, C.F. Shen, C.M. Cheng, Combining point-of-care diagnostics and the internet of medical things (IoMT) to combat the COVID-19 pandemic. Diagnostics (Basel) **10**, 224 (2020)
64. M.N. Mohammed, N.A. Hazairin, H. Syamsudin, S. Al-Zubaidi, A.K. Sairah, S. Mustapha, E. Yusuf, 2019 novel coronavirus disease (Covid-19): Detection and diagnosis system using IoT based smart glasses. Int. J. Adv. Sci. Technol. **29**(7 Special Issue), 954 (2020)
65. J. Bright, R. Liao, Chinese startup Rokid pitches COVID-19 detection glasses in the US (2020)
66. T. Tamura, M. Huang, T. Togawa, Current developments in wearable thermometers. Adv. Biomed. Eng. **7**, 88–99 (2018)
67. M.N. Mohammed, N.A. Hazairin, S. Al-Zubaidi, S. AK, S. Mustapha, E. Yusuf, Toward a novel design for coronavirus detection and diagnosis system using IoT based drone technology. Int. J. Psychosoc. Rehabil. **24**(7), 2287–2295 (2020)
68. S.D. Chamberlain, I. Singh, C.A. Ariza, A.L. Daitch, P.B. Philips, B.D. Dalziel, Real-time detection of COVID-19 epicentres within the United States using a network of smart thermometers. medRxiv (2020)
69. A. Dubov, S. Shoptaw, The value and ethics of using technology to contain the COVID-19 epidemic. Am. J. Bioeth. **20**, 1–5 (2020)
70. D.G. McNeil, Can smart Thermometers track the spread of the coronavirus? The New York Times (2020)
71. M.N. Mohammed, H. Syamsudin, S. Al-Zubaidi, R.R. AKS, E. Yusuf, Novel COVID-19 detection and diagnosis system using IOT based smart helmet. Int. J. Psychosoc. Rehabil. **24**(7), 2296 (2020)
72. N.W. Ruktanonchai, C.W. Ruktanonchai, J.R. Floyd, A.J. Tatem, Using Google location history data to quantify fine-scale human mobility. Int. J. Health Geogr. **17**(1), 28 (2018)
73. S. Ghosh, Police in China, Dubai, and Italy are using these surveillance helmets to scan people for COVID-19 fever as they walk past, and it may be our future regular. Business Insider (2020)
74. G. Fortino, D. Parisi, V. Pirrone, G. Di Fatta, BodyCloud: A SaaS approach for community body sensor networks. Futur. Gener. Comput. Syst. **35**, 62–79 (2014)
75. G. Fortino, G. Di Fatta, M. Pathan, A.V. Vasilakos, Cloud-assisted body area networks: State-of-the-art and future challenges. Wirel. Netw. **20**(7), 1925–1938 (2014)

Chapter 9
Remote Human's Health and Activities Monitoring Using Wearable Sensor-Based System—A Review

M. Parimala Devi, T. Sathya, and G. Boopathi Raja

9.1 Introduction

Enhancements in the development of wearable sensors have improved monitoring healthcare conditions of humans. In recent research studies, with the arising of technology, new and tremendous increase in the usage of modern devices such as smart watches, smartphones, and wearable sensor-based embedded devices can be connected with wired or wireless means of communication, and hence, the attention of the next-generation human health is concerned with a detailed analysis through Internet of Medical Things (IoMT). The various sensors are connected to the parts of a human to receive the biopotential, which is an indication of clinical disorders. The clinical data collected by those sensors are periodically stored as electronic medical records and electronic health records collected from healthcare workers like physicians, nurses, and paramedical workers. The data that are collected are vital for many pharmaceutical companies, researchers, and academicians for clinical data Analysis. The Big Data Analysis is mandatory to deal with an enormous amount of biological datasets collected from associated wearable sensors. Smart Health care has introduced an increased demand for biomedical datasets, which periodically generates signals by sensors planted on the embedded devices. The novel technical challenges are also created alongside with innovation and emerging business prospects [1, 2].

The signals generated by the embedded wearable sensors are in huge volume, and the rate of receiving the signals is dealt with the velocity of signal reaching the storage space. Numerous sensors collect the data from multiple nodes in human body to provide a stream of data in large volume continuously to characterize the clinical data of patients in Smart healthcare technology [3, 4]. The embedded wearable sen-

M. P. Devi (✉) · T. Sathya · G. B. Raja
Department of Electronics and Communication Engineering,
Velalar College of Engineering and Technology, Erode, India

© The Author(s), under exclusive license to Springer Nature Switzerland AG 2021   203
C. Chakraborty et al. (eds.), *Efficient Data Handling for Massive Internet of Medical Things*, Internet of Things,
https://doi.org/10.1007/978-3-030-66633-0_9

sors are interconnected with either gateways to the smartphones, and the resultant data could be very huge, and hence, those big data are analyzed by the data analysts. The necessary information could be retrieved by the machine learning using a neural network. The data with useful information are extracted by collecting the real-time data from the wearable sensors in the available and manageable time with few innovations. The boundless number of healthcare data can be analyzed by storing those data in the cloud services like Microsoft Azure, Google cloud, etc.

This chapter is structured as follows: Section 9.1 describes the introduction about the wearable sensor and remote monitoring of patients. Section 9.2 deals with the challenges faced by the wearable sensors through integration for online monitoring. Section 9.3 describes Internet of Things (IoT) and Internet of Medical Things (IoMT) for collecting patient data through internet. Section 9.4 describes role of wearable sensors in modern healthcare systems. This chapter is further classified in terms of three major disease monitoring for diabetes, heart, and Alzheimer. Section 9.5 deals with blood glucose monitoring and diabetes management through online. Section 9.6 deals with cardiac monitoring and its associated issues. Section 9.7 discusses about the online monitoring of Alzheimer patients under Active Assisted Living. Section 9.8 deals with Samrt Healthcare system through big data analytics. Section 9.9 gives the conclusion on the integration of sensors and data handling in the online healthcare monitoring.

9.2   Challenges and Issues in Integration of Data From Wearable Sensors for Online Healthcare Monitoring

Data gathered from multiple sensors vary in quality and integrity. Data format also varies due to the absence of common approach for gathering data from different types of physiological variables. Data gathering and analysis methods vary depending upon the wearable sensor manufacturers.

Data analysis could be done on board directly from the incoming data streams, or data stream is taken and analyzed using a secondary data acquisition system. Methods for analyzing data vary upon the factors like quality, integrity, type of dataset, etc. Structured approaches are required for validating the data from wearable sensors and analyzing data and feedback from the data analysis. Common approaches are required for data acquisition, transmission, and integration and processing.

9.2.1   Challenges in Building a System Integrated with Multisensor-Based Wearables

Big Data play an important role in the massive growth of wearable technology in which speed and reliability are important parameters. Big Data speaks about the enormous variety of data collected and their velocity and volume. The constant data stream calls for huge data processing and storage capabilities. The real Challenge arises with computation limitations and multitasking requirements.

A robust strategic system is required for integrating multisensor inputs. The steps involved in integrating the data from wearable are as follows:

1. Identification of the type of disease present in the patient
2. Identify the types of sensors based on the patient's health record. Type of sensor must be precise enough to get the physiological parameters pertained to the nature of the disease.
3. Identification of the methods for analyzing the data (Different approaches are to be analyzed depending upon the quality of output of the system).
4. Integration of different datasets from different sensors.
5. Analyzing datasets of different sensors and indication of the output parameters.
6. Measures taken to treat the nature of disease.
7. Methods to store and reproduce datasets as and then depending upon the requirement.

Acceptance of wearable sensor technology is based on the ease of usage of software and hardware devices, ease of usage, area occupied by the system, total eight of the devices, and power consumption of the battery. Superior performance, accurateness in measurements, and higher suitability for a variety of applications in health care are important. Major constraints are the absence of universal platform and interoperability. Safety, confidentiality, and ethics are other needs of concern. Common safer methods of storage and authentication techniques are present and realized successfully in many systems. Privacy and ethical principles are handled in an ad hoc way, and advantage could be obtained by applying universal frameworks that are available with different vendor.

Body Sensor Networks (BSNs) have emerged as a revolutionary technology in many application domains in health care, fitness, smart cities, and compelling Internet of Things applications. In particular, BSNs have demonstrated great potential in health care. These systems hold the promise to improve patient care/safety and result in significant cost savings. Recent years have seen considerable research demonstrating the potential of BSNs in a variety of physical activity monitoring applications [5–8].

9.3 Internet of Things

The Internet of Things can be illustrated as networking of a variety of embedded gadgets such as sensors and transducers interacting with each other to communicate themselves like machine to machine communication for provision of grouping and exchanging of data among them [1, 9–11]. The Internet of Things and its associated technology not only enable the automation of industries but also play an inevitable role in the medical stream, which aims at allowing for the collection of big clinical data. IoTs are extensively used for intelligent structural health monitoring [12–14].

9.3.1 Internet of Medical Things

Nowadays, Internet of Things plays a major role in healthcare sector. It provides various services as Internet of Medical Things (IoMT). It serves the public by providing user interface Health mobile app, smart watch, Blood Glucose monitor, smart wheel chair, Respiratory belt, etc. Figure 9.1 shows the pictorial illustration of Real-time IoMT services in healthcare industry.

The Internet of Medical Things (IoMT) permits a device-to-device intercommunication and relies on providing solutions for real-time applications that have an ability to modify health care and enhance delivery and reliability in the upcoming

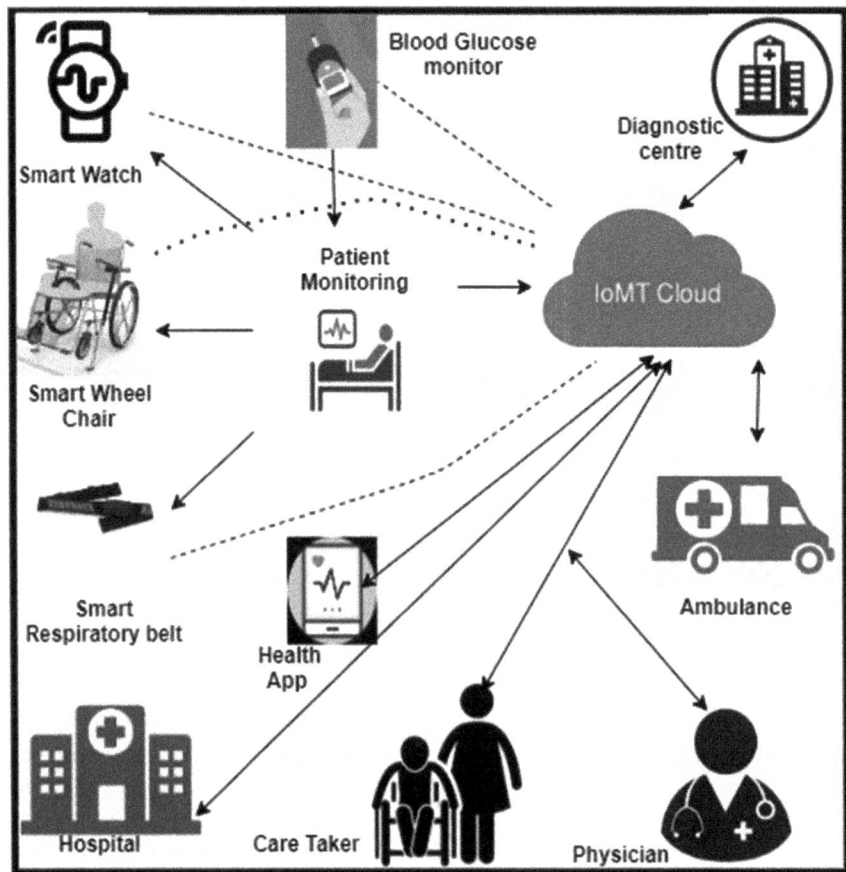

Fig. 9.1 Illustration of Real-Time IoMT services

era. IoMT supports the interaction of the sensors and large wireless networks through technologies like Body Area Networks (BAN), Wireless sensor network (WSN), Near-Field Communication (NFC), and Long-Range wide area networks (LoRa). Additionally, increase in the patient engagement in decision-making will enhance the healthcare service compliances.

9.4   Roles of Wearable Sensors in Healthcare

An enormous development in the field of construction and use of wearable (e.g., wellness trackers, wearable sensors for biometric applications etc.) change the way by which the data are collected and analyzed [15, 16]. Figure 9.2 shows the wearable sensors used by humans to monitor the physiological parameters continuously.

Internets of Medical things associated with wearable-embedded sensor technologies have improved the life style of each and every human. It can provide intelligent and reliable healthcare systems that are necessarily responsible for not only tracking but also managing the health of human under all circumstances. The improved fea-

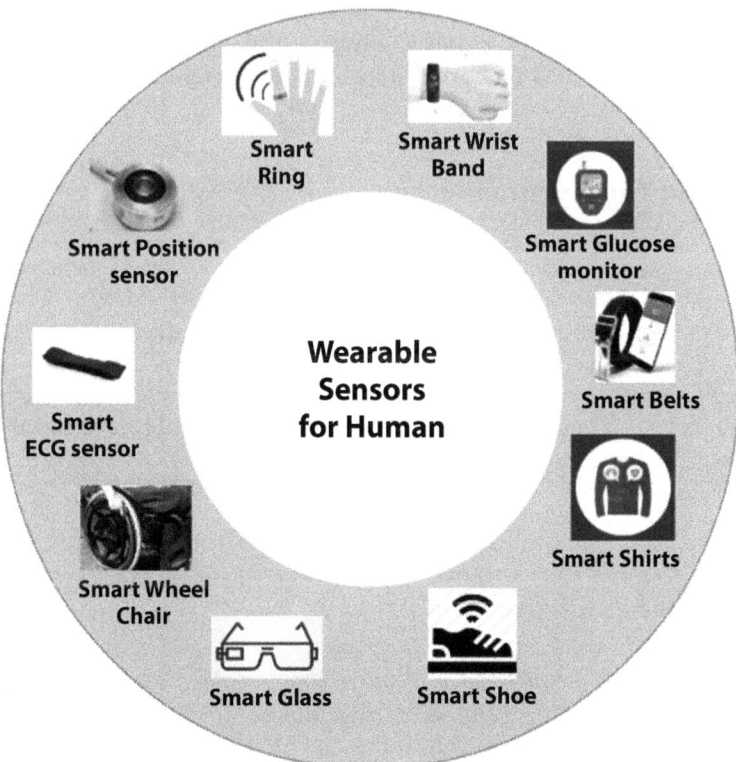

Fig. 9.2 Wearable Sensors for Humans

tures such as near-field communication and wireless technologies enable the transmission and analysis of biological data by healthcare professionals based on identification of earlier symptoms of many chronic diseases[15–17]. Improving the overall efficiency and cost-effective smart health care is one of the rights of every citizen in the developed as well as developing countries.

The wearable sensors support everyone to do their routine life. If the sensed information deviates from the threshold level of normal range, then it indicates the person to go for clinic. These sensors are popular because these are embedded into anyone of the wearable things such as smart wrist band, smart belt, smart shirt, smart shoe, smart glass, etc [18, 19]. In some cases, these sensors are linked with special devices as smart glucose monitor, smart wheel chair, smart ECG sensor, smart position sensor, etc.

9.4.1 Motivation for Smart Healthcare System

Internet of things provides better solution for remote smart health monitoring because of the numerous benefits associated with it. In a few implementations, IoT healthcare systems extend the best solution for chronic diseases including diabetes, cardiac diseases, and Active Assisted Living (AAL) for physically challenged and elderly persons. While these technical advancements meant for a huge range of applications, they are robustly linked through the usage of available resources.

9.5 Blood Glucose Monitoring

Continuous real-time Glucose Monitoring of diabetes patient helps them to correct insulin injection level and avoid accidental overdose. Smart wearable device displays the glucose level and alerts the doctor and patient on their mobile phone using Internet of Things (IoT) platforms. These wearables keep track of insulin dosage and glucose level in cloud platform and give visualization to the doctors for proper prescription [20]. The smart glucose monitoring device could be embedded in the wristbands, watches, and even in shoes of the patients. The doctors can give virtual care to patients easily.

9.5.1 Diabetes Management

Diabetes mellitus, commonly stated as diabetes, is one of the worldwide epidemics. Diabetes is a long-standing metabolic disorder that occurs due to variation in blood glucose level due to the absence of secretion of insulin. There is a tremendous increase in the number of diabetes patients due to aging, huge population growth in countries like India, and increase in obesity because of physical inactivity. It is caused by either insufficient insulin production in the human body or inability of human body to utilize insulin produced in human body. Type 1 diabetes is caused in human because of destruction of β-cells, which usually leads to deficiency in absolute insulin (T1D). Type 2 diabetes is caused because of lower secretion of insulin, which can possibly cause defect in the background of insulin resistance (T2D).

Gestational diabetes mellitus (GDM) is also common in highly populated countries, which can be diagnosed during the pregnancy [21]. It is impossible to provide suitable healthcare need for diabetes patients for the entire population in developing countries, which seems quite cumbersome. Also, entire population could not afford the low-cost diabetes medication especially the insulin. Due to various reasons such as family environment, poor diet control, and malnutrition, diabetes is common in many countries. Because of the limited resources, the population has to focus on high-calorie protein-rich foods that cause diabetes often.

The modern healthcare technology with right communication ability can be utilized to monitor the diabetes patients. Because of the advances in the available healthcare technologies and wearable sensors, continuous monitoring of a patient's condition in real time is possible and one can manage the diabetes continuously and efficiently [22].

Glucose level monitoring of the diabetic patients using a real-time system in the blood was proposed in Ref. [23]. The proposed system enables the diabetic patients to check manually and obtain the blood glucose level at the regular time intervals. The existing system checks the unusual levels of blood glucose and also blood glucose count that is missed. It not only analyses abnormality in the blood glucose level but also make decision on its own to indicate, and the notification will be sent to the patient themselves as well as family members and the emergency healthcare persons such as nurses, doctors, etc. Even though this system is feasible, it can be additionally improved by the automation of measurements of blood glucose level.

Wearable Sensor technology enables a professional way of monitoring the diabetic patients, and hence, personal health of the individuals can be improved. Ganjar et al. proposed a personalized healthcare monitoring system that constitutes low energy-based bluetooth sensor devices to analyze data in real-time domain by using machine learning-techniques to assist diabetic patients to handle their health conditions [24].

9.6 Cardiac Monitoring

Heart rate is a primary factor in the identification of health of patients for long time. Since people all over the world are paying extensive awareness on their health and fitness, monitoring of heart rate for long term is an essential part of early diagnosis of plenty of illness. Persons like athletes, Sports persons, and elderly people who suffer from diabetes and high pressure require continuous monitoring of heart rate. In view of these needs, it is essential and vital procedure to devise and manufacture system that is appropriate for monitoring of heart rate on long-term basis, which should also be free from noises. The embedded and wearable sensors are used for this purpose.

The wearing device should be compatible and cost-effective for daily use to measure heart rate regularly. Numerous conventional methods have been proposed previously to calculate heart rate, which are usually based on electrocardiogram (ECG or EKG) [25], Photoplethysmography (PPG) (PPG), [26] and piezoelectric effect-based devices [27–29]. Many other techniques for measurement of heart rate have been proposed, demonstrated, and verified by some researchers [30–32]. By analyzing the methods already proposed for examining heart rate monitoring, ECG is the most commonly used technique. It is often the standard diagnosis method for heart rate measurement in healthcare centers, but a specific kit is required for use in household applications. Heart rate monitors based on wearable technology using ECG technique are available in the market, but chest strap transmitters are generally required, which are not suitable for daily usage.

Recently, a few research projects are aiming to combine the well-known benefits of Wireless Body Sensor Network (WBSN) technologies to monitor the HRV continuously and noninvasively. Currently, few research prototypes based on BSNs exist that allow for heart rate variability analysis. Many BSN applications need handling of multiple sensor signals at the same time, which is sometime referred to as sensor data fusion and context awareness [33–35].

9.6.1 Principles of the ECG

The ElectroCardioGram (ECG) is nothing but the recording of the electrical activity performed by the heart. An electrical recording can be produced by using one myocardial muscle cell. Each myocardial cell will record an action potential, that is, the electrical movement that happens when the cell is invigorated. The electrical activity of the heart is recorded in the form of the vector whole, i.e., the mixture of every single electrical sign for the activity possibilities of the myocardium, and generates a consolidated trace.

During resting state, the potential difference developed across the myocardial membrane is around -90 mV. This is because a higher concentration of intracellular potassium may be kept up by the sodium/potassium pump. Depolarization of a cardiovascular cell happens when there is an abrupt change in the permeability of the layer to sodium. Sodium floods into the cell, and the negative resting voltage is lost. Calcium continues the sodium, the slower calcium diverts bringing about authoritative between the intracellular proteins actin and myosin, which brings about withdrawal of the muscle fiber.

The depolarization of a myocardial cell causes the depolarization of neighboring cells, and in the typical heart, the depolarization of the whole myocardium follows in a coordinated design. During repolarization, potassium moves out of the phones and the resting negative layer potential is reestablished.

These existing methods deploy a distant observing diagnostic system to identify abnormal heart conditions in real time, which facilitates in staying away from heart diseases in early stages, and treatment of the patients makes progressing from cardiac diseases.

An existing model identifies the heart attacks with a help of sensor, signal processing unit, and a conventional antenna in Ref. [36]. ECG picks up the heart rate, which is the processed by a microcontroller. The actuating signal from microcontroller is transmitted to smartphone by using Bluetooth. The signal is then plotted in the smartphone or recorder. The authors identified that building up software for predicting heart attack will improve the system. Even more the improvements could be made by measuring the signals such as respiratory rate, so as to predict the heart attack in earlier stages [37].

Figure 9.3 shows the block diagram of IoT-based ECG signal processing module. It consists of three units. They are

1. Sensing Unit
2. Processing Unit
3. Master Data Management

Usually, sensing unit consists of physiological sensors to capture the bioelectric potential of human. For ECG recording, there are several electrodes used to capture the raw ECG signal. The obtained raw ECG signal is then processed and analyzed in Processing unit. In this, Signal conditioning and communication module are used

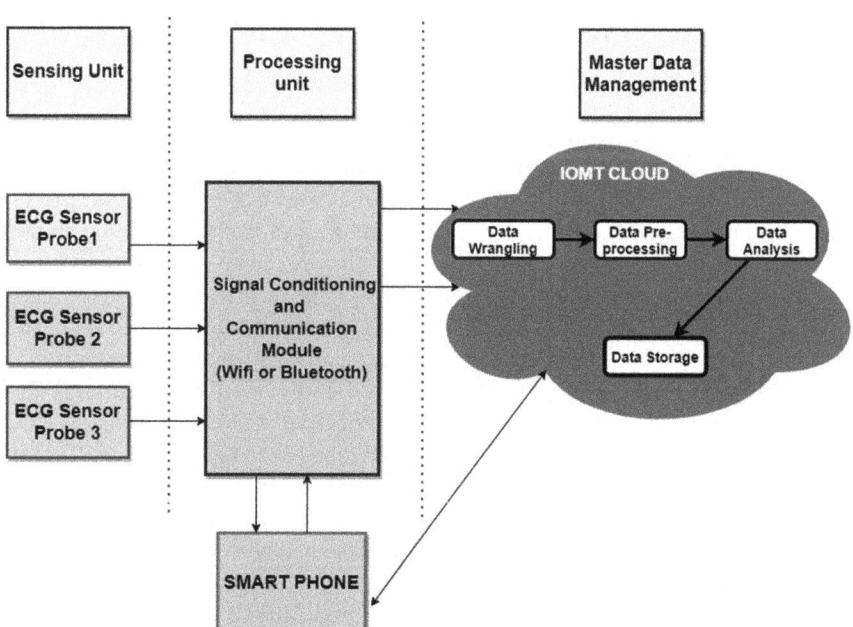

Fig. 9.3 IoT-based ECG Signal processing module

for ECG signal processing and communicating with external interface. The processed ECG signal is stored in IoMT cloud for future reference.

9.6.2 ECG Monitoring in Theater

Heart-Related Diseases/Wearable Watch Strap monitors continuously the health status of a patient's heart and displays the captured data through a mobile app. Electrocardiogram (ECG) is the key sensor for Heart rate monitoring and to identify serious medical conditions such as stroke and heart attacks. It gives the patient accurate information about the heart health.

ECG wearables have optical monitoring device inside them. There are watch-based and chest-based ECG wearables that measure 20 million data points in a day. If the captured data detect any possibility of heart arrhythmia, this device prompts the user to start the recording of electrical activity of heart, that is, ECG signals. This allows the patient to study their own ECG anytime and anywhere they want without having to go to any specialist, any lab, or emergency room. Also, it saves both time and money for the patients and their healthcare provider.

The regular CRO-based ECG is considered as one of the most broadly utilized anesthetic screens. In addition to monitoring arrhythmias, it can also be utilized to diagnose the myocardial ischemia, electrolyte imbalanced characteristics, and to evaluate pacemaker work. A 12-lead recording is one of the standard lead systems to record Electrocardiogram. It will give significantly more data about the electrical activity of the heart than is accessible on a theater ECG screen. This should be conceivable and received preoperatively for any patient with suspected heart sickness.

Electrocardiography (ECG) is a pictorial portrayal of electrical conduction and myocardial excitation in the heart. As action potential travel through the heart, they produce a positive current (depolarization) that is quickly trailed by a flood of negative current (repolarization). Finally, it results in the fact that the ECG recognizes and records Placement of the leads, which may provide positive or negative deflections in various regions of the heart.

The recording of the electrical action of the heart was stated as ECG. It doesn't provide any information about the pumping activity of the heart. Also, it cannot be utilized to assess cardiovascular output or pulse. Heart work under sedation is normally evaluated utilizing continuous estimations of circulatory strain, end tidal $CO2$ concentrations, pulse rate, saturated oxygen level, and peripheral perfusion. Cardiac performance is once in a while estimated straightforwardly in theater utilizing catheters or Doppler procedures, in spite of the fact that this is exceptional.

The ECG monitor ought to consistently be associated with the patient with prior acceptance of sedation and/or establishment of a provincial square. It will permit the anesthetist or specialist to recognize some modification or adjustment in the presence of the cardiogram complexes during anesthesia.

9.6.3 Connecting an ECG Monitor

Even an ECG signal might be acquired from placed electrodes connected in changes with positions. Expectedly, these electrodes are placed in a standard position each and every time so that the variations from the norm are simpler to recognize. Most of the recordings have 3 electrode leads, and they are associated as follows:

- Electrode lead in Red color is placed in Right Arm, that is, second intercostal space on the privilege of the sternum.
- Electrode lead in Yellow color is placed in Left Arm that is located in second intercostal space on the left of the sternum.
- Electrode lead in Black or Green color is placed in Left Leg that is located more frequently in the area of the summit beat.

These may permit the Lead I, II, and III setups to be chosen to monitor the ECG waveform. Among all 3-lead setup, Lead II was considered as the most widely preferred in the medical field.

The connectivity link from the electrodes is ordinarily end in a solitary link. It is connected to the port on the ECG screen.

A better electrical connectivity among the patient and the electrodes is achieved to limit the electrical resistivity of the skin. Hence, gel cushions or suction cups with electrode gel were preferred to link the electrodes with the patient's skin. Suppose if the skin is sweat-soaked, the electrodes cannot be placed well, and it may lead to an insecure follow. At this point, suppose the electrodes are in short supply, they might be reused frequently by soaking with saline or gel before being taped to the patient's chest.

Once again, a void 1000 milliliters of IV mixture bag might be sliced open to permit it to a bit level (as a level bit of plastic) on the patient's chest. In this activity, 3 little openings are formed with 3 of the corner's terminals. It might be placed on one side of the plastic, permitting the electrode gel to reach the skin. Thus, the gadget can be washed toward the finish of the activity. It may be placed on the following patient, permitting electrodes to be utilized over and over.

9.6.4 Lead Positions

The ECG might be utilized in two distinct categories. This 12-lead standard ECG system might be analyzed, which examines the heart electrical action from various electrodes situated on the limbs and over the chest. A major scope of variations from the norm might be distinguished including arrhythmias, myocardial ischemia, and left ventricular hypertrophy.

The Electrocardiogram might be checked by utilizing just 3 (or sometimes 5) electrodes during anesthesia, which give a progressively confined examination of the cardiovascular electrical movement and can't give a similar measure of data that might be uncovered by using the standard bipolar 12 lead system. "LEAD" in ECG corresponds to the following of the voltage difference between two of the electrodes and is truly what is conveyed by the ECG machine.

9.6.5   Graphical Recording

ECG wave is recorded on a paper in a period size of 0.04 seconds/mm. Also, in the paper, the center point and a voltage affectability of about 0.1 mv/mm are compared to the vertical hub. In like manner, on normal ECG recording paper, 1 minimal square corresponds to 0.04 seconds. The one large square relates 0.2 seconds duration in ECG. In the normal ECG waveform, the P wave relates to atrial depolarization and the ventricular depolarization is represented by QRS complex and the ventricular repolarization by T wave.

- The P–R length is taken from the earliest starting point of the P wave to the start of the QRS complex. It is the time taken for depolarization to go from the SA hub by methods.
- The QRS relates to the time taken for depolarization to experience the His-Purkinje structure and ventricular muscles. It is deferred with infection of the His-Purkinje system.
- The Q–T range is taken from the earliest starting point of the QRS complex to the uttermost furthest reaches of the T wave. This addresses the time taken to depolarize and repolarize the ventricles.
- The S–T partition is the period between the completion of the QRS complex and the start of the T wave. The ST area is changed by pathology, for instance, myocardial ischemia or pericarditis.

9.7   Monitoring Patients Under Active Assisted Living (AAL)

The population in all countries has increasing tremendously due to the availability of advanced medical facilities. There is also an increase in the number of elderly people in each country who require additional care, [18, 19] which is also increasing. Even in the well-developed countries, the materialization of an ageing people is rapid and the measures are to be taken to closely monitor the public health. The price of health care and service is rapidly increasing to meet the quality of services, which is not in proper concern in modern societal developments [38].

The only solution is to ensure the remote and real-time health monitoring to overcoming the existing challenges. Periodic smart health monitoring of the elderly and needy people can be achieved by using wearable devices and smartphones.

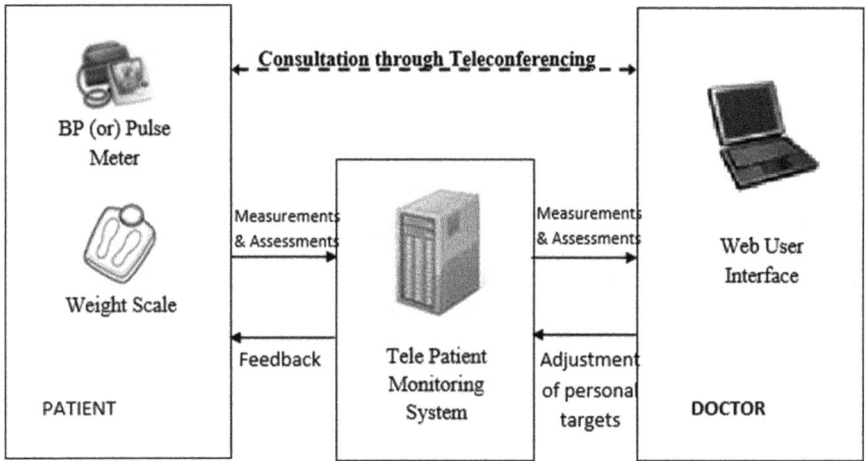

Fig. 9.4 Basic setup for Teleconsultation

Figure 9.4 shows the basic setup used for teleconsultation. This is possible through videoconferencing. From last decade, this type of consultation becomes more popular among the healthcare sector.

The Project SPHERE [39] aims at monitoring the elderly and physically challenged persons, which includes wearable sensors and vision (i.e., camera) sensors for monitoring the regular daily activities and also for monitoring their health. The ultimate aim of this model is to help the elderly and chronically ill patients to lead their life with full comfort at their homes, and the mean time of their health is also regularly monitored without any discomfort. The patients under the critical illness will be on utmost care by nurses, caregivers, and doctors if there exist abnormalities. Academicians and researchers are working for improving the project using machine learning since the machine learning is advantageous for providing better results and taking decisions regarding the health care of patients.

Figure 9.5 shows the pictorial description of one healthcare setup used to observe the daily health care of the elderly aged people. They used wireless sensor network (WSN) to collect the health information in this technique. Each sensor node is placed along with Elderly people home. These nodes collect the health information and store in the cloud database. The stored information is retrieved from the cloud and continuously monitors the health status in the monitoring unit.

9.7.1   Alzheimer's Disease

Alzheimer's disease and dementias can be noticed during earlier periods by observing the changes in the behavior of the person who is suffering from that disease. Alzheimer Patients experience difficulties like loss in memory for short intervals of

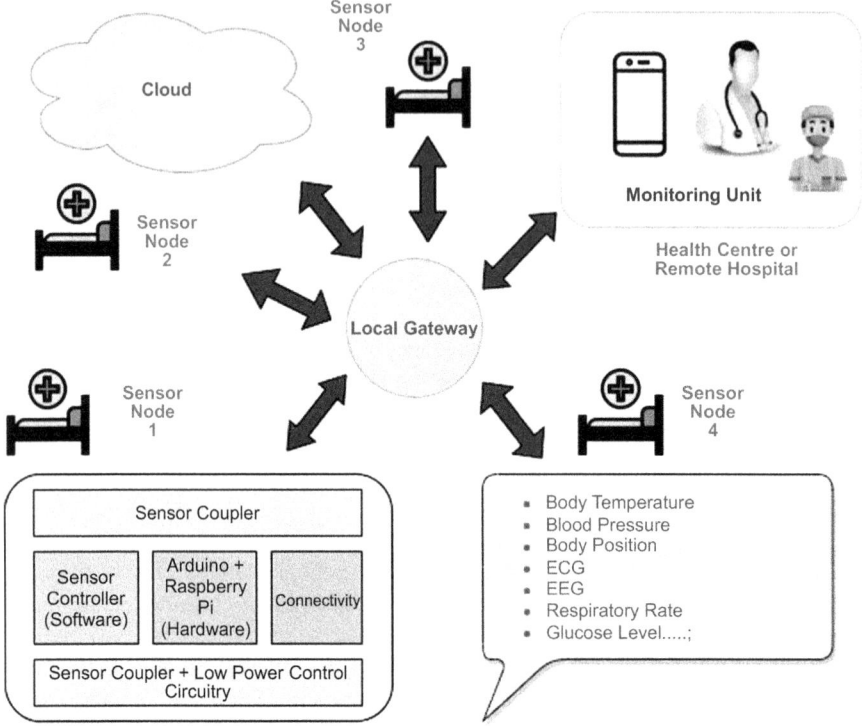

Fig. 9.5 WSN-based Healthcare setup for Elderly people

time, learning of subjects, counting numbers, and confusion in the process of decision-making. Alzheimer's disease affects the patient's abilities mentally. Individual symptoms of this disease might vary from person to person, depending on the person's personality, routine life style, and overall health condition of the patients. Alzheimer's disease is divided into three stages, namely,

1. Early Stage
2. Mild Stage
3. Advanced Stage.

All patients do not know-how a progression has occurred from one stage to another. The transition from one stage to another stage will happen several years. During the early stages, activities like speech, memory, socializing skills, judgment, thinking logically, and mobility are affected. All senses and skills get worsened where a substitute can be used to eliminate problems. During the mild stages, activities like speech, memory, socializing skills, judgment, thinking logically, and mobility are affected. Symptoms of mild stage include loss of the ability of the people to take care of themselves. Lose in the ability in decision-making and the orientation starts deteriorating.

Activities affected in the advanced stages are capability to do difficult tasks (expressing them self) is reduced, and the patient is in need of caretakers and members from family. Difficulty in movement is noticed and becomes often bed-bound patient. Symptoms of advanced stage are requiring assistance for fulfilling routine actions as well as the ability to speak, walk, sit, and stand. Patients will lose the communication abilities with other people.

The wearable devices can be used to send patient location of Alzheimer's Patients data over an Internet of Thing cloud network to a caretaker. The device can produce alerts to the caretaker if the patient goes outside of a selected "safe" zone. The device provides a safety measure for the patients and a relief for the caretakers, thus enabling the patients to stay in their home without moving to hospitals. Innovations are to be included in assistance, and monitoring for Alzheimer's Patients helps them to attain the independent and comfortable life.

Increase in population and unhealthy and stressful lifestyle in turn increases Alzheimer's disease in Indian population. Numerous technological solutions are provided for people suffering with dementia and Alzheimer's disease. Technology-assisted living improves the day-to-day life of these people. The patients with Alzheimer disease in rural areas do not have access to assistive technology like the patients living in urban areas. Training the caretakers and staff members involving with the patient plays a vital role in the success of this technology-assisted living. Security concerns over the use of wireless technology, legal, privacy, and ethical issues are also need to be considered before choosing the method of implementation.

9.8 Hexagon Chart of Smart Healthcare System Through Big Data Analysis

Device Connectivity is a major issue since the patients may or may not aware of the signals collected from the wearable sensors. If more than 10 to 15 sensors are needed for elderly people who are affected by Alzheimer's disease, then connectivity will be achieved by some routers with the help of some near-field communication devices such as RFID, Wireless Area Networks, and Body Area Network.

Figure 9.6 shows the hexagon diagram of smart healthcare system through big data analytics. It consists of six phases. These phases are listed as follows:

1. Connectivity of devices
2. Sensing and Collecting of data
3. Transport and access of data
4. Data Analytics
5. Actions defining data values
6. Human values, applications, and experiences.

Data that are sensed by different sensors may be of different varieties. For example, the blood sugar level is a real valued data ranging from 70 mg/dL to

Fig. 9.6 Hexagon Chart of Smart Healthcare System through Big Data Analysis

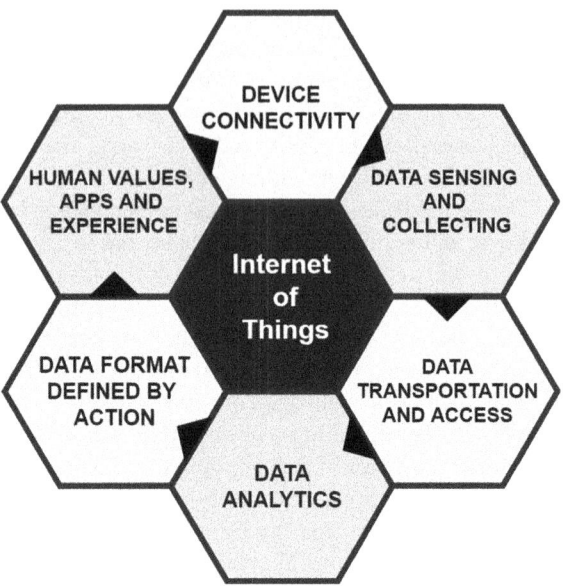

maximum 500 mg/dL. The data that are collected from ECG may be pulse rate that is a real valued number or graphical form such as ECG, which is 2-dimensional images. If the data are taken from Alzheimer's patient, it is necessary to obtain the clear color image of the patient, also the real-time values for position monitoring, etc. The collection and integration of these data can be done by various sensors that are also wearable. These wearable sensors must be chosen such that they are compatible with the patient under monitoring to ensure the proper transmission of data from sensors to the servers.

Data transportation can be done by any of the suitable and affordable Near-Field Communication networks like Wire Networks or Body Area Networks. There should be a sufficient number of Access points needed for each and every sensor to ensure proper connectivity.

In order to analyze the data that are stored in remote server could be very large since these data were stored periodically to monitor the patients under observation. Because of increase in the modern healthcare technologies, the prevention of many chronic diseases was possible and the mortality rate could be considerably reduced. Since the data collected are streaming with high velocity, variety, and huge volume, they are analyzed using deep learning. Before applying any deep learning algorithm, the data wrangling and data cleansing have to be done and the best optimization has to be done to choose the neural network to learn data from the available sensors.

Neural network analyses data by preprocessing and involve in training the available data types for a sufficient number of times. The processed data have to be sent to the end user for further processing of clinical data. Hence, the patient with abnormal values should be immediately handled by the healthcare persons like doctors, nurses, or caretakers. In order to enable quick accessibility of the patient, these data have to be sent to the healthcare person's mobile through well-organized mobile application. Hence, the data that are collected from the patients may be immediately transmitted to the family persons also in the case of emergency or healthcare persons through mobile applications in a presentable form.

9.8.1 Data Analytics

Data Analytics play a vital role in analyzing the data associated with healthy and unhealthy patients who suffer from different diseases. Analyzing the data of both healthy and unhealthy might be helpful to predict the risk factors and complications of various drugs for future reference. Data mining in healthcare data follows some rules and regulations. By following rules, disease management is possible by which one can get best treatment and health insurance.

The sensor output is compared with available model using regression algorithm or decision tree algorithm in healthcare analysis. Association rules are designed to evaluate the health of the patient. Positive and negative association rule generation and creating associative rule-based classifier are needed for the prediction analysis in health care.

The medical data should be accompanied by personal information, and medical test results, etc., are essential to predict the probability of occurrence of a certain disease. It might be used for physicians and also for the patients' caretaker regarding the probable risk of certain disease.

9.8.2 Data Mining in Healthcare

Data mining is one of the most inevitable popular techniques that is necessary to observe the health care of the patients. Since there is a huge increase in essential healthcare data, Data mining would be preferable one. There will be huge benefits available not only for healthcare industries, but the right healthcare facilities can be afforded for many needy patients.

The huge amounts of complex data that include patient database, hospital resources, diagnosing capability, electronic record of the patients, and medical devices were to be analyzed continuously. The wearable sensor provides various datasets that are to be integrated to create a medical database. That database makes a lucid depiction of the whole data that may be useful for the medical information system.

Enormous amount of data extracted and transmitted from the wearable sensors is a major resource for data processing. The analysis and extraction of knowledge enable support for decision-making. Data mining algorithms are used to extract information or patterns from raw data.

9.8.3   Data Classification

Classification deals with predicting a label and regression to predict a quantity. Once multiple data are received in the medical data base management system, it is necessary to extract the useful data from the available set of data. The classification enables the prediction of data to create discrete class label output from the received medical datasets. The regression enables the prediction of a continuous data as output.

9.8.4   Predictive Modeling

The predictive modeling enables to develop a new model from historical data to make a new set of predictions when the data are new within a received set of the time and resources available.

9.8.4.1   Sample Data

Data that are received from sensor are a real valued function. From the available Datasets, we need to classify the data that are required to identify the disease from the whole set of data. For diabetes patients, the blood sugar level will be in the range of 60–100 mg/dl. This range is taken as the label. Since the predictable data are known, they are considered as labeled data that can be implemented using supervised learning technique. The goal is to take some data with a known relationship so as to create a model of the required relationships. The learning is done by the supervised learning algorithm as shown in Figure 9.7. The model is able to learn the relationships.

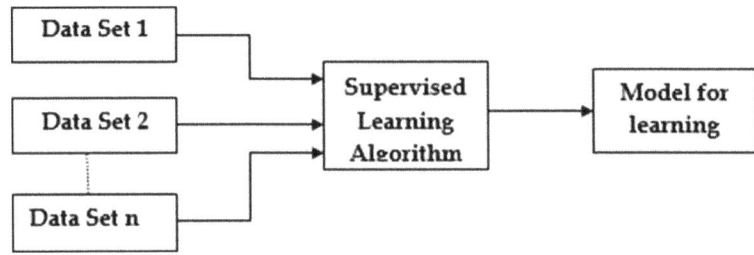

Fig. 9.7 Model for supervised learning algorithm

9.8.4.2 Making Predictions

The model will read the raw data observed by the wearable sensors and perform comparisons with model to make a prediction about real data that are necessary for the end user. If the sample data are good, a robust model learns from the data and it will provide the accurate result.

9.8.4.3 Predictive Modeling in Wearable Sensors

There are two protocols used in predictive modeling. The Classification and regression are the two-modeling algorithm that is used for analyzing the health-care data. The function is developed from the available input to develop a discrete output dataset. Labels are given for the output data. The activation function thus predicts the signal from the wearable sensors.

A classification of data from wearable sensors requires that data to be classified into required set of classes. A data classification could be done for real-valued or discrete variables. If the given sensors involve two classes of data, then they are referred to as binary classification. During classification, continuous values from different sensors are predicted by obtaining the probability of each set of classes. Ones belonging to good data are termed as 'confident' data, and other belonging to error are 'bad' data. A predicted value can be converted into strongest class when it has highest probability. If a probability values of confident data, which are labeled as 'good data,' have the probability of 0.1, the other data are grouped as 'false data,' which have the probability value of 0.9.

The estimated predicted value will assure the best classification accuracy. The classification accuracy is properly classified with all set of predictions made. If a classification predictive model made 10 predictions, out of them 4 were correct and 6 were incorrect predictions.

$$\text{Prediction Accuracy} = \frac{\text{Correct predictions}}{\text{Total number of predictions}} \times 100$$

$$\text{Prediction Accuracy} = \frac{4}{6} \times 100$$

$$\text{Prediction Accuracy} = 66.66\%$$

A classification algorithm learns with a classification predictive model to get wearable sensor data with good accuracy.

9.8.4.4   Regression Predictive Modeling

Regression predictive modeling algorithms like k-Nearest Neighbors, Decision Tree algorithms, Support Vector Machines, and MultiLayer Perceptron are used to generate the best data output from available input variables. A continuous data output variable mentioned here is the data that are received from sensors from patients. When it is a real value, such as an integer or floating-point value, then Root mean Square would be calculated while training a set of predicted data. A regression predictive model would predict a best quantity from the available set of data, and it could generate root mean squared error. For example, if a regression predictive model could produce 2 predictions, one of that would be 1.3, where the expected value is 1.0 and another prediction is 3.8, and the expected value is 3.0, then the Root Mean Square Error is calculated as mentioned below.

$$\text{Root Mean Square Error} = \sqrt{\text{Average}\,(\text{Error})^2}$$
$$\text{Root Mean Square Error} = \sqrt{\frac{(1.0-1.3)^2 + (1.0-1.3)^2}{2}}.$$
$$\text{Root Mean Square Error} = \sqrt{\frac{0.09 + 0.64}{2}}.$$
$$\text{Root Mean Square Error} = \sqrt{0.73}.$$
$$\text{Root Mean Square Error} = 0.854.$$

The Root Mean Square Error has the same unit as the predicted data. Among Classification and Regression algorithm, Regression algorithm could provide a better result.

9.8.5   Data Format for Wearable Sensors

9.8.5.1   MQTT (Message Queuing Telemetry Transport)

The Publish/subscribe messaging scheme was enabled by MQTT protocol. It is a specific lightweight protocol used for connecting things at remote places. It handles minimal code as well as communication network bandwidth. MQTT-SN stands for Message Queuing Telemetry Transport for Sensor Networks. The important feature of this protocol is open type. Also it provides lightweight publish/subscribe protocol. It is designed specifically for machine-to-machine communications and mobile applications, and because of this, it is used in wearable sensors.

MQTT clients are very small, and hence, it requires minimal resources. It can be used even on small and low cost microcontrollers. Since the headers of the MQTT message are quite small, it will reduce the bandwidth. This protocol allows messaging between IOT device and cloud and vice versa. It leads to better broadcasting to deliver the information to needful places through IOT. This protocol is used for connecting millions of devices. The important factor in IOT is reliability of message delivery. MQTT accomplishes reliability by means of defined quality of service levels. Many IOT devices are connected to unreliable cellular network, but the MQTT supports for persistent and reliable way of connecting things to cloud. MQTT protocol encrypts the message using TLS and accomplishes authentication to the service provider.

9.8.5.2   Communication Protocol for IOT-Enabled Wearable Sensors

The Websocket API is one of the advanced powerful technologies. It enhances a two-way interactive communication among the server as well as application end user browser. This API sends frames of messages and receives responses from the connected devices without any acknowledgement from the server as shown in (Fig. 9.8).

9.8.5.3   *Internet Protocol*-IPv6

The term IPv6 stands for Internet Protocol version 6 (IPv6). IPv6 is a latest Internet Layer protocol. It is implemented for providing packet-switched networking devices. IPv6 assigns and operates with end-to-end data connection in the available IP networks. It ensures identification and location of connected devices on networking platform. It handles the routing and traffic across the Internet connection. A unique IP address is utilized for each device connected through the Internet.

9.8.5.4   802.1x/EAP-TLS-Based Access Control

An authenticated network access is provided by 802.1X. It is an IEEE standard for network to ensure security for wired Ethernet networks and wireless 802.11 net-

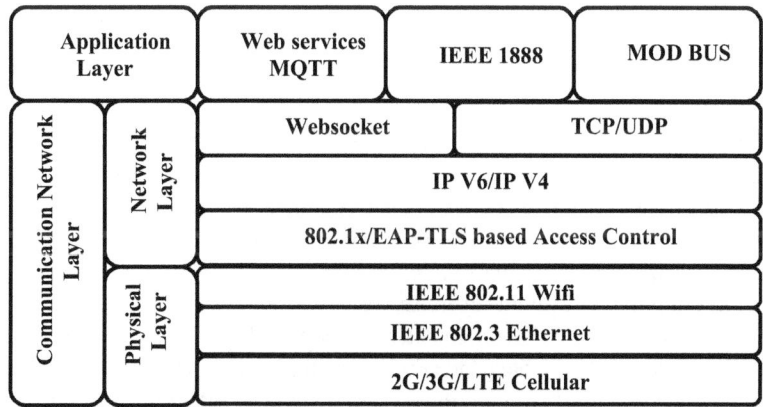

Fig. 9.8 Communication Protocol for IOT*7.52 Websocket API*

works. It enhances security by identifying the user with the help of dynamic key management.

9.8.5.5   IEEE 802.11 WiFi

WiFi otherwise called wireless local area network uses the IEEE 802.11 standard whose operating frequency ranges from 2.4 GHz UHF and 5 GHz. WiFi enables secured Internet access to the connected devices of range about 66 feet from access point. It is an affordable way of secure connection between IOT devices and Cloud where the huge device data are stored periodically. The connection could also be controlled with proper control unit. Wi-Fi is always Access point centered where its client-server connection could be implemented via router with many access points. WiFi is useful for connecting many Internet of Things sensors or devices, but such connections typically should be connected to an external cloud-server. Its usage is limited for battery-powered devices due to its relatively high power consumption. WiFi requires high speeds of internet connectivity as network access could be made with the help of an n number of access nodes.

9.8.5.6   IEEE 802.3 Ethernet

IEEE 802.3 Ethernet cable supports networking among wired systems and devices. It is used for supporting network with higher bit rates. It is used for connecting many nodes for short and long distances too. If an advanced networking system is needed, it can also be replaced by Token ring, ARCNET, etc. The devices connected with Ethernet divide a particular data stream into many frames. Every data frame contains source address and destination addresses in all the frames. It also has dedicated error-checking capability. The damaged frames could be identified and eliminated among the device in the network.

9.8.6   *IOT Cloud Platform*

Amazon Web Services (AWS) is a managed cloud service that not only provides connectivity but also helps to exchange the secured data among the connected IoT devices. AWS can support millions of devices connected in IoT. It communicates among the things with messages between AWS end points and other devices with high-end security. The wearable sensors are connected to AWS Cloud Platform. It tracks and communicates with all those wearable sensors for even a second even though there is no live internet connectivity. AWS gathers the data in regular time interval, and it analyzes the data and acts according to predefined data that are set in the control algorithm. It does not require additional infrastructure to manage the Big Data received by the sensors in real time.

The huge amount of data that are expected to be generated by BSNs requires a powerful and scalable storage and processing that is able to support both online and offline analyses of data streams. Such requirements can be met by an integrated platform based on Cloud computing [23] with the following characteristics: (a) the ability to utilize heterogeneous sensors; (b) scalability of data storage; (c) scalability of processing power for different kinds of analysis; (d) global access to the processing and storage infrastructure; (e) easy sharing of results; and (f) pay-as-you-go pricing for using BSN services [40, 41].

9.8.7 Analysis of Big Data

Data are aggregated in sequential time and analyzed by a fully managed service. It is very easy to analyze the massive volume of big data received by the wearable sensors connected in IoT. The usage of AWS cloud platform is available at low cost and least complexity to build a medical Internet of Things in a real time. It takes accurate and precise decisions in the absence of human with the help of advanced machine learning techniques. The wearable sensors provide the data of huge volume and different variety. Hence, traditional data analytics is replaced by special built-in intelligence to process the structured and variable data. The data received might have noises, corrupted data, and assumption of readings. They should be cleaned periodically to ensure the third-party access. AWS used in built data analytics filters and transforms, which could enrich IoT data. In a regular time instance, the series of sensor data are stored in a cloud of Amazon and it could be retrieved when it is necessary.

It is possible to set up the service to receive the required data with respect to the need and availability. It is possible to schedule queries of the stored data by utilizing the built-in SQL query engine. The complex data analytics might be done using a specialized machine learning algorithm by implementing the same with prebuilt models for common IoT use cases. It is possible to customize the data analytics with respect to the users need by tools such as MATLAB or Octave.

9.9 Conclusions

Wearable technology has motivated human being toward monitoring health and wellness. This review work focuses on the data analytics part in the wearable sensor and includes review on diabetes management, heart rate monitoring, and Alzheimer patient monitoring. This work summarizes techniques and devices materialized over the past few years and highlights on current methods using wearable sensor systems and systems in the area of clinical applications. The significance of researchers for tracking applications of wearable sensor-based systems has created a change in the field of wearable technology from the progress of sensors to the design of systems. Data analysis methods play an important role in the integration of wearable sensors for a variety of diseases. Integration of inputs from the different sensors helps the researchers to develop a model for remote monitoring of patients in home and hospitals. Researchers have developed methods to integrate multiple sensors in the remote monitoring systems so that monitoring could be carried in home itself. In future, robotics will be integrated into patient care monitoring systems to achieve the goal of establishing a telepresence in the home environment. Remote monitoring of patients in undergoing treatments will soon face challenges regarding the establishment of a variety of models to cover up the costs incurred for the whole process. The implementation problems will be important to promise that wearable sensors and systems communicate on their promise of improving the superiority of care provided to patients who are suffering from chronic diseases and ailments via monitoring of wellness remotely from home and hospitals.

Battery lifetime constraints play a vital role in determining the success of wearable sensors. Challenges encountered in interfacing machine with other machines as well as human need to be rectified. Security is key factor in present IOMT deices as huge data are handled in cloud. Connectivity issues while networking needs to be taken care. Data handling has to be enhanced by utilizing advanced machine learning algorithms. Sampling rate and speed of conversion should be taken care during the transmission of data through online.

References

1. D.V. Dimitrov, Medical Internet of Things and Big Data in healthcare. Healthcare Inform. Res. **22**(3), 156–163 (2016)
2. W. Raghupathi, V. Raghupathi, Big Data analytics in healthcare: Promise and potential. Health Inform. Sci. Syst **2**(1), 3 (2014)
3. D. Apiletti, E. Baralis, G. Bruno, T. Cerquitelli, Real-time analysis of physiological data to support medical applications. IEEE Trans. Inform. Technol. Biomed **13**(3), 313–321 (2009)
4. R. Dautov, S. Distefano, R. Buyya, Hierarchical data fusion for Smart Healthcare. J. Big Data **6**, 19 (2019). https://doi.org/10.1186/s40537-019-0183-6
5. R. Gravina, P. Alinia, H. Ghasemzadeh, G. Fortino, Multi-sensor fusion in body sensor networks: State-of-the-art and research challenges. Fusion **35**, 68–80 (2017)
6. G. Fortino, R. Giannantonio, R. Gravina, P. Kuryloski, R. Jafari, Enabling effective programming and flexible management of efficient body sensor network applications. IEEE Trans. Human-Machine Syst **43**(1), 115–133 (2013)
7. G. Fortino, A. Guerrieri, F. Bellifemine, R. Giannantonio, Platform-independent development of collaborative wireless body sensor network applications: SPINE2, IEEE international conference on systems, man and cybernetics, 2009.
8. S. Iyengar, F.T. Bonda, R. Gravina, A. Guerrieri, G. Fortino, A. Sangiovanni-Vincentelli, A framework for creating healthcare monitoring applications using wireless body sensor networks, Proceedings of the ICST 3rd international conference on Body area networks, 2010.
9. Y.J. Fan, Y.H. Yin, L.D. Xu, Y. Zeng, F. Wu, IoT based smart rehabilitation system. IEEE Trans. Ind. Inform **10**(2), 1568–1577 (2014)
10. S.M.R. Islam, D. Kwak, H. Kabir, M. Hossain, K.-S. Kwak, The Internet of Things for health care: A comprehensive survey. IEEE Access **3**, 678–708 (2015)

11. G. Fortino, P. Trunfio, *Internet of Things Based on Smart Objects: Technology, Middleware and Applications* (Springer Science & Business Media, Cham, 2014)
12. T.C. Arcadius, B. Gao, G. Tian, Y. Yan, Structural health monitoring framework based on Internet of Things: A survey. IEEE Internet Things J **99**, 1 (2017)
13. C. Savaglio, M. Ganzha, M. Paprzycki, C. Bădică, M. Ivanović, G. Fortino, Agent-based Internet of Things: State-of-the-art and research challenges. Futur. Gener. Comput. Syst **102**, 1038–1053 (2020)
14. G. Fortino, W. Russo, C. Savaglio, W. Shen, M. Zhou, Agent-oriented cooperative smart objects: From IoT system design to implementation. IEEE Trans. Syst. Man Cybernet. Syst **48**(11), 1939–1956 (2018)
15. L. Angelini, S. Carrino, O. AbouKhaled, S. Riva-Mossman, E. Mugellini, Senior living lab: An ecological approach to foster social innovation in an ageing society. Futur. Internet **8**(4), 50 (2016)
16. P. Bonato, Wearable sensors and systems. IEEE Eng. Med. Biol. Mag **29**(3), 25–36 (2010)
17. M. Zheng, P.X. Liu, R. Gravina, G. Fortino, An emerging wearable world: New gadgetry produces a rising tide of changes and challenges. IEEE Syst. Man Cybernet Mag **4**(4), 6–14 (2018)
18. S. Patel, H. Park, P. Bonato, L. Chan, M. Rodgers, A review of wearable sensors and systems with application in rehabilitation. J Neuroeng. Rehabil **9**(1), 21 (2012)
19. M. Pham, Y. Mengistu, H.M. Do, W. Sheng, Cloud-Based Smart Home Environment (CoSHE) for home healthcare, in *2016 IEEE International Conference on Automation Science and Engineering (CASE)*, (IEEE, 2016), pp. 483–488
20. Standards of medical care for patients with diabetes Mellitus, American Diabetes Association. Diabetes Care **26**(suppl 1), s33–s50 (2003). https://doi.org/10.2337/diacare.26.2007
21. C. Chinmay, Computational approach for chronic wound tissue characterization. Elsevier: Inform. Med. Unlocked **17**, 1–10 (2019). https://doi.org/10.1016/j.imu.2019.100162
22. S.H. Chang, R.D. Chiang, S.J. Wu, W.T. Chang, A context-aware, interactive M-health system for diabetics. IT Prof **18**(3), 14–22 (2016)
23. G. Alfian, M. Syafrudin, M. Fazalljaz, M.A. Syaekhoni, N. LatifFitriyani, J. Rhee, A personalized healthcare monitoring system for diabetic patients by utilizing BLE-based sensors and real-time data processing. Sensors (Basel) **18**(7), 2183. Published online 2018 Jul 6 (2018). https://doi.org/10.3390/s18072183
24. J.S. Lee, J. Heo, W.K. Lee, Y.G. Lim, Y.H. Kim, K.S. Park, Flexible capacitive electrodes for minimizing motion artifacts in ambulatory electrocardiograms. Sensors **14**, 14732–14743 (2014)
25. J.A.C. Patterson, D.C. McIlwraith, G.-Z. Yang, A flexible, low noise reflective PPG sensor platform for ear-worn heart rate monitoring, in *Proceedings of the Sixth International Workshop on Wearable and Implantable Body Sensor Networks*, (Washington, DC, USA, 3–5 June 2009), pp. 286–291
26. S. Yoon, Y.-H. Cho, A skin-attachable flexible piezoelectric pulse wave energy harvester. J. Phys. Conf. Ser. **557**, 012026 (2014)
27. Y.M. Chang, J.S. Lee, K.J. Kim, Heartbeat monitoring technique based on corona-poled PVDF film sensor for smart Appare l application. Solid State Phenom **124-126**, 299–302 (2007)
28. D. Buxi, J. Penders, C. van Hoof, Early results on wrist-based heart rate monitoring using mechanical transducers, in *Proceedings of the Annual International Conference of the IEEE Engineering in Medicine and Biology Society, Buenos Aires, Argentina, 31 August–4 September 2010*, pp. 4407–4410
29. G. Lu, F. Yang, Y. Tian, X. Jing, J. Wang, Contact-free measurement of heart rate variability via a microwave sensor. Sensors **9**, 9572–9581. Sensors 2015, 15 3234 (2009)
30. E. Suaste-Gómez, D. Hernández-Rivera, A.S. Sánchez-Sánchez, E. Villarreal-Calva, Electrically insulated sensing of respiratory rate and heartbeat using optical fibers. Sensors **14**, 21523–21534 (2014)
31. A. Sa-Ngasoongsong, J. Kunthong, V. Sarangan, X. Cai, S.T.S. Bukkapatnam, A low-cost, portable, high-throughput wireless sensor system for phonocardiography applications. Sensors **12**, 10851–10870 (2012)

32. A. Andreoli, R. Gravina, R. Giannantonio, P. Pierleoni, SPINE-HRV: A BSN-based toolkit for heart rate variability analysis in the time-domain, in *Wearable and Autonomous Biomedical Devices and Systems for Smart Environment*, (Springer, Berlin, 2010), pp. 369–389

33. R. Gravina, G. Fortino, Automatic methods for the detection of accelerative cardiac defense response. IEEE Trans. Affect. Comput **7**(3), 286–298 (2016)

34. Y. Zhang, R. Gravina, H. Lu, M. Villari, Giancarlo Fortino, Parallel electrocardiogram-based authentication for smart healthcare systems. J. Netw. Comput. Appl **117**, 10–16 (2018)

35. G. Wolgast, C. Ehrenborg, A. Israelsson, J. Helander, E. Johansson, H. Manefjord, Wireless body area network for heart attack detection [Education Corner]. IEEE Antennas Propag. Mag **58**(5), 84–92 (2016)

36. M.A. Cretikos, R. Bellomo, K. Hillman, J. Chen, S. Finfer, A. Flabouris, Respiratory rate: The neglected vital sign. Med. J. Aust **188**, 657–659 (2008)

37. G. Fortino, A. Guzzo, M. Ianni, F. Leotta, M. Mecella, Exploiting marked temporal point processes for predicting activities of daily living. ICHMS, pp. 1–6, 2020.

38. N. Zhu, T. Diethe, M. Camplani, L. Tao, A. Burrows, N. Twomey, D. Kaleshi, M. Mirmehdi, P. Flach, I. Craddock, Bridging e-Health and the Internet of Things: The SPHERE Project. IEEE Intell. Syst **30**(4), 39–46 (2015)

39. R. Gravina, C. Ma, P. Pace, G. Aloi, W. Russo, W. Li, G. Fortino, Cloud-based activity-a a service cyber–physical framework for human activity monitoring in mobility. Futur. Gener. Comput. Syst **75**, 158–171 (2017)

40. G. Fortino, D. Parisi, V. Pirrone, G. Di Fatta, Body Cloud: A SaaS approach for community Body Sensor Networks. Futur. Gener. Comput. Syst. **35**, 62–79 (2014)

41. M. Parimala Devi, G. Boopathi Raja, V. Gowrishankar, T. Sathya, (2020) IoMT-Based Smart Diagnostic/Therapeutic Kit for Pandemic Patients. In: Chakraborty C., Banerjee A., Garg L., Rodrigues J.J.P.C. (eds) Internet of Medical Things for Smart Healthcare. Studies in Big Data, vol 80. Springer, Singapore. https://doi.org/10.1007/978-981-15-8097-0_6

Chapter 10
A Healthcare Resource Management Optimization Framework for ECG Biomedical Sensors

Ammar Awad Mutlag, Mohd Khanapi Abd Ghani, and Mazin Abed Mohammed

10.1 Introduction

Healthcare is a vital aspect of life, offering various services such as medication, illness diagnosis and prevention, infections, accidents, and epidemic problems. There is a very long history of contact between technology and healthcare. With the assistance of technology, many healthcare apps are built to change our lives. Remote monitoring is one of the important features of healthcare which has many applications like telemedicine, electronic health (eHealth), and ambient assisted living (AAL). These applications provision remote monitoring and patient tracking for those who are living alone, those who are staying at hospitals, and those who are living in rural areas. Health parameters can be monitored through sensor devices which could be implanted or wearable sensors. Vital signs like heart pulses, body temperature, and the rate of respiratory can be conducted by wearable sensors in order to specify the situation of the patient either normal or critical. Other signs also can be conducted from the patients by sensors such as blood oxygen and blood pressure. Fall detection sensors can be implemented to detect patients. All these signs conducted by sensors will be sent wirelessly to be processed [1].

A. A. Mutlag · M. K. A. Ghani
Biomedical Computing and Engineering Technologies (BIOCORE) Applied Research Group,
Faculty of Information and Communication Technology, UniversitiTeknikal Malaysia
Melaka, Durian Tunggal, Malaysia
e-mail: khanapi@utem.edu.my

M. A. Mohammed (✉)
College of Computer Science and Information Technology, University of Anbar, Anbar, Iraq
e-mail: mazinalshujeary@uoanbar.edu.iq

Cloud computing provides powerful ICT services. Cloud computing technology has the ability to improve healthcare services. Cloud computing enables healthcare applications to implement infrastructure services to huge numbers of stakeholders with dynamic and assorted changing requirements [2]. Cloud computing has been developed in recent years in order to support many applications such as healthcare applications. While some healthcare application constraints have been overcome by cloud computing, some other challenges have been met by the cloud itself. The distance between the cloud and the end devices, which is not suitable for delay-sensitive applications and also results in high connectivity costs, is one of these challenges. Fog computing has been implemented in literature to deal with these problems, putting the services and resources at the edge of the network. Fog nodes, on the other hand, suffer from resource heterogeneity, instability, and dispersion, as well as processing, storage, and memory limitations. Therefore, to use these resources optimally, there is a need for a proper task scheduling strategy [3].

In this study, HRMO framework has a contribution in providing three levels of processing: edge, fog, and cloud. MAS plays the role of communicating among all processing levels. We provide a preprocessing in the edge of the network using personal agents to overcome the limitation of sensor processing. Then, the next level of processing is handled by fog node agents at fog level, in which each fog node has an agent responsible for prioritizing, scheduling, and processing. The third level of processing will be handled by cloud data centers for the normal tasks, and when all fog nodes are busy, critical tasks will be processed in cloud.

The rest of this paper is organized as follows: Section 10.2 is the literature review which consists of explanation of health monitoring importance and critical health-care tasks and a background of cloud computing and its limitation in healthcare applications and presents fog computing as a solution to cloud computing limitation, the implementation of a multi-agent system in cloud and fog computing, and the related work of using fog computing resource management. Section 10.3 presents the illustration of HRMO framework and the possible example scenario. Section 10.4 presents the research conclusion.

10.2 Literature Review

10.2.1 Health Monitoring

Many types of health monitoring in healthcare applications are implemented to provision a healthy life and increase wellness. The ratio of the aging population is increasing significantly. Health monitoring systems (HMS) have quickly grown in smart environments and turned to be a worthy alternative solution to traditional healthcare. The purpose of HMS is to provision e-health services on time to people who want to sustain their health. HMS help elderly people to prevent any connection with a hospital or home nursing and decrease health system demand. There are many types of health monitoring. The following are a few types:

- Heart disease prediction is a challenging task in the traditional healthcare system. Health monitoring system makes use of the data acquired from patient sensor devices via electronic health records (EHR). Monitoring the rate of heart pulses and blood pressure in real time by wireless sensors shows the situation of the heart in order to prevent heart attacks. ECG requires uninterrupted remote monitoring in order to save patient's life if adequate action is taken. Therefore, patients need to be monitored and transmitted to the hospital [4].
- Breathing disorders require reliable monitoring of long-term diagnosis in earlier phase to provision an enhancement of quality of life, life expectations, and medical history. Hence, real-time monitoring of breathing and its parameters is a crucial demand in healthcare applications [5].
- IoT wireless hospital sensor network (WHSN) integrated with a body area network (BAN) facilitates the mobility of patients and enhances their autonomy [35]. Wireless sensing for fault detection of various health attributes can be done through monitoring [6].

Real-time health attribute sensing for trainees can also be done through monitoring techniques to specify the factors that affect their health that may be affected by the environment that surrounds them. Coordination of multiple tasks is a popular challenge in complex environments and various domains such as healthcare. For example, assume the workflow of an emergency medical system that is responsible for a triage zone in a large smart city. The key roles for which the medical system is responsible for are, but not limited to, the triage of patients; the assessment of acute and non-acute patients; the drafting of medical order forms, blood tests, and imaging studies; the review of test results; the supervision of junior doctors; the coordination of treatment plans with other healthcare professionals, in both local and remote area; and the recording of findings. The medical system must recognize the tasks, describe task characteristics, define the relative significance of the tasks, and schedule them for execution. This is particularly crucial in complicated life-critical healthcare settings, which have many conditions where there are multiple tasks and limited resources for processing all tasks. The responsibility of the resource manager is to coordinate the emergency medical system resources while dealing with healthcare sensor tasks. In fact, it monitors, manages, and deploys the resources and infrastructures that provide solutions to healthcare. It can share, schedule, and balance the resources depending on the workload, task demand, and context. It also ensures a higher degree of resource access control. Furthermore, the resource manager specifies resource dependencies such that they can be run and executed in a suitable order. Various task scheduling procedures are implemented such as earliest deadline first (EDF), weighted fair queuing (WFQ), and first come first service (FCFS). FCFS enables high-speed task processing without additional computation, but it is unproductive as small-size tasks may be required to wait for the large ones to be completed and critical data may not be immediately processed due to the processing procedure that is based on the order of arrival time. Also, the EDF and WFQ scheduling scheme, which is usually used in the environment of IoT, face the problem of task termination because of the failure that may occur to the low-priority task. Moreover, it is difficult to decide on the proper task priority value [7].

10.2.2   Cloud and Fog Computing

The most important applications of cloud computing are healthcare. The information produced from healthcare is confidential, and in order to deliver superior healthcare quality, healthcare stakeholders must exchange patient and clinic information securely. Because healthcare data is a large data set in many different formats, the cloud computing environment is a powerful way to process and save the data. There are many types of healthcare data that are supported by cloud computing and provide numerous facilities, such as electronic health records (EHR). EHR includes information summary about patient care like progress notes, medications, demographics, diagnosis, vital signs, immunizations, imaging reports, laboratory data, and medical history. These data are accessible through several sites, making healthcare easily accessible for the patients [8]. Electronic medical record (EMR) is a reliable source of medical knowledge; it consists a comprehensive data of patient's health in an electronic style that the clinical decision support (CDS) can use. EMR data contain rich medical information like medical history, clinical diagnosis, treatment plans, radiology images, and results of lab tests [9].

Despite the numerous advantages of cloud computing, there are some limitations such as high delays [10]; it is also not possible to address the growing demands for real-time or latency-sensitive applications and limit network bandwidth by using only cloud computing.

Cloud computing has become a successful way to process, store, and retrieve certain information. Challenges, however, can still not be overcome by using only cloud computing, such as the increasing demands of applications responsive to real time or latency and the restriction of network bandwidth. The paradigm of cloud computing is a centralized computing model, with most computations taking place in the cloud. This means that it is necessary to transfer all data and requests to a centralized cloud. While the speed of data processing has increased exponentially, there is no sufficient increase in the network bandwidth. So, with such a large amount of data, the bandwidth of the network is the bottleneck of cloud computing. Long latency can result from this. Depending on the network speed and server loads, cloud computing can take a long time. The delays may be even longer, especially for mobile devices, because the wireless network bandwidth is relatively poor. For latency-sensitive applications such as healthcare applications, data transfer to a remote cloud will result in an unreasonable delay, especially if data analysis is designed to cause a real-time local response [11].

In recent decades, centralized or decentralized computational models have been debated depending on two main groups of issues: first, efficiency versus effectiveness to find a solution based on a rationalistic strategy and second, organization and resource politics. The centralized cloud computing paradigm has been adopted at the start of the 2000s. There is a need to transfer computation from centralized to a novel decentralized to overcome high latency, location awareness, etc. that may occur in a centralized approach. Shifting from centralized to decentralized introduced the term fog computing. The infrastructure paradigm of fog computing was first announced by Cisco Systems in 2012 [12]. Fog computing shifts the cloud services near to end user and provides computation, communication, and storage to edge network devices. Fog computing will perfectly fit the latency-sensitive or real-time application in which it will enable and increase mobility, privacy, protection, low latency, and network bandwidth. In ubiquitous healthcare systems, with mobility, energy consumption, scalability, and reliability problems, a fog-assisted device architecture can solve many challenges [13].

10.2.3   Multi-agent Systems

There is no unique definition for the agents. All agent definitions are inherited from the technology of agent (computer science, software engineer, artificial intelligence, cognitive science, etc.). The main idea of the agent is simple. A system entity that is able to execute autonomous actions is an agent. The agent doesn't need to wait to get instructions to do any action [14]. The agent is embedded by a programmer with desire, intentions, and beliefs; by these feeling agents will have the ability to guide their actions. Potentially, agents have the ability to manage the allocation of resources, specifically in distributed systems taking into account processing of the request, cost optimization, and service composition as essential factors [15] (Fig. 10.1).

The main role of the cloud is to provide on-demand services for consumers via the Internet [16]. Scheduling is one of the critical services in cloud computing [17] propose a multi-agent architecture to solve the problem of scheduling in cloud computing. In the same field, cloud monitoring system using multi-agent is presented in [18] that support gathering, scheduling, and execution of tasks and improving security performance in large-scale environment.

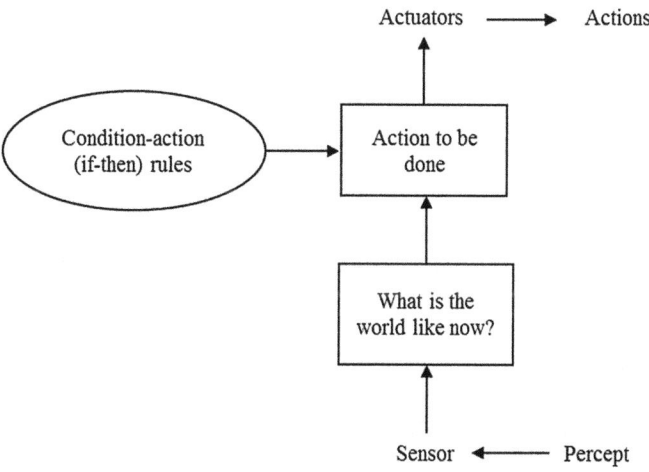

Fig. 10.1 An overview of an agent

Fog computing is a distributed computing framework that is front end that operates at the edge of networks, ensuring low execution time, scalability, energy consumption, latency, etc. [19] suggest a multi-agent system in mobile fogs for distributed computing offloading. Authors in [20] present a self-organizing agent-based model for rapid biological threat detection, which facilitates efficient monitoring of large-scale environments and precise detection of biological threats. An Open IoT fog agent was built in [21] in which the agent provides monitoring, link identification, autonomous action, and connection handling between the devices of the fog node and the container, whereas MAPS is an agent framework proposed in [22] for wireless sensor networks for the implementation of a real-time WBSN-based human activity monitoring system based on the Java-programmable Sun SPOT sensor platform.

10.2.4   Related Work

With the development of computing technologies, the connected devices in the world have increased in an unprecedented rate [23]. By 2030 the number of sensor-enabled objects connected to the network will rise to 75 billion, according to the International Data Corporation (IDC), and from 50 billion to 1 trillion connected devices [24]. There are different types of computers, sensors, and artifacts in fog computing, and all of them generate a huge amount of data that need to be processed; some of them are in a critical situation. Devices, sensors, and objects' requests will make full use of resources. In fog computing, therefore, resource management is indeed necessary, which must be treated carefully.

Resource management in fog computing improves the performance of healthcare applications, especially in emergency cases. Few studies have been carried out on fog computing resource management [25] propose two fog computing resource management schemes: fog resource reallocation and fog resource reservation. In the same context, [26] focus on resource allocation and management using seamless handover scheme with efficient algorithm. Similarly, [27] proposed a refinement of resource management technique to improve resource management by considering execution time. In the same vein, [28] propose a resource management simulator, called iFogSim. Application scheduling and application placement are the main job of this simulator. iFogSim provides an environment of fog computing and IoT and evaluates the effect of resource management in energy consumption, latency, cost, and network congestion, whereas [29] argue task distribution, virtual machine placement, and base station association by integrating MCPS with fog computing (FC-MCPS).

Stackelberg sub-game has been applied in the proposed framework for the interaction between DSOs and ADSSs. For DOSs and FNs interaction, moral hazard modeling has been used, and student project allocation matching sub-game has been applied in [30]. An integration of spare resources called crowd-funding is presented in fog computing structure by [31], whereas [32] propose a scheme in fog computing called MIST, to support crowd sensing, and for limited resource cost provisioning, the authors investigate task distribution, a data consumer association, and virtual machine.

Similarly, with [31], a virtual resource tool has been created by collecting limited resources with distributed devices called "crowd-funding" [33] and developed a game prototype to get the number of optical devices that contribute perfectly through Nash equilibrium feedback. A new scheduling algorithm was proposed in [34], and the future theoretical game plan is designed to solve the issue of application admission control management and dynamic vehicle resources. The decentralized algorithm is designed in [35] using game theoretical tools to coordinate device decisions with periodic tasks and manage the computing and communication resources for computation offloading in fog computing. Multi-agent fog computing (MAFC) model was proposed in [36], in which MAS was employed to offer a scheduling optimization among fog and cloud.

10.3 Healthcare Resource Management Optimization Framework

In this section, the healthcare resource management optimization (HRMO) framework is presented. It contains three tiers: global area network, fog tire, and cloud tire. The main contribution of this framework is the employment of fog computing to overcome cloud computing resource management limitation and provision of a superior response, especially to critical healthcare tasks. Fog computing has the ability to provide links to the cloud [37]. The architectures of fog move communication, storage, computer, decision-making, and control to the edge of the network where information is generated to resolve current infrastructure constraints to allow mission-critical, data-dense use cases [38]. In contrast to the centralized cloud, fog offers geo-distributed environment through fog nodes. The fog tier has the power of distributing the analytics and data processing throughout the network and enabling the system, due to its widely distributed deployments, to provide basic locally critical services, and a distributed system that is controlled locally in order to offer high quality of services. In this framework, fog computing nodes will be connected in order to share computing resources (Fig. 10.2).

(a) *User tier: personal agents*

In this layer, all patient's wearable sensors are connected to the network. Each sensor group is linked to the nearest node through a wireless connection. The first layer in the HRMO framework is the global area network; it consists of sensors and personal agents. Each sensor group is linked to a single personal agent. This tier has two main tasks:

- Sensing: Sensing signals will be handled by the sensors. It will include the software and hardware components and the responsibility of gathering data

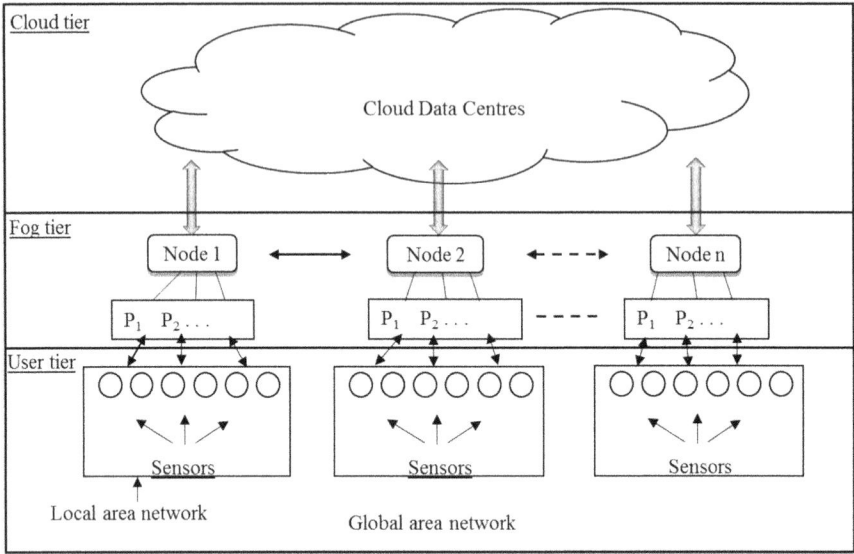

Fig. 10.2 The HRMO framework

from patients. For row sensed data for each group of patients, a PA will sort the incoming signals according to their criticality, in which the normal patient signal is transmitted to the cloud and abnormal signals are transmitted to the fog tier in order to operate a pre-processing.

- Perception: The observed data by the sensor of a signal from the perception of the patient situation. According to sensed data, the personal agent will attach the appropriate task and forward it to the fog tier.

(b) *Fog tier*

As mentioned above, fog computing tier is employed to overcome cloud computing limitations as well as provide a superior response for healthcare critical tasks. A number of nodes compose this layer, each node responsible for a group of sensors. Fog nodes responsible for processing critical healthcare tasks, in which tasks will be divided into normal and abnormal tasks. Normal tasks will be forwarded immediately to cloud computing, whereas abnormal tasks will be handled by fog nodes, and the result of processing critical tasks will be sent to the cloud in order to update patient's record. The micro datacenter in fog computing having a group of servers will distribute all the tasks to handle the load of the arrived requests, allowing dynamic load balancing in a fog domain between fog nodes upon the arrival and exit of a task. So, in this framework, we propose that fog computing nodes are connected to each other in order to share their resources. If an overload occurs in any fog node, then the incoming tasks will be forwarded to the nearest node according to available resources at that node.

(c) *Cloud tier*

The top tier of the proposed work is cloud tier, in which all the signals that are sensed by the sensors in user tier "global area network" will be stored permanently; by that EHR for each patient will be updated. Cloud tier will support fog computing tier in two things: First, processing tasks in case all the nodes in fog computing tier are busy. Second, cloud tire will provide EHR for each patient to fog computing tier in order to schedule the tasks.

10.3.1 Multi-agent System Role in HRMO Framework

MAS' job contributes the response to the situation of an abnormal patient. Sorting the tasks according to each patient's priority would then greatly enhance reducing response time, as well as saving the entire life of the patient with a highly critical situation. On the other hand, MAS handles the resources of the network wherein the cost of constructing enormous resources is reduced. Agents will assume responsibility for communicating between third parties. A group of personal agents (PAs) can manage the patient's sensor signals. Each sensor group is linked to a single personal agent. The primary task of PAs is to prioritize incoming signals by defining the normal and abnormal tasks. Normal tasks are forwarded to the cloud stage, and abnormal tasks are immediately forwarded to the fog node agent (FNA).

10.3.1.1 Personal Agents (PAs)

A group of personal agents (PAs) will handle the patient's sensor signals. Each sensor group is linked to a single personal agent. The primary task of PAs is to prioritize incoming signals by defining the normal and abnormal tasks. Normal tasks are forwarded to the cloud stage, and abnormal tasks are immediately forwarded to the fog node agent (FNA). Following are explanation of each tier in the model. Following are the PAs' algorithm.

Algorithm 1 forming a local task list based on PAs' priorities.
Input: sensed tasks T from connected sensors
Output: list of sorted critical C and normal N data

if T = C then do,

      update priority list (P)
else,

      set T as N
end if

10.3.1.2   Fog Node Agents (FNAs)

It has three main components:

- Task prioritization module: All the data and its tasks type will arrive tasks prioritization module with their priorities from many personal agents. Task prioritization module has a global view of the tasks, in which a re-evaluation process will re-evaluate all the tasks from different personal agents according to their priority. Task prioritization module will receive the cost from cost function in order to dynamically reprioritize the tasks. Algorithm 2 shows the prioritization steps.

Algorithm 2 forming a global task list based on FNA priorities.
Require (input): algorithm 1 // criticality C of every task in Personal Agent (PA)
Ensure (output): Priority Decision Table (PDT)

1. The C of T is calculated for all PAs // reprioritization globally among all PAs
2. The normal (N) of T is calculated for all PAs
3. Empty priority list (P) and stack (S)
4. Push the C into stack S in decreasing order
5. While the stack S is not empty do
6. If top (S) is not the highest critical C then
7. S ← the highest critical C
8. Else
9. P ← top (S)
10. pop top (S)
11. End if
12. End while

- Task scheduling module: Three main decisions will be produced by this module: execute locally, execute in neighbor, and execute in the cloud. Task scheduling module will get the cost and available resources from cost function, according to the cost and the history of each patient; through EHR from the cloud, tasks are scheduled. Algorithm 3 shows the steps of scheduling.

Algorithm 3 scheduling-based priority and resource availability
Input: Priority Decision Table (PDT)
Output: Property Tasks

1. // call algorithm 2 to form the list of tasks based on priorities
2. Get local node Available Resources
3. Get local node Used Resources

(continued)

5. Get global nodes available resources
6. Get global nodes used resources
7. Get cloud available resources
9. Resource Availability Decision Table (RADT) is created
10. Load Balancing Decision Table (LBDT) is created
11. Check for appropriate resources

> If,
> Found in local node available resources
> Then
> Deploy task
> Deployed = true

12. Else if,

> Global Resources Able to Host Extra Task then
> Deploy task
> Deployed = true

13. Update local and global available and used resources
14. Else

> Cloud Resources Able to Host task then
> Deploy task
> Deployed = true

15. End if
16. If deployed then
17. Return successful

- Task processing module: each fog node agent has its own processing module with predefined processing resources. Current workload is sent to cost function.

10.3.2 Example Scenario of the HRMO Framework

The following scenario example shows the contribution of the HRMO framework in responding to critical healthcare tasks by providing on-demand resources. A patient's ECG signal is used in this scenario. ECG signal is a complex signal, and it affects the patient's life. QRS is the high frequency of ECG signals. The period of the QRS complex indicates that the ventricles are working suitably. If there are any problems associated with the heart, QRS may become shorter or widened when ventricles of the atria have more muscle mass. QRS5 complex is greater than the P wave [32–34]. Figure 10.3 shows the QRS complex.

Heart rate, R-R interval, and QRS duration are the main parameters used to QRS complex analysis; all these parameters are described in the following sections.

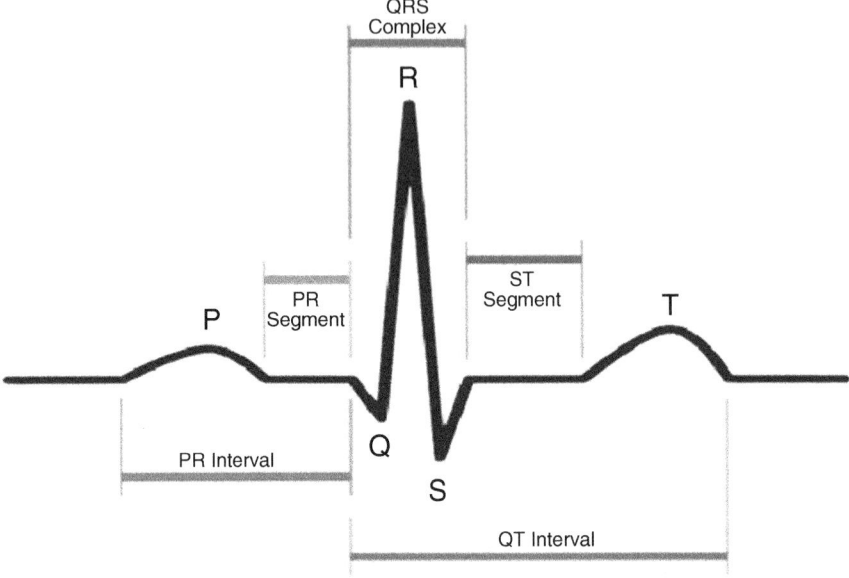

Fig. 10.3 The QRS complex

Heart rate is the rate of heart pulses that can be calculated using the following equation:

$$\text{Heart rate} = 60 / \text{RR interval in second} \qquad (10.1)$$

R-peak is the largest peak in the ECG signal. The number of samples can be divided between two peaks of R to calculate R-R interval and signal frequency sampling. Using this procedure, the abnormalities of the signal can be calculated.

QRS duration: In order to find QRS complex duration of ECG, the number of samples is divided between signal frequency sampling and QRS complex. By calculating duration, the signal can be recognized as normal or abnormal. 0.6–0.10 seconds is the range of normal ECG signal.

In this part, the smart city deployment scenario will be explained to demonstrate the fluency of the work and the efficiency of the work proposed. When at the smart city, IoT sensor connectivity is usually given through the sensor's Bluetooth connection and patient's Internet access. Each group of homes is connected to the nearest fog node. The personal agent will be responsible to collect, detect, and send the critical tasks to fog node. Normal tasks are transmitted immediately to the cloud.

10.3.3 Example Use Case for Deployment Scenario

In this section, we show smart home example of typical healthcare use cases and its deployment. Figure 10.4 shows the HRMO use case architecture.

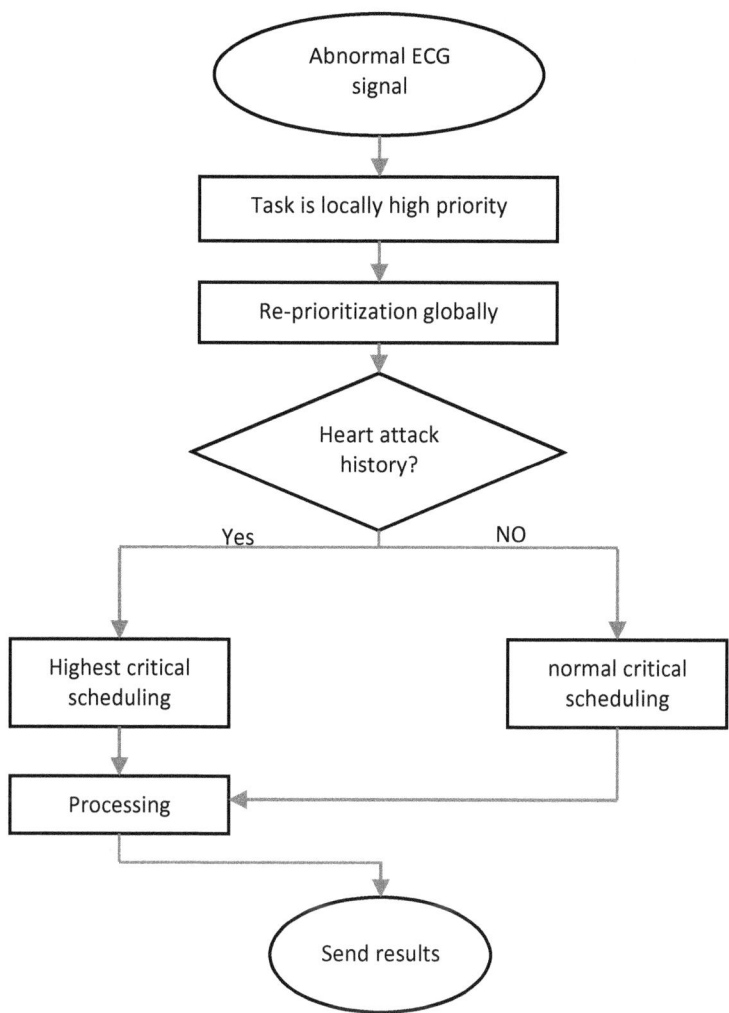

Fig. 10.4 HRMO use case architecture

- Smart home: Monitoring a patient's ECG signals is an example of IoT smart home deployment scenario. A fog node is located on the LAN tier of the network. Fog computing is used to receive, save, and process sensors' critical raw data, before transferring it to the cloud for permanent storage. The main contribution of fog computing is to reduce latency and network traffic.

Let as assume that 100 elderly patients are living in smart city. Each 25 patients are connected to the nearest fog node. Patients are equipped with ECG wearable sensors. When 5 out of 25 patients have unstable ECG signals, the personal agent will attach these signals with local high priority and forward them to fog node agent.

Table 10.1 RR, heart rate, and QRS of ECG signals

Signal	RR interval (sec.)	Heart rate (beats/min)	QRS duration (sec.)	Condition
Normal signal	0.791	75.84	0.094	STANDARD
Signal 1	0.877	68.41	0.093	NORMAL
Signal 2	0.911	65.83	0.088	NORMAL
Signal 3	1.059	56.65	0.238	ABNORMAL
Signal 4	0.80	75.00	0.080	NORMAL
Signal 5	0.516	116.07	0.197	ABNORMAL
Signal 6	0.78	76.90	0.083	NORMAL
Signal 7	0.45	133.33	0.162	ABNORMAL

In fog node agent, task prioritization module will reprioritize in global view among all attached personal agent tasks. Local, neighbor, and cloud workloads will be provided continuously by cost function. Task scheduling module will schedule the tasks according the following conditions:

(a) If the patient has a history of heart attack, they will be scheduled as critical. If not, the patient with a history of attack will be scheduled first.
(b) If the cost function shows that the local workload has enough resources, then processing will be done locally. If not, by collaborative function, scheduling module will check the neighbor workload and decide either sending to a neighbor or putting in waiting list according to available resources and job completion time. If not, it will do the same procedure with the cloud workload. The RR interval, heart rate, and QRS duration are calculated in Table 10.1.

10.4   Conclusion

This research aims to establish a resource management framework for healthcare applications. Subsequently, this study proposes the employment of fog computing as an intermediate layer. Fog computing has been used in order to overcome cloud computing limitation, especially in resource management, and to provide a superior response to healthcare critical tasks. A deployment smart home scenario has been explained to show the contribution of the proposed framework in the management of complex healthcare environment. In the future, we will enhance the framework to process all the types of vital signs at the same time.

Acknowledgments This research has been supported by BIOCORE research group of Universiti Teknikal Malaysia Melaka, Malaysia.

Conflict of Interest "The authors declare no conflict of interest."

References

1. T. Nguyen Gia et al,. Low-cost fog-assisted health-care IoT system with energy-efficient sensor nodes, 2017 13th international wireless communications and mobile computing conference IWCMC 2017, pp. 1765–1770, July, 2017.
2. A. Abdelaziz, M. Elhoseny, A.S. Salama, A.M. Riad, A machine learning model for improving healthcare services on cloud computing environment. Meas. J. Int. Meas. Confed **119**, 117–128, 2018 (2017)
3. M.R. Alizadeh, V. Khajehvand, A.M. Rahmani, E. Akbari, Task scheduling approaches in fog computing: A systematic review. Int. J. Commun. Syst **2019**, 1–36 (2019)
4. G. Yang et al., A Health-IoT platform based on the integration of intelligent packaging, unobtrusive bio-sensor, and intelligent medicine box. IEEE Trans. Ind. Inform **10**(4), 2180–2191 (2014)
5. A.R. Fekr, K. Radecka, Z. Zilic, Design and evaluation of an intelligent remote tidal volume variability monitoring system in E-health applications. IEEE J. Biomed. Health Inform **19**(5), 1532–1548 (2015)
6. O. Salem, Y. Liu, A. Mehaoua, R. Boutaba, Online anomaly detection in wireless body area networks for reliable healthcare monitoring. IEEE J. Biomed. Health Inform **18**(5), 1541–1551 (2014)
7. L.H. Barg-Walkow, W.A. Rogers, Modeling task scheduling in complex healthcare environments: Identifying relevant factors. Proc. Hum. Factors Ergon. Soc **61**, 772–775 (2017)
8. B. Aldosari, Patients' safety in the era of EMR/EHR automation. Inform. Med. Unlocked **9**, 230–233 (2017)
9. C. Zhao, J. Jiang, Y. Guan, EMR-based medical knowledge representation and inference via Markov random fields and distributed representation learning. Artif. Intell. Med. **87**, 49 (2017)
10. H. Abbas, S. Shaheen, M. Elhoseny, A.K. Singh, M. Alkhambashi, Systems thinking for developing sustainable complex smart cities based on self-regulated agent systems and fog computing. Sustain. Comput. Inf. Sys **19**, 204–213 (2018)
11. Z. Musa, K. Vidyasankar, A fog computing framework for Blackberry supply chain management. Procedia Comput. Sci. Elsevier B.V **113**, 178–185 (2017)
12. F. Bonomi, R. Milito, J. Zhu, S. Addepalli, Fog computing and its role in the internet of things, in *MCC'12 - Proceedings of the 1st ACM Mobile Cloud Computing Workshop*, (2012), pp. 13–15
13. A.A. Mutlag, M.K. Abd Ghani, N. Arunkumar, M.A. Mohammed, O. Mohd, Enabling technologies for fog computing in healthcare IoT systems. Futur. Gener. Comput. Syst. **90**, 62–78 (2019)
14. G. Fortino, W. Russo, E. Zimeo, A statecharts-based software development process for mobile agents. Inf. Softw. Technol. **46**(13), 907–921 (2004)
15. G. Fortino, A. Garro, W. Russo, Achieving Mobile Agent Systems interoperability through software layering. Inf. Softw. Technol. **50**(4), 322–341 (2008)
16. G. Fortino, A. Guerrieri, W. Russo, C. Savaglio, *Internet of Things Based on Smart Objects* (Springer, Cham, 2014)
17. Y. Liu, L. Wang, Y. Wang, X.V. Wang, L. Zhang, Multi-agent-based scheduling in cloud manufacturing with dynamic task arrivals. Procedia CIRP **72**, 953–960 (2018)
18. D. Grzonka, A. Jakóbik, J. Kołodziej, S. Pllana, Using a multi-agent system and artificial intelligence for monitoring and improving the cloud performance and security. Futur. Gener. Comput. Syst. **86**, 1106–1117 (2018)
19. M.G.R. Alam, Y.K. Tun, C.S. Hong, Multi-agent and reinforcement learning based code offloading in mobile fog, International conference on information networking, pp. 285–290, 2016.
20. M. Al-Zinati, Q. Al-Thebyan, Y. Jararweh, An agent-based self-organizing model for large-scale biosurveillance systems using mobile edge computing. Simul. Model. Pract. Theory **93**, 65 (2018)

21. S. Hoque, M.S. De Brito, A. Willner, O. Keil, T. Magedanz, Towards container orchestration in fog computing infrastructures. Proc. Int. Comput. Softw. Appl. Conf. **2**, 294–299 (2017)
22. F. Aiello, F.L. Bellifemine, G. Fortino, S. Galzarano, R. Gravina, An agent-based signal processing in-node environment for real-time human activity monitoring based on wireless body sensor networks. Eng. Appl. Artif. Intel. **24**(7), 1147–1161 (2011)
23. G. Fortino, D. Parisi, V. Pirrone, G. Di Fatta, BodyCloud: A SaaS approach for community Body Sensor Networks. Futur. Gener. Comput. Syst. **35**, 62–79 (2014)
24. M. Mukherjee, L. Shu, D. Wang, Survey of fog computing: Fundamental, network applications, and research challenges. IEEE Commun. Surv. Tutor, 1–1 (2018)
25. J. Li, C. Natalino, P. Van Dung, L. Wosinska, J. Chen, Resource management in fog-enhanced radio access network to support real-time vehicular services, Proceedings of the 2017 IEEE 1st international conference on fog and edge computing ICFEC 2017, pp. 68–74, 2017.
26. H.A.M. Name, F.O. Oladipo, E. Ariwa, User mobility and resource scheduling and management in fog computing to support IoT devices, 7th international conference on innovative computing technology INTECH 2017, pp. 191–196, 2017.
27. G.C. Jana, S. Banerjee, Enhancement of QoS for fog computing model aspect of robust resource management, 2017 International conference on intelligent computing, instrumentation and control technologies ICICICT 2017, vol. 2018-Janua, pp. 1462–1466, 2017.
28. H. Gupta, A. Vahid Dastjerdi, S.K. Ghosh, R. Buyya, iFogSim: A toolkit for modeling and simulation of resource management techniques in the Internet of Things, Edge and Fog computing environments. Softw. - Pract. Exp. **47**(9), 1275–1296 (2017)
29. L. Gu, D. Zeng, S. Guo, A. Barnawi, Y. Xiang, Cost efficient resource management in fog computing supported medical cyber-physical system. IEEE Trans. Emerg. Top. Comput. **5**(1), 108–119 (2017)
30. H. Zhang, Y. Zhang, Y. Gu, D. Niyato, Z. Han, A hierarchical game framework for resource management in fog computing. IEEE Commun. Mag. **55**(8), 52–57 (2017)
31. Y. Sun, N. Zhang, A resource-sharing model based on a repeated game in fog computing. Saudi J. Biol. Sci. **24**(3), 687–694 (2017)
32. H.R. Arkian, A. Diyanat, A. Pourkhalili, MIST: Fog-based data analytics scheme with cost-efficient resource provisioning for IoT crowdsensing applications. J. Netw. Comput. Appl **82**, 152–165, 2017 (2016)
33. Y. Sun, F. Lin, Non-cooperative differential game for incentive to contribute resource-based crowd funding in fog computing. Bol. Tech. Bull. **55**(8), 69–77 (2017)
34. J. Klaimi, S.M. Senouci, M.A. Messous, Theoretical game approach for mobile users resource management in a vehicular fog computing environment, 2018 international wireless communications and mobile computing conference IWCMC 2018, pp. 452–457, 2018.
35. S.Dana Jošilo, G. Dán, Poster abstract: Decentralized fog computing resource management for offloading of periodic tasks, pp. 1–2, 2018.
36. A.A. Mutlag et al., MAFC: Multi-agent fog computing model for healthcare critical tasks management. Sensors (Switzerland) **20**(7), 1853 (2020)
37. P. Tirumala Rao, S. Koteswarao Rao, G. Manikanta, S. Ravi Kumar, Distinguishing normal and abnormal ECG signal. Indian J. Sci. Technol. **9**(10), 1 (2016)
38. A. Kishor, C. Chakraborty, W. Jeberson, Reinforcement learning for medical information processing over heterogeneous networks. Multimedia Tools Appl.. Springer (2021). https://doi.org/10.1007/s11042-021-10840-0

Chapter 11
Diabetes Detection and Sensor-Based Continuous Glucose Monitoring – A Deep Learning Approach

G. Swapna and K. P. Soman

11.1 Introduction

Diabetes is a disease that makes the body incapable of metabolizing glucose effectively and leads to hyperglycaemia (presence of abnormally large amount of glucose in the blood). Hyperglycaemia means raised blood sugar. Two reasons can lead to diabetes. One is because the pancreas does not generate sufficient insulin. Second is due to the inability of the cells to react to this generated insulin. The insulin hormone, produced by beta cells in the pancreas, regulates the metabolism of fats, proteins and carbohydrates contained in our food and promotes blood glucose absorption to the liver.

Diabetes types are types 1 and 2 and gestational diabetes. General diabetic symptoms are frequent urination, increased hunger and thirst and deficiencies in vision. But these indications are not that pronounced at the early stages of diabetes. They become visible only after some period. By that time, there exists a possibility that diabetes might have worsened to the stage of complications. Hence, it is very important that diabetes have to be diagnosed at the start itself. Diabetes, if not managed, causes severe damages to body organs like the heart, kidneys, blood vessels, eyes and nerves over time.

According to the statistics of the World Health Organization (WHO), the number of diabetes-affected people was 108 million in 1980, whereas in 2014, it was 422 million. Globally, 4.7% of the adults in 1980 had diabetes, while it increased to 8.5% in 2014. There was a 5% increase in premature mortality due to diabetes in 2000–2016 period. In 2020, according to the International Diabetes Federation

G. Swapna (✉) · K. P. Soman
Center for Computational Engineering & Networking (CEN), Amrita School of Engineering,
Coimbatore, Amrita VishwaVidyapeetham, Coimbatore, India
e-mail: kp_soman@amrita.edu

© The Author(s), under exclusive license to Springer Nature Switzerland AG 2021
C. Chakraborty et al. (eds.), *Efficient Data Handling for Massive Internet of Medical Things*, Internet of Things,
https://doi.org/10.1007/978-3-030-66633-0_11

(IDF), diabetes has affected 463 million (9.3% of the total population) people worldwide. This may reach 10.2% (578 million) by 2030 and 10.9% (700 million) by 2045. Out of the 463 million people, 88 million belong to Southeast Asia region. Of this 88 million people, 77 million belong to India. Underdeveloped countries are still more affected. Taking USA as an example of developed countries, about 34.2 million US people (10.5% of the US population) have diabetes as per the National Diabetes Statistics Report 2020. Of the above, around 21.4% did not even know that they have diabetes (undiagnosed diabetes). Taking India as a case of developing countries, India (which has the second largest diabetes population in the world) has 8.9% of its total population affected by diabetes. Kerala is its state with the highest number of diabetic people. The prevalence of diabetes in Kerala is about twice that of national average. Related to diabetes-caused consequences, the WHO has stated that in 2015, diabetes was the cause for 1.6 million deaths globally.

Commonly used diabetes detection method is the clinical means of conducting a blood test which is invasive. Allowable levels of fasting blood sugar are in the range 70–110 mg/dL. Below 70 condition is hypoglycaemia. Glucose level can rise above 110 in the case of food intake. But in the case of normal persons, blood sugar will not exceed 180 however much food is taken. The above 180 condition is hyperglycaemia, which indicates diabetes.

There are two other diabetes detection management-related tests – oral glucose tolerance test (OGTT) and haemoglobin A1c (HbA1c) test. OGTT detects the presence of gestational diabetes in pregnant woman. After oral intake of required quantity of sugar contained drink, blood test is conducted at the prescribed time intervals. Above 200 value of blood glucose indicates diabetes. HbA1c test is an important test which tells how good the diabetes management is. It gives information about the overall blood glucose management levels for the past 2–3 months. It measures the amount of blood sugar associated with haemoglobin. Haemoglobin carries oxygen from the lungs to the remaining parts of the body. HbA1c means glycated haemoglobin. Haemoglobin, when attached to blood glucose, is known as glycated haemoglobin or haemoglobin A1c. HbA1c value larger than 6.5% is indicative of diabetes.

Popular diabetes detection test is an invasive test of taking blood sample from a person suspected of diabetes and testing it [51].

Diabetes detection by analysing HRV is a novel automated method which achieved very high accuracy of above 90%. Initially machine learning (ML) techniques were employed for that task. Machine learning came before deep learning (DL). In ML, feature engineering and employment of the best of classifiers are essential which demanded complete domain knowledge of the system. In deep learning, there is no need of much domain knowledge as no features need to be explicitly extracted. With the advent of deep learning era, a wide variety of DL architectures like CNN, LSTM and autoencoder were developed which were very effective in analysing vast amount of data and arriving at conclusions with high accuracy and very less processing time. Since diabetes is a condition without cure, just like timely detection, effective management is also of same or of more importance.

Before the deep learning networks are ready for testing/analysing new data, these networks are to be trained. In particular, analysis of biomedical data which is highly complex and highly dimensional and with a possibly heterogeneous and unstructured mix of vital data components is a very challenging task for which the best tool is deep learning architectures. One of the constraints in employing deep learning networks in healthcare is the insufficient availability of labelled test data. But the research progressing on the networks which are capable of handling semi-supervised and unsupervised data and concepts like reinforcement learning are making DL applications more and more feasible in biomedical area. Piccialli et al. [49] give valuable information on applications of deep learning methods in medicine.

Diabetes management is extremely important, especially in those patients showing large variations of blood glucose values. Ten years back, only about 7% of type 1 diabetes patients used CGM sensor-based devices. In recent times, due to the technological advancement in various aspects like cost and size along with improved accuracy in the measured values, CGM use has increased considerably, especially in developed countries.

CGM devices, in general, and depending on their lifetime too, have a store of gigantic amount of data, analysis of which can be only done by employing deep learning techniques. Fast and accurate analysis of data is extremely beneficial especially in acute diabetic patients with high hyperglycaemia and for those showing huge variations of blood glucose values to avert life-threatening hypoglycaemic events and for giving a notice when very high BG values are recorded.

Technology has developed to the extent of combining an insulin pump with CGM so as to give a controlled flow of insulin into the body based on CGM values. Deep learning networks have a great role to play in making the decisions very accurate and very fast. Specialized deep learning networks have the capability of predicting near future critical events by the analysis of the temporal behaviour of the data. Almost every healthcare-related data analytics is moving to deep learning. Deep learning has a great role to play in sensor-based devices in healthcare and especially in sensor-based diabetes management.

This chapter reviews two main aspects of diabetes – diabetes management using sensors and non-invasive detection of diabetes using HRV. Real-time monitoring and analysis of the vast data collected by CGM devices can even save the life of patient by being capable of giving timely alerts on occurrences of dangerous hypo-/hyperglycaemic events. In latest systems, information can reach in real time to doctors through email or to his mobile. Wireless technologies are also used in an adjunct manner with CGM devices.

Managing and analysing vast amount of CGM data, that too may be at multiple levels of hospital/doctor/caretaker/patient, in a distributed and parallel manner, is a challenging task which can be effectively handled by deep learning. Another direction of research is the aggregation of CGM data from various CGM devices of specific group of people. A different requirement is combining CGM data along with important patient specific information from health records and/or other medical devices/sensors ultimately aiming at the creation of a data management system, analysis of which can give valuable information to further steps needed for diabetes management (Fig. 11.1). The accurate and varied analysis of this complex gigantic data can be performed only by deep learning networks.

One main constraint in employing deep learning, especially in diabetes care-related healthcare system, is the necessity of having large amount of labelled data to train the network before we feed the actual data as input. As said before, instead of such supervised learning methods, research is also advancing to semi-/unsupervised learning methods. Active research is also going on to produce low-cost CGM devices and make them successfully work in non-adjunctive manner. Once the minimally invasive nature of CGM sensor and the need for frequent calibrations are done away with, the use of CGM devices will increase manifold. This book chapter touches some important aspects of the above topics.

In CGM systems, detection of anomaly and prediction of future anomalies in a fast manner are the main requirements. In this context, we discuss how deep learning networks/algorithms are used to detect diabetes non-invasively using HRV data taking into consideration the fact that the popular and commonly used clinical method of diabetes detection is the invasive blood test method. Deep learning methods achieve very high accuracy of above 95% in the non-invasive detection of diabetes. We discuss briefly the related machine learning/deep learning works on that topic.

In this chapter, Sect. 11.2 discusses in detail diabetes management under which continuous glucose management (CGM) and different devices for CGM and connected topics are covered. Section 11.3 discusses the format and analytics of CGM data. Section 11.4 discusses diabetes detection using HRV making use of machine learning and deep learning methods, along with brief details of works which establishes the dependence of diabetes-cardiac health-HRV. Section 11.5 gives brief details about deep learning techniques used in the detection of diabetes and which can be used in analysis of CGM data in diabetes management. Section 11.6 tells of challenges in CGM sensors along with a brief description of a few non-CGM sensors used in healthcare. Section 11.7 concludes the chapter.

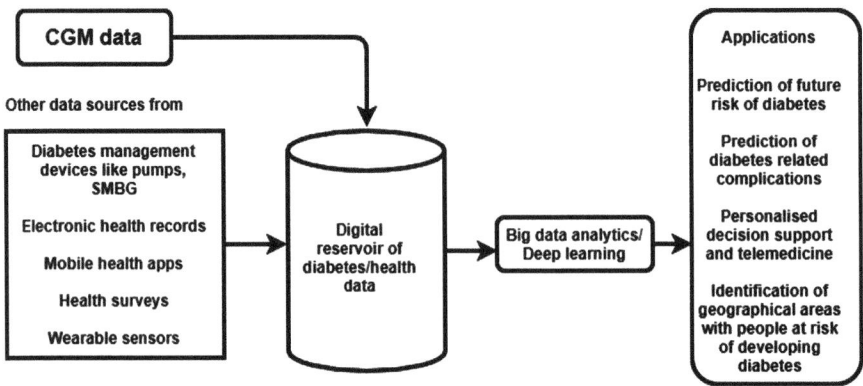

Fig. 11.1 Aggregation of CGM data with other data sources to form useful applications

11.2   Management of Diabetes

Diabetes is incurable. Hence, proper management by means of medication, food and physical activity is essential in order to make the blood glucose (BG) values close to normal levels. In acute cases, management of diabetes is extremely difficult.

Diabetes variability and HbA1c are two important metrics showing effectiveness of diabetes management. Diabetes variability indicates the fluctuation of important parameters around the average value over the designated time duration. Diabetes variations can only be known by continuous measurements similar to what is done in CGM devices. To monitor whether diabetes is under control, people who have diabetes have to undergo HbA1c test regularly to see if their BG levels are staying within allowable range.

The management of diabetes took a big leap in 1921 with the discovery of insulin. When diabetes progresses beyond that can be managed by oral medication, subsequent step is subcutaneous multiple-dose insulin therapy which means injection of insulin subcutaneously many times daily. For still acute patients or possibly for the acute category of type 1 diabetic patients, the controlling method is subcutaneous continuous insulin therapy (also known as insulin pump). This is an insulin delivery technique which uses a battery-operated medical device to infuse insulin in a continuous manner into the diabetic person. This device contains battery and internal processing unit to control the insulin delivery.

Closed-loop insulin therapy (also known as artificial pancreas) can be considered as the next modification of insulin pump. This is a closed-loop system, and it integrates insulin pumps with CGM system. Information from the real-time glucose data is of potential use to control insulin dispensed through insulin pump. In this chapter, we concentrate on the diabetes management involving CGM systems.

Self-monitoring of blood glucose (SMBG) is an important process used in diabetes management. Here diabetic people measure their BG themselves using glycaemic reader (glucose metre). Portable blood glucose metres where current BG values are found out by testing small amount of blood from the fingertip are called glucometers. Patient can thus adjust their treatment (medication, diet, exercise etc.) based on this readings. Traditional self-monitoring of blood glucose is done through a glucometer. Sensors have no role to play here.

Now, we will move into discussing CGM in detail. They are relatively new techniques to measure glucose levels involving detection of interstitial glucose. Continuous glucose monitoring (CGM) or flash glucose monitoring (FGM) both make use of sensors. Flash glucose monitors will give the BG value and its trends only when its sensor is scanned. FGM technology is sometimes known as intermittent continuous glucose monitoring (iCGM). FreeStyle Libre belongs to the category of FGM device. CGM sensors are capable of providing BG values almost continuous for several days, and it can be said with conviction that CGM sensors have revolutionized diabetes management.

Sensors for continuous glucose monitoring Continuous glucose monitoring is essential for effective diabetes management to reduce the risks of shooting up of glucose levels on one hand and the dipping to the case of hypoglycaemia on the other hand. It provides BG details every 1–5 minutes, thus giving the information of possibility of BG variations and trend. CGM provides hypo-hyper-glycaemic events whose details are not evident in SMBG.

Glucose-oxidase-based sensing is the commonly used sensing technique in CGM sensors. A platinum electrode is doped with glucose-oxidase. Needle with the electrode fitted at its end is then inserted in the tissue just beneath the skin. Glucose oxidation is triggered resulting in the formation of hydrogen peroxide and gluconolactone. Finally, this glucose concentration is measured as variations of electrical current by means of a calibration process using a glucose metre reading corresponding to sample blood samples of the patient itself (as part of SMBG process). Calibrations are needed for maintaining the accuracy level of glucose sensors. Calibration of the device is done using a few SMBG samples collected by the patient [1]. Calibrations which are needed to be done on daily basis are cumbersome and lead to the development of some sensors which don't require calibration at this rate.

The most common parameter used to rank CGM devices' accuracy is mean absolute relative difference (MARD). MARD is computed using the difference between the CGM readings and the values measured at the same time by the reference measurement system.

CGM sensors The first real-time CGM system which the diabetes patient can use personally is Guardian Real-Time CGM system by Medtronic which gave BG value for every 5 minutes for 3 days with MARD of 15%. Lifetime was more (7 days) for Dexcom SEVEN Plus with a MARD of 16.7%. Abbott Freestyle Navigator by Abbott Diabetes Care is a glucose sensor. Though with low lifetime of 5 days, it has a MARD of 12.8%.

More recent sensors are as follows.

Enlite CGM system by Medtronic has a wear time up to 6 days with MARD of 13.6%. It is compact in size and weight and waterproof. Further, it had the memory capacity to store up to 10 hours of BG data. Freestyle Navigator II, by Abbott, was another CGM system which could give BG readings every minute with a MARD of 12.3%.

G4 Platinum by Dexcom has a sensor-based CGM which has a lifetime of 7 days with a MARD of 13% which was later improved to 9%. Dexcom later introduced G5 mobile which has the same MARD and lifetime as G4 Platinum with the additional improvement of being capable to transmit the BG data to the user's cellphone. The Dexcom G5 mobile system is the first CGM system to receive FDA approval for non-adjunctive use (i.e. to make CGM-based treatment decisions).

FreeStyle Libre by Abbott with a MARD of 11.4% and 14 days lifetime and more improvements like the absence of need of fingerstick while wearing the sensor-based device. It needs no calibrations, but gives a performance similar to devices which require calibrations to the extent of minimum twice per day (Freestyle Navigator and G4 Platinum). It belongs to flash glucose monitoring FGM device category that gives glucose information when it is sought by the patient but continuously measures glucose values. G6 by Dexcom (in 2017) has a lifetime of 10 days, needs no calibrations and has accuracy the same as G5 Mobile. Guardian Sensor 3 by Medtronic (2017) has a lifetime of 7 days. It is small sized with an accuracy of 10.6% and MARD of 9.1% and a shorter startup time [13] (Table 11.1).

In the 90-day lifetime Eversense CGM system, the interstitial glucose value is computed every 5 minutes using fluorescence and radio-frequency-based technology. The values and/or alerts (when values go above and below thresholds) can be transmitted to the patient/doctor's smartphone through Bluetooth by the demountable transmitter attached to the sensor over the skin [14]. A variety of parameters can be computed from this vast 90-day-long glucometric data. Some important parameters are the mean, coefficient of variation (CV), median, standard deviation (SD) and interquartile range (IQR). These parameters are computed for different conditions (e.g. for different glucose ranges). Figure 11.2 below shows a sample CGM device being worn by a patient.

Alarms in CGM Alarms in CGM are very essential as an intervening feature to prevent extreme hypo- and hyperglycaemic events. Characterization of CGM alarm performance is not as easy as it may appear at first thought as alarms are dependent on threshold set. Alarms are to be quickly cross-checked for false alarm alerts with SMBG devices. The alarms can be in audible or in vibration mode,

Table 11.1 Some features of CGM devices

CGM type	Manufacturer	MARD (%)	Lifetime (days)	Remarks
Guardian Real-Time	Medtronic	15	3	BG value given every 5 minutes
SEVEN Plus	Dexcom	16.7	7	
Freestyle Navigator	Abbott	12.8	5	
Enlite	Medtronic	13.6	6	Can store up to 10 hours of BG data
Freestyle Navigator II	Abbott	12.3	5	BG value given every minute
G4 Platinum	Dexcom	Initially 13%, later reduced to 9%	7	
G5 Platinum	Dexcom	9	7	Cellphone of the user can get the BG data directly from the CGM device
FreeStyle Libre	Abbott	11.4	14	No calibration required, FGM device
G6 (2017)	Dexcom	10	10	No calibration required
Guardian sensor 3 (2017)	Medtronic	9.1	7	Shorter startup time
Eversense (2016)	Senseonics	11.4	90	Very large lifetime, no calibrations needed, optical sensing based

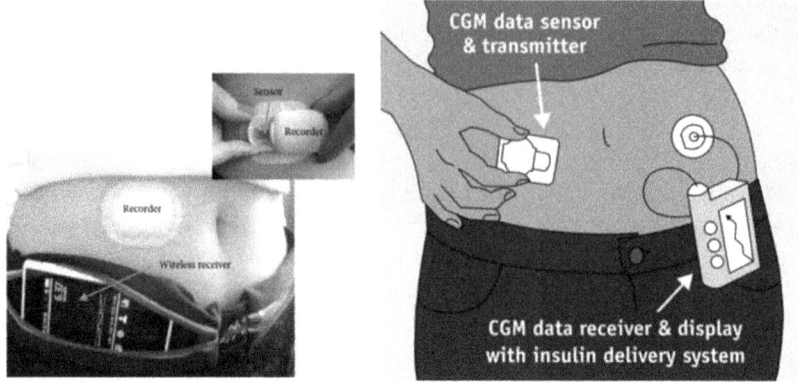

Fig. 11.2 A patient with CGM device. (Left side figure courtesy: Cai et al. [12], Right side figure courtesy: U.S. Food and Drug Administration)

according to the preference and need of patient. It is a topic which can bring in much improvization for the benefit of patient like increasing the volume depending on time like day/night. Another feature may be the facility to send a very fast alert to the doctor as a part of remote monitoring system.

There are two important modes of data collection from CGM sensors: retrospective analysis and real-time analysis.

Blinded data collection and retrospective data analysis Here the continuous data collected by the CGM sensors are not displayed to the patients wearing it, but the doctor/caretaker can review the data at the end of the monitoring period. Examples of such sensors are FreeStyle Libre Pro system by Abbot and IPro2 by Medtronic. At the end of the monitoring period, retrospective data analysis can be conducted to extract important parameters and glycaemic variability patterns can be studied to fix the diabetic management therapy needed by the patient.

Ambulatory glucose profile (AGP) can be placed under this section. AGP is a standardized one-page report which provides daily glycaemic pattern variations and summary statistics. Several software exist for providing retrospective data analysis. Some examples are Medtronic CareLink, LibreView and Dexcom Clarity. It includes summary statistics including glucose profile graph.

Real-time data collection There are another set of CGM systems which allow the individual/patient (whose blood glucose is measured by the device) to view in real time information of BG and its trends on suitable receiver or in a smartphone application. Examples are Medtronic's Guardian and Enlite and Dexcom's G5 Mobile and G6. Even the Eversense (by Senseonics) which primarily does the retrospective data analysis has the provision to alert the patient when the BG level crosses allowable upper and lower limits to detect dangerous hypo-/hyperglycaemic events. Newly introduced FGM systems also have alerts.

11.3   CGM Data – Format and Analytics

As the technology of CGM progressed, several improvements are incorporated; one such improvement is on the longevity of the sensor. It is in June 2018 that Eversense CGM system, with 90-day lifetime sensor, got Food and Drug administration (FDA) approval. It is a huge leap achieved in sensor lifetime and a big relief to patients considering the fact that present CGM sensors are minimally invasive. From the measured glucose values corresponding to the 90-day wear period, several parameters can be extracted out of it. Sanchez et al. [53] had given a listing of some of these extracted parameters in his study to highlight the benefits of the Eversense CGM device. Examples of these parameters are mean, glucose measurement index (GMI), coefficient of variation (CV), standard deviation and median interquartile range of the measured glucose values provided by the CGM sensor to mention a few. These parameters are calculated for different times like for 24-hour period, for night time, for 30-day wear period. All are patient-specific parameters extracted from the CGM data.

Vettoretti et al. [62] have given examples of many parameters that can be extracted from the CGM data. Excluding those mentioned above, some others are minimum and maximum of all sensor glucose values, the number of glucose values greater than a fixed set threshold value, the total duration of time the glucose values were above a set threshold value, below another set threshold value, minutes spent in the range of 70–180 mg/dl, same measure as a percentage of the total time CGM device was worn and the approximate area under the glucose curve.

This is the general case for CGM devices. It records glucose values continuously, say for every 5 minutes, day and night, for the entire wear period of the sensor (sensor lifetime dependent). From these glucose data, a variety of patient-specific parameters as mentioned above can be extracted. In addition to that, certain parameters which tell about the credibility of the CGM device like sensor reinsertion rate, safe data, sensor accuracy and transmitter wear time can also be assessed. These CGM device parameters tell us how reliable, accurate and safe are the measured glucose values.

A variety of glucometric reports like AGP can give a better representation of diabetes management. Figure 11.3 gives a sample AGP report. It contains glycaemic trends represented by a graph along with his health index parameters like heart rate, blood pressure etc. In addition, the report contains patient-specific input data of his food intake and insulin administration dose and time.

In order to know the regular trends, the day-to-day glucose values are superimposed to obtain a variation pattern. Figure 11.4 gives a sample of such a superimposed CGM value curve.

Figure 11.5 shows the sample of an average curve obtained from the scattered curves collected on all the days corresponding to wear time of the sensor. The average curve values are clinically very useful to ascertain the condition of the patient.

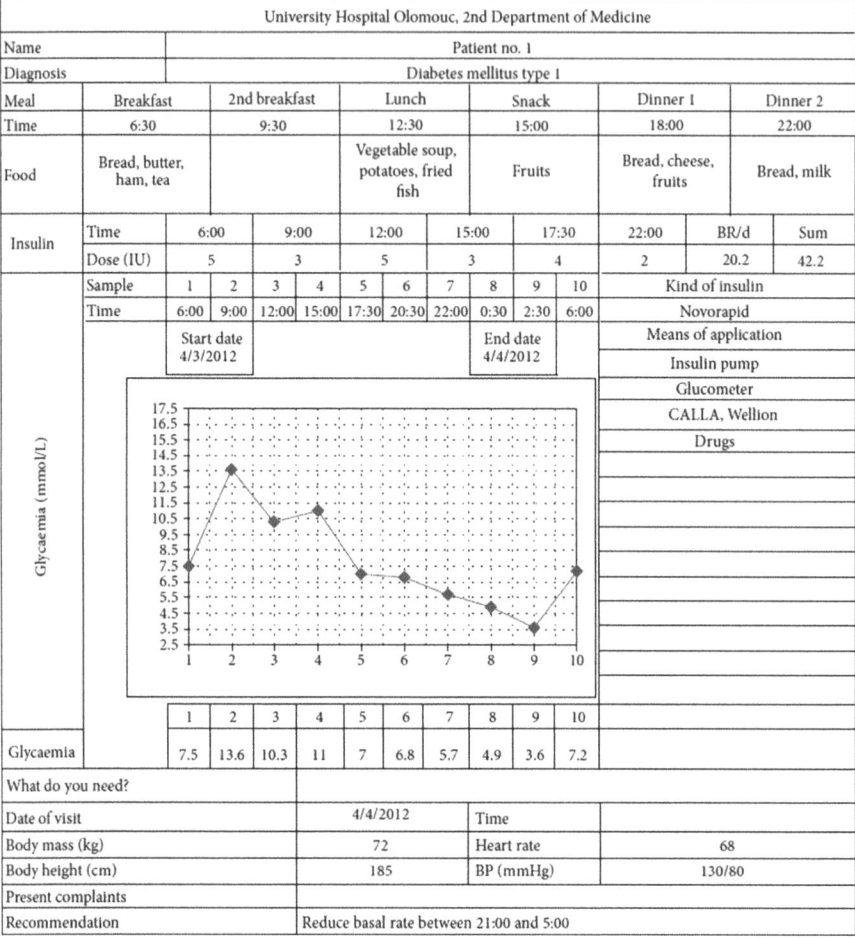

Fig. 11.3 Sample AGP report. (Courtesy: Chlup et al. [16])

11.4 HRV-Based Diabetes Detection and Related Works

ECG is a recorded biosignal which is obtained based on the fact that when the myocardial tissue (cardiac muscular tissue) is electrically depolarized, a minute current
is produced which can be captured by electrodes placed on the body. Electrical
representation of the heart's working is ECG. Typical ECG waveform is generated
as follows: sinoatrial (SA) node activates atrial depolarization to give rise to P wave.
Next is depolarization through atrioventricular (AV) node and then followed by the
activation of bundle of His and Purkinje system leading to ventricular depolarization producing the QRS component. Since the muscle content of ventricles is much
larger than that of atria, the QRS complex is much dominant and large compared to

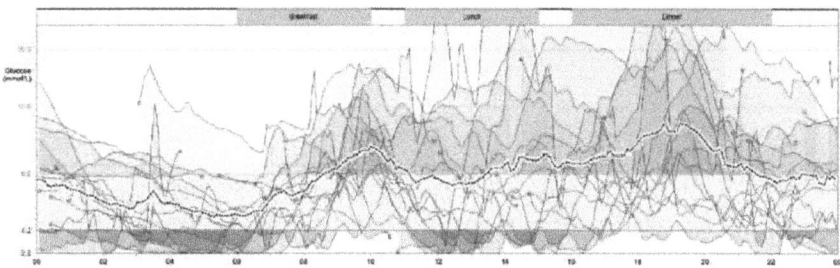

Fig. 11.4 Superimposed CGM traces. (Courtesy: Hammond [34])

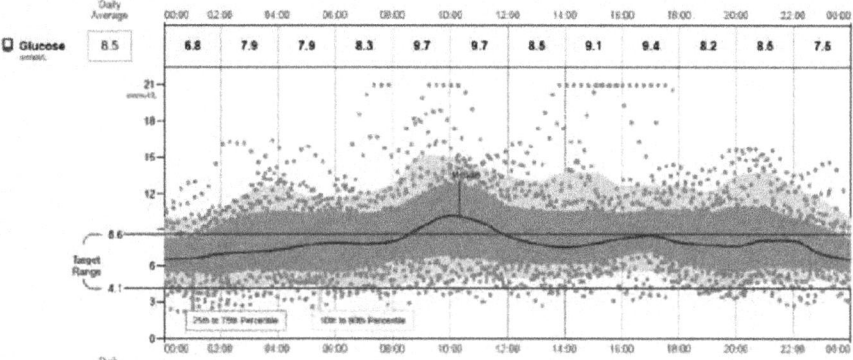

Fig. 11.5 Clinically relevant average values obtained from scattered data points. (Courtesy: Hammond [34])

P wave. PR interval indicates the duration of AV nodal conduction. Atrial repolarization hasn't been found connected to any ECG wave component, while ventricular repolarization gives rise to T wave. The complete duration of ventricular depolarization and repolarization represents the QT interval.

Diabetes causes changes in ECG signal and thus in HRV too. ECG is the PQRST waveform as shown in below Fig. 11.6. Normal ECG is the 12-lead ECG generated using 10 electrodes attached to the skin.

ECG reflects the role of autonomic nervous system (ANS) in controlling the heart's rhythm. The deformities in ST segment, QRS and P-wave in ECG waveform are indicators of disease affecting the heart.

Cardiovascular autonomic neuropathy (CAN), which negatively affects the normal functioning of the ANS, is a diabetes-related complication. CAN due to diabetes can cause ECG deviations such as ST-T and HRV alterations, left ventricular hypertrophy, long QTc, sinus tachycardia and QT dispersion. It is observed that there is correlation between QT duration in ECG and amount of coronary calcium. In diabetes-affected people, fibrotic changes in the basal area of the left ventricle have been very frequently observed even at the stage when cardiac abnormalities are not clinically evident. Gravina and Fortino [29] used ECG signals to assess even

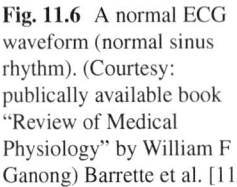

Fig. 11.6 A normal ECG waveform (normal sinus rhythm). (Courtesy: publically available book "Review of Medical Physiology" by William F Ganong) Barrette et al. [11]

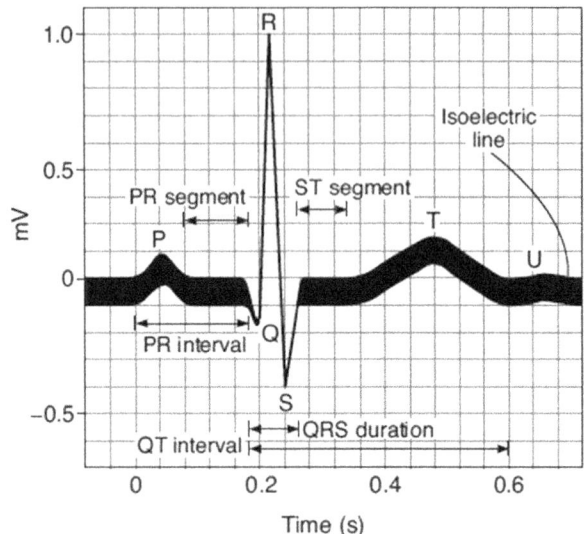

the emotional states like fear by detecting cardiac defence response. Zhang et al. [66] proposed a parallel ECG-based authentication system with improved authentication stability using ECG feature extraction and analysis methods.

The difficulty in ECG analysis is due to the fact that the morphologies of ECG waveform can show vast differences even when it is connected with the same person. Because of this, the performances of many biosignal analysis techniques which use ECG signals as input aren't up to the mark. Osowski et al. [46] showed that higher-order spectrum (HOS) techniques are less sensitive to ECG morphological variations. An ECG recognition system using HOS features and support vector machine (SVM) was developed by them. Instead of using the original ECG signal as input, Engin [23] used features that were a combination of autoregressive model coefficients, higher-order cumulant and wavelet transform variances as input to the fuzzy hybrid neural network classifier they developed for the analysis of ECG. Here, the non-stationary information was captured by the wavelet transform section, and non-Gaussian information was analysed by the HOS part, and together they could reduce the effect of variations due to ECG morphological changes.

Instead of ECG, we discuss the role of HRV signals extracted from ECG for analysing cardiac health. Unlike the analog ECG signal, HRV is a discrete data where shape parameter is irrelevant. HRV is the time sequence data indicative of the heartbeat variations. It corresponds to the instantaneous heart rate. HRV represents the cumulative changes happening in ANS because of hyperglycaemia caused by diabetes. HRV signals are simple, reproducible and accurate and can be easily processed. Thus, analysing HRV is like conducting a test to know the health of cardiac system and correctness in the working of ANS which in turn is responsible for normal heart rate. Andreoli et al. [7] used HRV time domain analysis in their body sensor network-based tool kit which can serve as a useful aid to cardiologists.

Diabetes and its effect on heart rate   SA node is the natural pacemaker of the heart producing heartbeat. But the heart rate is influenced also by the effect of both parasympathetic and sympathetic nervous systems (PNS, SNS). SA node operates at its intrinsic rate in the absence of any of inputs from SNS and PNS. Normal resting heart rate is decided by the parasympathetic vagus nerve. Increased parasympathetic effects lead to decreased heart rate, while increased sympathetic effects increase heart rate.

Diabetic neuropathy causes considerable morbidity and increases mortality by damaging the nervous system due to effect of the high blood glucose condition of diabetes. The chance of incidence of heart diseases and stroke will be double for diabetes patients compared to those without diabetes. Diabetes promotes atherosclerosis (hardening of arteries) due to hyperglycaemia. Microvascular complications (diabetic microangiopathy) manifest in the form of thickened capillary basement membrane and increased vascular permeability. Large blood vessel (macrovascular) complications of diabetes lead to mortal events like coronary artery diseases.

The time duration between two consecutive QRS complexes is termed as NN or RR interval. The continuous time series of these non-uniform values is the heart rate (HR) signal. These RR or NN intervals are given the name heart rate variability (HRV) data. HRV represents variations in instantaneous heart rate. HRV data, which is thus a true representation of ANS, is now widely used as a non-invasive tool, analysis of which accurately represents the ANS health.

The following three Tables 11.2, 11.3, and 11.4 give the summary of all works relating diabetes-cardiac health-HRV (Table 11.5).

11.5   Deep Learning for Diabetes Detection and Management

Insulin pumps can work better when integrated with CGM sensors, and such integrated devices have started coming commercially since 2006. Such combined systems can, for example, discontinue insulin inflow into the body when BG values

Table 11.2 Summary of works on diabetes and cardiac health

Author of study	Result
ARIC study (1987–1989) [7]	Found that autonomic cardiac function worsened in a progressive manner in diabetic patients throughout the 9-year period they investigated
Stamler et al. [59] Coutinho et al. [19]	Confirmed the relationship between fasting value of blood sugar and cardiovascular issues
Di Carli et al. [20]	Explains how hyperglycaemia promotes vasoconstriction
Di Carli et al. [20] Gresele et al. [33]	Explains how hyperglycaemia leads to endothelial impairments and aggregation of platelets
Victor et al. [63]	Explains how hyperglycaemia leads to cardiovascular malfunctioning independent of presence of influencing factors like abnormally high cholesterol or fat levels, high blood pressure and overweight

Table 11.3 Summary of works on the reproducibility of HRV and its significance in analysing cardiac health (with input signal as HRV)

Author	Method	Result obtained
Goldberger and West [32] Pincus [50]	Theory of chaos and nonlinear dynamics	Quantified the dynamics related to heart rate variations
Kleiger et al. [41] Ge et al. [31]	–	The reproducibility of HRV measurements and the easiness by which it can be conducted
Emily et al. [22]	Time-related parameters like SDNN	HRV can detect cardiac autonomic dysfunctions at a much earlier stage compared to clinical autonomic function tests
Allyson et al. [6]	Nonlinear parameter detrended fluctuation analysis (DFA)	DFA can reflect changes in HRV. Their study was to identify cardiac disease (those which are quite undetectable by clinical means) using HRV
Sun et al. [60] Mohammed et al. [44] Acharya et al. [2] Chua et al. [17]	Nonlinear techniques using ECG signal instead of HRV	Developed cardiac arrhythmia detection algorithms
Chua et al. [18]	HOS and SVM	Accurate classification of HRV signals to normal category and 4 different arrhythmia categories

Table 11.4 Summary of works on the significance of HRV for analysis of diabetes-induced CAN and diabetes (using HRV as input signal)

Author	Method	Result
Pfeifer et al. [48] Singh et al. [55] Villareal et al. [64]	RR variations SDNN, high and low frequency power Linear and nonlinear dynamics of HRV	Showed declined parasympathetic autonomic activity in diabetes patients much before clinical tests gave those indications thus emphasizing the connection between diabetes and HRV data
Mackay [43]	–	HR variation was noticeably diminished in diabetic patients compared to normal people
Kirvela et al. [40]	Time/frequency parameters	All time domain/frequency parameters of HRV were significantly reduced
Awdah et al. [10]	Time domain features like NN50, SDRR etc.	Significant reduction in parameters values for those with diabetes
Herbert et al. [35]	Tone entropy (TE) feature	TE feature reduction in diabetic people (with absent early history of cardiac disease)
Chemla et al. [15]	Autoregressive spectral analysis	Depressed HRV in diabetic people
Emily et al. [22]	Time domain parameters like RR interval, SDNN etc.	All parameters showed lower value in diabetic people than nondiabetic people
Ahamed Seyd et al. [54]	Many time/frequency domain features	Parameters reduced for diabetic people
Trunkvalterova et al. [61]	Multiscale entropy method, RR variability features (e.g. RMSSD)	Type 1 diabetes young patients' minute cardiovascular impairments were detected
Robert et al. [52]	Total RR variability	Features showed reduction for type 1 and type 2 diabetes patients

Table 11.5 Automated diabetes detection works using HRV data as input

Author	Techniques/parameters	Accuracy (%)
Acharya et al. [3]	Nonlinear (CD, RQA)	86
Swapna et al. [56]	Higher-order spectrum	90.5
Jian and Lim [39]	Higher-order spectrum	79.93
Acharya et al. [4]	Nonlinear	90.0
Acharya et al. [5]	DWT	92.02
Pachori et al. [47]	EMD	95.63
Swapna et al. [57]	Deep learning (DL)	95.1
Swapna et al. [58]	DL	95.7
Yildirim et al. [65]	DL	97.62

are predicted to reduce to threshold preset values in another half an hour. The prediction algorithm performs glucose prediction 15 minutes earlier the event is supposed to occur, making use of Kalman filter working on model-based algorithm using concept of risk function, and arrive at the required attenuation levels for insulin infusion in the event of predicted hypoglycaemia (i.e. if the BG concentration is below 80 mg/dL) [36]. The prediction of future values based on the analysis of a sequence of past data can be done very effectively by deep learning network (e.g. LSTM). If the prediction algorithm is very accurate, then a patient with fluctuating BG values can be treated at home under real-time conditions rather than in clinic under controlled conditions.

The sensor-based wearable devices like CGM systems collect a lot of data. The need of this vast data analysis has led to the development of automated systems which can analyse and arrive at accurate decisions in no time. These decision-making tools are developed so as to make diabetes disease management more effective [45]. If more real-time processing capabilities are added to the devices, quick action can be taken by the patients/doctors. The employment of deep learning techniques can make that 'quick' really to 'super-quick'. Decision support systems (DSS) for diabetes have been a developing area in diabetes management. Deep learning which is highly effective in automated collection, aggregation and analysis of loads of sensor-collected data is fast gaining prominence in healthcare and in diabetes management. When clubbed with transmission through wireless modes, tele-monitoring systems are developed which can serve as a great assisting tool specially in the case of young type 1 diabetic (T1DM) patients to prevent hypo-/hyperglycaemic events [38]. Diabetes management using DSS is a substitute to artificial pancreas (AP) (a closed-loop system). The artificial pancreas is not presently widely accepted by patients as they are not fully confident that the device that specially incorporates insulin pump is foolproof. Many patients prefer DSS-assisted open loop systems. The popularization of deep learning techniques can be used for building up patients' confidence level on closed-loop systems.

Different types of deep learning architectures are available. Researchers have used these architectures for a variety of tasks involving biosensors, starting from anomaly detection to prediction (Table 11.6).

Table 11.6 Some important deep learning architectures

Description	Special features	Architecture
Recurrent neural network (RNN) – RNN makes use of the sequential nature of data	RNN is useful in analysing time series data like text, speech etc. where an element of the sequence are dependent on the elements that appeared before it. This is achieved by a hidden memory in RNN	RNN and unfolded RNN
Long short-term memory (LSTM) – a variant of RNN resistant to vanishing gradient problem	LSTM is capable of learning long-term dependencies by the inclusion of 4 interacting layers and 3 gates (input, forget and output gates)	Memory units of RNN (left) and LSTM (right)
Gated recurrent unit (GRU) – variant of RNN. GRU is also resistant to vanishing gradient problem	3 gates of LSTM replaced by 2 gates – update gate and reset gate. Simpler internal structure, faster training time and lesser number of needed computations compared to LSTM	
Convolutional neural network (CNN) – CNN makes use of the spatial geometry of the input	It mainly applies convolutional and pooling operations and are applied along time dimension for audio and text data and along 2 dimensions for images	
Autoencoder (AE) – unsupervised learning based, used for dimensionality reduction	AE tries to recreate the input as its target (output). Encoder part converts the input to a compact form, while decoder recreates the input from this compact form	

The deep learning works for diabetes detection using HRV is mentioned earlier. The sample architectures of two researches in automated diabetes detection with HRV as input using deep learning network is given in the below diagram. In the work of Swapna et al. [57], CNN-LSTM combination gave the maximum accuracy of 95.1% (Fig. 11.7 (left figure)), while Swapna et al. [58] showed an improved accuracy of 95.7% with SVM added (Fig. 11.7 (right figure)).

CGM has a great role in diabetes management, but randomly made measurements won't help much. Real benefit will be obtained by collecting large-scale data using CGM devices in home and analysis of this real data using efficient CGM data management systems.

11.6 Challenges, New Technologies and Sensor-Based Data Analytics

Body sensor network (BSN) (also known as body area network (BAN)) refers to wireless network of wearable computing devices in human body. Iyengar et al. [37] presented a framework of healthcare monitoring applications using BSN. Fortino et al. [24, 25] gave valuable information on the development of a variety of BSN applications. Fortino et al. [26] highlighted the software framework programming aspects and effective management of BSN applications. Fortino et al. [27, 28] proposed and detailed the latest technology and future challenges in cloud-assisted community BSN applications. Gravina et al. [30] gave the latest information on data fusion in BSN.

CGM sensors and its connected network fall under BSN. CGM sensors are minimally invasive. The difficulties associated can be further researched to be mitigated to possible lower levels. Glucose-oxidase-based electrochemical sensors generally don't exhibit a linear response corresponding to the relevant biological parameter ranges. The accuracy of the measured value depends on the availability of the biological enzyme surrounding the electrode surface inserted. Delays in measurement will not affect retrospective glucose data, but it will affect real-time analysis. Research is going on further improving desirable parameters like sensor lifetime, sensor size and other useful features.

Research on development of new modes of sensing methods instead of glucose-oxidase based is also progressing. Instead of the conventional electrochemical sensors, research is going on in the area of optical sensing. There are some hindrances in using optical fibres practically due to lack of biocompatible fibre materials, complex readout approaches, time-consuming fabrication processes and slow response of the system. Elsherif et al. [21] have demonstrated the quantification of glucose by smartphone-integrated fibre optics that overcomes existing technical limitations, and their system achieved a high sensitivity (2.6 μW mM-1), rapid response and high glucose selectivity in the physiological glucose range.

Until recently, CGM devices mostly were used along with SMBG. Confirmation of CGM readings was done by glucometer-based SMBG. Past CGM sensors suffered from accuracy problems due to plasma-to-interstitium kinetics, calibration-related issues and presence of artefacts and interfering material like acetaminophen. Presently CGM is fast approaching the state of being used independently without the backing of glucometer-based confirmation. MARD is reducing to below 10% levels. All these are paving way to non-adjunctive use of CGM devices. In 2014–2015, many CGM sensors like FreeStyle Libre, Dexcom

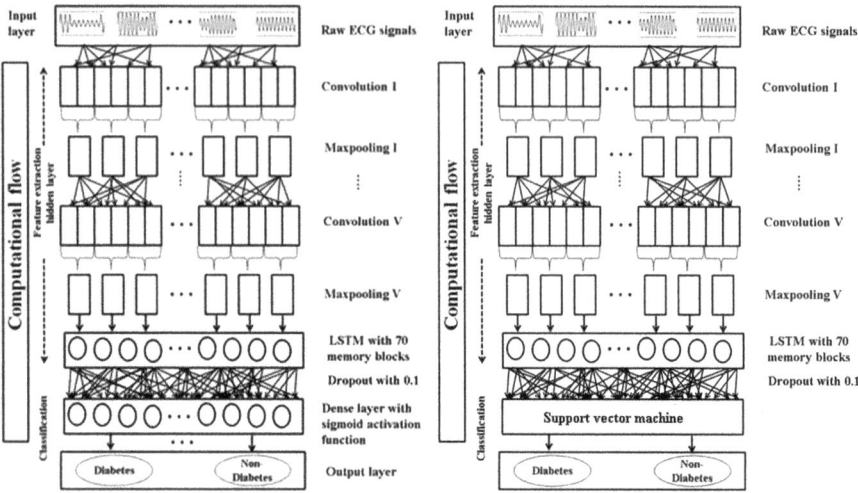

Fig. 11.7 Architectures of two deep learning-based automated diabetes diagnosis systems (left figure) for CNN-LSTM and (right figure) CNN-LSTM-SVM

G5 Mobile etc. were conferred the consent to operate in non-adjunctive manner in Europe. Dexcom G5 Mobile received it in 2016, FreeStyleLibre in 2017 and Dexcom G6 in 2018.

The vital information from CGM sensors can be used in insulin pumps. Insulin pump (subcutaneous continuous insulin therapy) gives the patients more flexibility over insulin injections. As said earlier, insulin pump, working in an integrated way with CGM system, is artificial pancreas. This battery-operated closed-loop device has a pump with controls, processing modules and insulin storage module along with tubing system for delivery and cannula for insertion. A specialist doctor can decide the flow rate of insulin upon detailed knowledge of the diabetic condition of the patient. Upon the knowledge of the BG provided by the CGM system every 5–15 minutes, the glucose monitor in the artificial pancreas decides on the amount of insulin injection. The control algorithm (based on which the closed-loop system runs) was mostly based on model predictive control [42] and fuzzy logic [9] to name a few. These algorithms can be replaced by deep learning algorithms when CGM devices with larger lifetime are used and when aggregation of data from several prevalent CGM devices is done for the purpose of obtaining crucial statistical information.

Optical sensing, mentioned earlier, if fully become successful, has the potential to turn CGM process from minimally invasive to non-invasive. For non-invasive optical sensors, concepts based on Raman spectroscopy, fluorescence sensing and near-infrared detection have been tried. Eversense by Senseonics is an implantable sensor (necessitating a simple surgical procedure) using fluorescence sensing method having 90 days as lifetime and MARD as 11.4%. The advancement in CGM devices mainly the huge leap in lifetime without compromising on the accuracy and credibility of measured values has been already discussed [53].

Eversense CGM system also throws light to the modern features/technologies used and new challenges to be addressed (as a representative of new advanced CGM devices).

- The volume of data handled is very high as interstitial glucose is measured every 5 minutes and sensor lifetime is very high.
- Measurement by using advanced fluorescence-based technology.
- Transmission of this glucose data to patient's mobile via Bluetooth, and this data can be shared by five additional people.
- Life-saving alerts, also in the form of body vibrations when actual and predictive glucose values touch low and high thresholds and when the glucose variation rates are above allowable threshold, and these data are also transported to the patient's smart phone.

CGM devices has a data management system (DMS) which stores the BG values along with some data inputs which are fed from patients' side like information about their meals, exercise, insulin, etc.

Another challenge to be tackled is ensuring the data security of CGM sensors. Sensors being more in wearable form and transmission being often in wireless mode, CGM data are prone to be hacked.

Sensors for cardiac health monitoring (non-CGM sensors) Diabetes affects cardiac system. Cardiac system parameter HRV is used for the non-invasive automated detection of diabetes. Hence a small peep into the electrogram (EGM), which is a visual representation of electrical potential difference measured between two points along time axis. ECG is the electrical display related to the working of the heart.

Intracardial electrograms For measuring electrical activity across two points, two electrodes are at minimum required. These electrodes can be considered as the sensing component since it is intracardial ECG and measures local activity of the parts of the heart. (Recall our earlier discussion regarding ECG-derived HRV input data-based automated diabetes diagnosis methods). The sensitivity of these electrode-based sensors should be really high considering the fact that the typical amplitude of the transvenous atrial and ventricular EGMs ranges between 1–5 mV and 5–20 mV, respectively, with a very low frequency level of 1–10 Hz [67].

Pacemaker Pacemaker (ICD – implantable cardioverter defibrillator) is a small device implanted under the skin in the chest through a surgical procedure. It helps to control heartbeat and make it regular in the case of a person with arrhythmia. Pacemaker uses a number of biosensors.

A pacemaker or ICD has three main parts: one is a pulse generator with a sealed lithium battery used to generate the electrical signals needed to make the heart beat. Most of them are also capable of receiving and responding to signals sent by the heart itself. Next are the leads which conduct electrical signals between the heart and the pulse generator. The third are the electrodes positioned in each lead. Pacemakers can 'sense' when the heart's natural rate falls below the rate that has been programmed into the pacemaker. The EGM signal collected by the electrode travels to the generator where it is amplified, filtered by electronic circuits and compared against threshold voltages which are generally programmed to fixed values like about 2 mV for ventricular channels and 0.3–0.6 mV for atrial channels [67].

11.7 Conclusion

To combat complications, efficient management of diabetes is essential. As diabetes progresses, its severity is likely to increase. This necessitates the need for self-assessment of glycaemic control in addition to the routine consultation at diabetes clinics. This is required more in general for type 1 diabetes people compared to type 2 cases. Diabetes management started with intermittent self-test of BG using glucose meters. People who are in need of better management are provided with sensor-based CGM devices for collecting minute details of daily glucose profiles. This data can be later analysed in diabetes clinic to review aspects of glycaemic control and hypoglycaemic episodes. One of the important advantages of CGM is its ability to reduce events of hypoglycaemia if the CGM device has great accuracy and has more real-time data processing capabilities. They will have the audio visual alerts also on episodes of hypoglycaemia which help users to take precautions. CGM devices are capable of capturing glycaemic fluctuations in a very fast manner. The real-time values of glucose concentration are made available to the patients/caretakers. Acute diabetic people, normally those with type 1 diabetes, have to be administered subcutaneous insulin therapy and, at a still progressed diabetes condition, need to be given closed-loop insulin therapy (insulin pump along with the CGM system). Deep learning techniques have a great role in making fast and accurate analysis of the vast CGM data based on which insulin pumps are controlled. Just like CGM sensors revolutionized glucose monitoring of type 1 diabetes mellitus patients and other acute diabetic patients, the blending of deep learning algorithms in sensor-based healthcare devices will make the devices very accurate and capable of real-time operation.

If CGM data could be analysed in a best way, that will prompt clinicians for preserving and storing the medical data. These data can be further used by the deep learning algorithms or other data analysis techniques to make predictions of acquiring diabetes in the future, to know the accurate trends of diabetes progression (so that complications can be prevented).

References

1. G. Acciaroli, M. Vettoretti, A. Facchinetti, G. Sparacino, Calibration of minimally invasive continuous glucose monitoring sensors: State-of-the-art and current perspectives. Biosensors (Basel) **8**, E24 (2018)
2. U.R. Acharya, J. Suri, A.E. Jos, S.M. Spaan Krisnan, *Advances in Cardiac Signal Processing* (Springer Verlag GmBh, Berlin Heidelberg, 2007)

3. U.R. Acharya, O. Faust, S. VinithaSree, D.N. Ghista, S. Dua, P. Joseph, A.V.I. Thajudin, N. Janarthanan, T. Tamura, An integrated diabetic index using heart rate variability signal features for diagnosis of diabetes. Comput. Methods Biomech. Biomed. Engin. **16**, 222–234 (2013)
4. U.R. Acharya, O. Faust, N.A. Kadri, J.S. Suri, W. Yu, Automated identification of normal and diabetes heart rate signals using nonlinear measures. Comput. Biol. Med. **43**(10), 1523–1529 (2013)
5. U.R. Acharya, S. Vidya, D.N. Ghista, L.W.J. Eugene, F. Molinari, M. Sankaranarayanan, Computer-aided diagnosis of diabetic subjects by HRV signals using discrete wavelet transform method. Knowl.-Based Syst. **42**, 4567–4581 (2015)
6. C.F. Allyson, H.F. Jelinek, M. Smith, Heart rate variability analysis: A useful assessment tool for diabetes associated cardiac dysfunction in rural and remote areas. Aust. J. Rural Health **13**, 77–82 (2005)
7. A. Andreoli, R. Gravina, R. Giannantonio, P. Pierleoni, SPINE-HRV: A BSN-based toolkit for heart rate variability analysis in the time-domain, Lecture Notes in Electrical Engineering 75:369–389, in *Wearable and Autonomous Biomedical Devices and Systems for Smart Environment*, (Springer, Berlin, 2010)
8. ARIC study (www.cscc.unc.edu/aric/)
9. E. Atlas, R. Nimri, S. Miller, E.A. Grunberg, M. Phillip, MD-logic artificial pancreas system: A pilot study in adults with type 1 diabetes. Diabetes Care **33**, 1072–1076 (2010)
10. A. Awdah, A. Nabil, S. Ahmad, Q. Reem, A. Khidir, Time-domain analysis of heart rate variability in diabetic patients with and without autonomic neuropathy. Ann. Saudi Med. **22**, 5–6 (2002)
11. K.E. Barrett, M.S. Barman, S. Boitano, H. Brooks, *Ganong's Review of Medical Physiology* (McGraw-Hill Companies)
12. L. Cai, W. Ge, Z. Zhu, X. Zhao, Z. Li, Data analysis and accuracy evaluation of a continuous glucose-monitoring device. Hindawi J. Sensors **2019**, Article ID 4896862 (2019)
13. G. Cappon, M. Vettoretti, G. Sparacino, A. Facchinetti, Continuous glucose monitoring sensors for diabetes management: A review of technologies and applications. Diabetes Metab. J. **43**, 383–397 (2019)
14. C. Chakraborty, B. Gupta, S.K. Ghosh, Identification of chronic wound status under tele-wound network through smartphone. Int. J. Rough Sets Data Anal, Special issue on: Medical Image Mining for Computer-Aided Diagnosis 2(2), 56–75 (2015). https://doi.org/10.4018/IJRSDA.2015070104
15. D. Chemla, J. Young, F. Badilini, B.P. Maison, H. Affres, Y. Lecarpentier, P. Chanson, Comparison of fast Fourier transform and autoregressive spectral analysis for the study of heart rate variability in diabetic patients. Int. J. Cardiol **104**(3), 307–313 (2005)
16. R. Chlup, B. Doubravova, J. Bartek, J. Zapletalova, O. Krystynik, V. Prochazka, Effective assessment of diabetes control using personal glucometers. Dis. Markers. Hindawi Publishing Corporation Disease Markers **35**(6), 895–905 (2013)
17. K.C. Chua, V. Chandran, U.R. Acharya, C.M. Lim, Computer- based analysis of cardiac state using entropies, recurrence plots and Poincare geometry. J. Med. Eng. Technol **32**(4), 263–272 (2008)
18. K.C. Chua, V. Chandran, U.R. Acharya, C.M. Lim, Cardiac health diagnosis using higher order spectra and support vector machine. Open Med Inform J **3**, 1–8 (2009)
19. M. Coutinho, H.C. Gerstein, Y. Wang, S. Yusuf, The relationship between glucose and incidence cardiovascular events: A meta-regression analysis of published data from 20 studies of 95783 individuals followed for 12.4 years. Diabetes Care **22**, 233–240 (1999)
20. M.F. Di Carli, J. Janisse, G. Grunberger, J. Ager, Role chronic hyperglycemia in the pathogenesis of coronary microvascular dysfunction in diabetes. J. Am. Coll. Cardiol. **41**, 1387–1393 (2003)
21. M. Elsherif, U. Hassan, H. Butt, Hydrogel optical fibers for continuous glucose monitoring. Biosens. Bioelectron. **137**, 25 (2019)

22. B.S. Emily, E.C. Lloyd, L. Duanping, J.P. Ronald, W.E. Gregory, D.R. Wayne, W.E. Gregory, D.R. Wayne, H. Gerardo, Diabetes, glucose, insulin, and heart rate variability, the Atherosclerosis Risk in Communities (ARIC) study. Diabetes Care **28**(3), 668 (2005)
23. M. Engin, ECG beat classification using neuro-fuzzy network. Pattern Recogn. Lett. **25**(15), 1715–1722 (2004)
24. G. Fortino, A. Guerrieri, F. Bellifemine, R. Giannantonio, Platform-independent development of collaborative wireless body sensor network applications: SPINE2, IEEE international conference on systems, man and cybernetics, 2009
25. G. Fortino, A. Guerrieri, F.L. Bellifemine, R. Giannantonio, SPINE2: Developing BSN applications on heterogeneous sensor nodes, IEEE international symposium on industrial embedded systems, pp. 128–131, 2009
26. G. Fortino, R. Giannantonio, R. Gravina, P. Kuryloski, R. Jafari, Enabling effective programming and flexible management of efficient body sensor network applications. IEEE Trans. Human-Machine Syst **43**(1), 115–133 (2013)
27. G. Fortino, D. Parisi, V. Pirrone, G. Di Fatta, BodyCloud: A SaaS approach for community body sensor networks. Futur. Gener. Comput. Syst. **35**, 62–79 (2014)
28. G. Fortino, G. Di Fatta, M. Pathan, A. Vasilakos, Cloud-assisted body area networks: State-of-the-art and future challenges. Wirel. Netw **20**(7), 1925–1938 (2014)
29. R. Gravina, G. Fortino, Automatic methods for the detection of accelerative cardiac defense response. IEEE Trans. Affect. Comput. **7**(3), 286–298 (2016)
30. R. Gravina, P. Alinia, H. Ghasemzadeh, G. Fortino, Multi-sensor fusion in body sensor networks: State-of-the-art and research challenges. Inf. Fusion **35**, 68–80 (2016)
31. D. Ge, N. Srinivasan, S.M. Krishnan, Cardiac arrhythmia classification using autoregressive modeling. Biomed. Eng. Online **1**(1), 5 (2002)
32. A.L. Goldberger, B.J. West, Application of non-linear dynamics to clinical cardiology. Ann. N. Y. Acad. Sci. **504**, 195–213 (1987)
33. P. Gresele, G. Guglielmini, M. Deangelis, et al., Acute short-term hyperglycemia enhances sheart stress-induced platelet activation in patients with type 2 diabetes mellitus. J. Am. Coll. Cardiol. **41**, 1013–1020 (2003)
34. P. Hammond, Interpreting the ambulatory glucose profile. Br. J. Diabetes **16**, S10 (2016)
35. H. Jelinek, A. Flynn, P. Warner, Automated assessment of cardiovascular disease associated with diabetes in rural and remote health practice, The national SARRAH conference, pp. 1–7, 2004
36. C.S. Hughes, S.D. Patek, M.D. Breton, B.P. Kovatchev, Hypoglycemia prevention via pump attenuation and red-yellow-green "traffic" lights using continuous glucose monitoring and insulin pump data. J. Diabetes Sci. Technol. **4**, 1146–1155 (2010)
37. S. Iyengar, F.T. Bonda, R. Gravina, A. Guerrieri, G. Fortino, A. Sangiovanni-Vincentelli, A framework for creating healthcare monitoring applications using wireless body sensor networks, Proceedings of the ICST 3rd international conference on Body area networks 2008, 1–2
38. P. Jia, P. Zhao, J. Chen, M. Zhang, Evaluation of clinical decision support systems for diabetes care: An overview of current evidence. J. Eval. Clin. Pract. **25**, 66–77 (2019)
39. L.W. Jian, T.C. Lim, Automated detection of diabetes by means of higher order spectral features obtained from heart rate signals. J. Med. Imag. Health Inf **3**, 440–447 (2013)
40. M. Kirvela, K. Salmela, et al., Heart rate variability in diabetic and non-diabetic renal transplant patients. Acta Anaesthesiol. Scand. **40**(7), 804–808 (1996)
41. R.E. Kleiger, J.T. Bigger, M.S. Bosner, M.K. Chung, J.R. Cook, L.M. Rolnitzky, et al., Stability over time of variables measuring heart rate variability in normal subjects. Am. J. Cardiol. **68**, 626–630 (1991)
42. J. Kropff, S. Del Favero, J. Place, C. Toffanin, R. Visentin, M. Monaro, M. Messori, F. Di Palma, G. Lanzola, A. Farret, F. Boscari, S. Galasso, P. Magni, A. Avogaro, P. Keith-Hynes, B.P. Kovatchev, D. Bruttomesso, C. Cobelli, J.H. DeVries, E. Renard, L. Magni, AP@home consortium. 2 month evening and night closed-loop glucose control in patients with type 1 dia-

betes under free-living conditions: A randomised crossover trial. Lancet Diabetes Endocrinol. **3**, 939–947 (2015)

43. J.D. Mackay, Respiratory sinus arrhythmia in diabetic neuropathy. Diabetologia **24**(4), 253–256 (1983). https://doi.org/10.1007/BF00282709

44. I.O. Mohammed, H. Ahmed, Abou-Zied, M. Abou-Bakr, Y.M.K. Youssef, Study of features of nonlinear dynamical modeling in ECG arrhythmia detection and classification. IEEE Trans. Biomed. Eng **49**(7), 733:6 (2000)

45. P.J. O'Connor, J.M. Sperl-Hillen, C.J. Fazio, B.M. Averbeck, B.H. Rank, K.L. Margolis, Outpatient diabetes clinical decision support: Current status and future directions. Diabet. Med. **33**, 734–741 (2016)

46. S. Osowski, L.T. Hoai, T. Markiewicz, Support vector machine-based expert system for reliable heartbeat recognition. IEEE Trans. Biomed. Eng. **51**(4), 582–558 (2004)

47. R.B. Pachori, M. Kumar, P. Avinash, K. Shashank, U.R. Acharya, An improved online paradigm for screening of diabetic patients using RR-interval signals. J. Mech. Med. Biol. **16**, 1640003 (2016)

48. M.A. Pfeifer, D. Cook, J. Brodsky, D. Tice, A. Reenan, S. Swedine, et al., Quantitative evaluation of cardiac parasympathetic activity in normal and diabetic man. Diabetes **3**, 339–345 (1982)

49. F. Piccialli, V.D. Somma, F. Giampaolo, S. Cuomo, G. Fortino, A survey on deep learning in medicine: Why, how and when? Inf. Fusion **66**, 111–137 (2021)

50. S.M. Pincus, Approximate entropy as a measure of system complexity. Proc. Natl Acad. Sci. USA **88**, 2297–2301 (1991)

51. S.H. Ralston, I.D. Penman, M.W. Strachan, R.P. Hobson, *Davidson's Principles and Practice of Medicine*, 23rd edn. (Book Elsevier, Edinburgh, 2018)

52. P.N. Robert, M.B.B. Susan, E.M. Adriana, H.C. Maggie, Sex-based differences in the association between duration of type 2 diabetes and heart rate variability. Diab. Vasc. Dis. Res **6**, 276 (2009)

53. P. Sanchez, S. Ghosh-Dastidar, K.S. Tweden, F.R. Kaufman, Real-world data from the first U.S. commercial users of an implantable continuous glucose sensor, diabetes technology & therapeutics. Diabetes Technol. Ther **21**(12), 677 (2019)

54. P.T.A. Seyd, V.T. Ahamed, J. Jacob, P. Joseph, Time and frequency domain analysis of heart rate variability and their correlations in diabetes mellitus. World Acad. Sci. Eng. Technol. **2**(3), 85 (2008)

55. J.P. Singh, M.G. Larson, C.J. O'Donell, P.F. Wilson, H. Tsuji, D.M. Lyod-Jones, D. Levy, Association of hyperglycemia with reduced heart rate variability: The Framingham heart study. Am. J. Cardiol. **86**, 309–312 (2000)

56. G. Swapna, U.R. Acharya, S. VinithaSree, J.S. Suri, Automated detection of diabetes using higher order spectral features extracted from heart rate signals. Intell. Data Anal **17**(2), 309–326 (2013)

57. G. Swapna, K.P. Soman, R. Vinayakumar, Automated detection of diabetes using CNN and CNN-LSTM network and heart rate signals. Procedia Comput. Sci **132**, 1253–1262 (2018)

58. G. Swapna, R. Vinayakumar, K.P. Soman, Diabetes detection using deep learning algorithms. ICT Express **4**, 243–246 (2018)

59. J. Stamler, D. Vaccaro, J.D. Neaton, D. Wentworth, Diabetes, other risk factors, and 12-year cardiovascular mortality for men screened in the multiple risk factor intervention trial. Diabetes Care **16**, 434–444 (1993)

60. Y. Sun, K.L. Chan, S.M. Krishnan, Arrhythmia detection and recognition in ECG signals using nonlinear techniques. Ann. Biomed. Eng. **28**(1), S-37 (2000)

61. Z. Trunkvalterova, M. Javorka, I. Tonhajzerova, J. Javorkova, Z. Lazarova, K. Javorka, M. Baumert, Reduced short-term complexity of heart rate and blood pressure dynamics in patients with diabetes mellitus type 1: Multiscale entropy analysis. J. Physiol. Meas **29**(7), 817 (2008)

62. M. Vettoretti, G. Cappon, G. Acciaroli, A. Facchinetti, G. Sparacino, Continuous glucose monitoring: Current use in diabetes management and possible future applications. J. Diabetes Sci. Technol. **12**(5), 1064–1071 (2018)
63. S. Viktor, I. Steven, D.I. Marina, N. Aleksander, M. Vojislava, Facta Universitatis, series. Med. Biol. **12**(3), 130–134 (2005)
64. R.P. Villareal, B.C. Liu, A. Massumi, Heart rate variability and cardiovascular mortality. Curr. Atheroscler. Rep. **4**(2), 120–127 (2002)
65. O. Yildirim, M. Talo, B. Ay, U.B. Baloglu, G. Aydin, U.R. Acharya, Automated detection of diabetic subject using pre-trained 2D-CNN models with frequency spectrum images extracted from heart rate signals. Comput. Biol. Med. **113**, 103387 (2019)
66. Y. Zhang, R. Gravina, H. Lu, M. Villari, G. Fortino, PEA: Parallel electrocardiogram-based authentication for smart healthcare systems. J. Netw. Comput. Appl. **117**, 10–16 (2018)
67. D.P. Zipes, P. Libby, R.O. Bonow, D.L. Mann, G.F. Tomaselli, *Braunwald's Heart Disease: A Textbook of Cardiovascular Medicine 2- Volume Set* (Elsevier, 2018)

Chapter 12
"Sensing the Mind": An Exploratory Study About Sensors Used in E-Health and M-Health Applications for Diagnosis of Mental Health Condition

Ahona Ghosh and Sharmistha Dey

12.1 Introduction

Depression is one of the major causes of losing lives of many people worldwide, irrespective of income status or age. According to a survey done by the World Health Organization, this silent killer can affect more than 264 million of people worldwide [1]. Unlike other physical illnesses, mental disorder can affect an individual heavily, resulting in a tendency for suicidal attempts.

Depression, unlike normal mood fluctuation, lasts long and becomes so severe that it can risk the life of an individual. Yearly near around 810,000 people expire because of suicide, caused by extreme depression. Suicidal death is one of the main reasons of death in teens as well as mature aged persons [1–3].

12.1.1 Depression Statistics in the World and in India

The rate of suicidal death due to stress and depression is increasing, nearly 810,000 per year. India, the USA, and China are among the countries around the world with most depressed people [4, 5]. This ratio varies country-wise or income wise. The following are some figures showing the rate of depression. Today, depression is one major problem for the developed as well the developing countries, and the overall statistics may vary according to country, age, sex, or different income groups. Following are some statistics.

It has been observed that the developed and highly developing countries, which live a very fast life and consume more alcohol and drugs, face the

A. Ghosh (✉) · S. Dey
Department of Computational Science, Brainware University, Kolkata, India

© The Author(s), under exclusive license to Springer Nature Switzerland AG 2021
C. Chakraborty et al. (eds.), *Efficient Data Handling for Massive Internet of Medical Things*, Internet of Things,
https://doi.org/10.1007/978-3-030-66633-0_12

problems of stress or depression. The below diagram shows depression statistics for some countries [6] (see Fig. 12.1).

We can also find income group-wise depression rate for analyzing the trend of depression [6, 8]. It has been observed that comparatively high- income group has higher side of depression index rather than low-income group, but lower-middle-income group shows a significant change in this rate. See the statistics in Fig. 12.2.

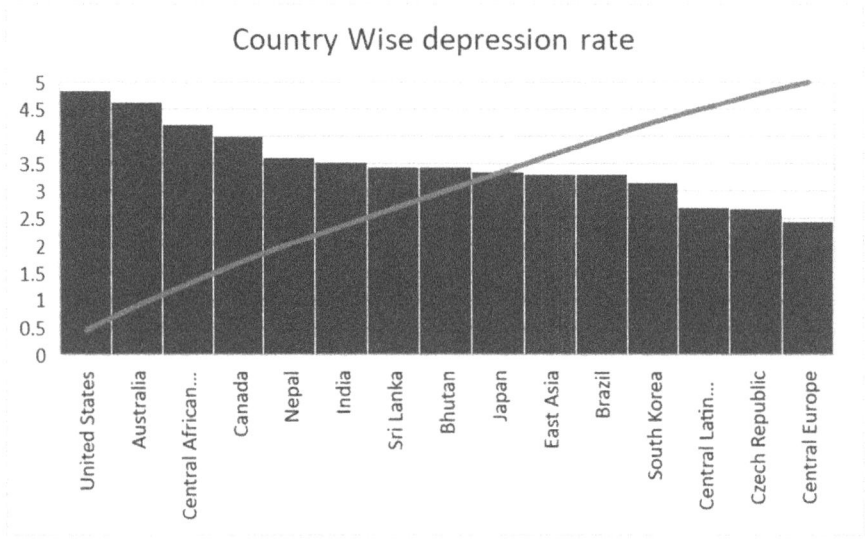

Fig. 12.1 Country-wise depression rate (major depressive disorder) 2000–2020

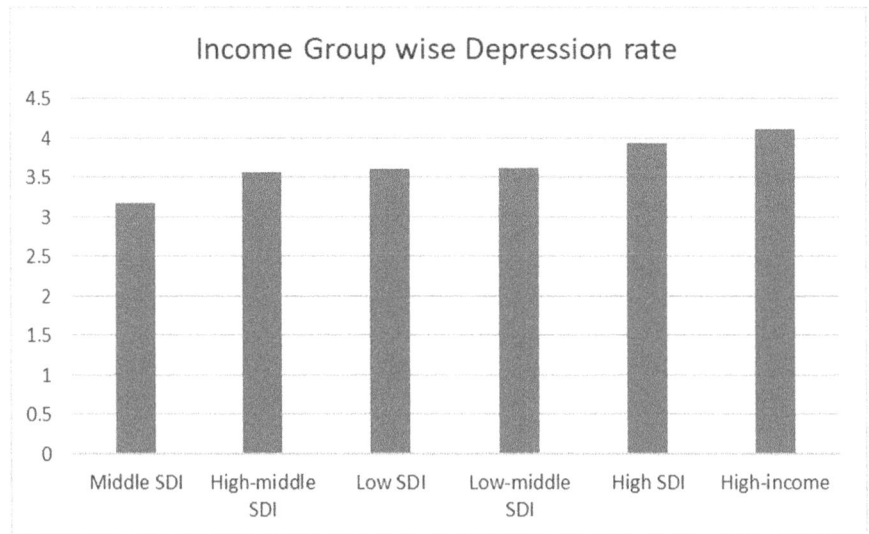

Fig. 12.2 Income group-wise depression rate

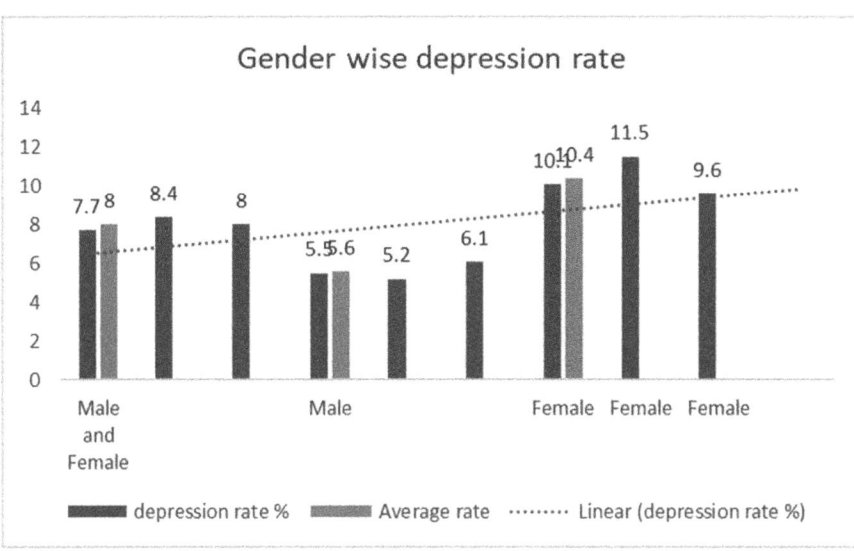

Fig. 12.3 Gender-wise depression rate (%)

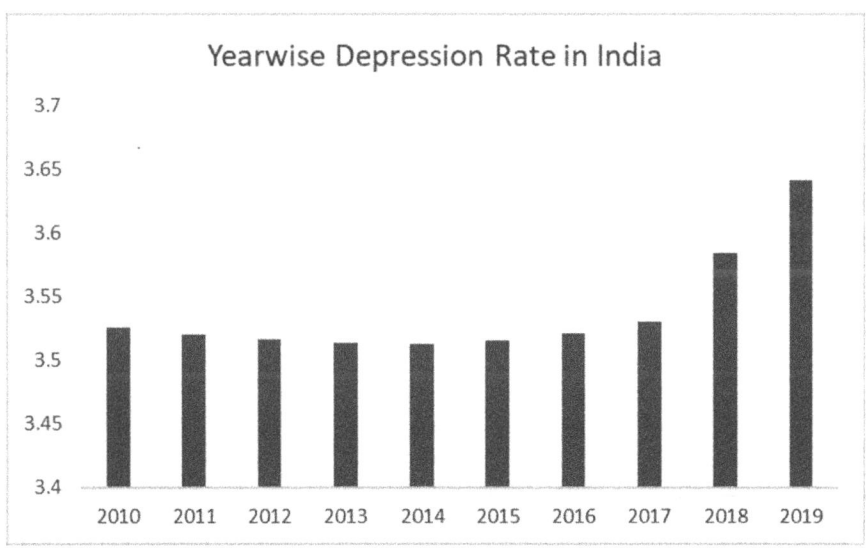

Fig. 12.4 Year-wise depression rate in India [77]

Figure 12.3 shows the sharp increase in depression rate and an increasing trend for females. Not only the so-called first-world countries like the USA, the UK, and China show high depression indexes but also India faces a high depression rate occupying the sixth position in the world. If we look at the statistics of depression rate in India, year-wise depression ratio is increasing. A sharp increase can be witnessed after 2017 (Fig. 12.4).

12.1.2   Different Depression Types

Depression has different types and symptoms. According to their severity, types, symptoms, and other side effects, depression is divided into several categories [7].

12.1.2.1   Major Depressive Disorder

It is one type of depression in which one person might feel depression for most of the time in a day and this persists for a long period unlike normal mood fluctuation [7]. This depression leaves some physical or other signals like reluctance of doing something, loss of interest to anything, being tired and lack of energy, and suicidal tendencies.

12.1.2.2   Bipolar Disorder

In this mental disorder, the mood shifts between too high and too low, i.e., highly energetic to highly depressed mood. Medication can resolve this issue. With the help of some mood stabilizer, the person can get temporary relief.

12.1.2.3   Persistent Depressive Disorder

It is also known as dysthymia, which creates a long-term depressive disorder. The main symptoms are lack of interest in doing anything, feeling hopeless, feeling low self-esteem, etc. The persistency may prolong for years. Since it is a clinical depression, medical consultancy is required [9].

12.1.2.4   Psychotic Depression

It is a major depression and a form of psychosis. Person having psychotic depression may have some illusions of listening to sound or seeing someone imaginary, unlike other clinical major depressive disorders [10].

12.1.2.5   Postpartum Depression

It is a special clinical depression usually developed after pregnancy [11]. The main symptoms are anxiety, sadness, and sleep trouble. Sometimes a suicidal tendency may develop for this [9]. There are certain physical and emotional issues developed in this stage, and this creates severe depression.

12.2 Literature Survey

IoT, being the market leader in the present era, has shown an excellent growth, especially in the healthcare domain. Along with some critical diseases like cancer, Alzheimer, or epilepsy, IoT devices are being used for detection for mental illness nowadays. Though mental health is a critical area in healthcare and diagnosis of proper symptoms are very much essential, sometimes people do not feel comfortable to open themselves up in front of a person. There are several mental disorders like post-traumatic stress disorder or personality disorder that researchers are continuously working on [12–14]. Usually doctors perform some clinical analysis based on a standard set of psychological questioners. But people often hesitate to visit a psychologist's chamber physically. So, telehealth could be one prominent area, and researchers have started their work in this field [25]. Though it is not very familiar to track mental health problem like depression, recently the introduction of IoT and sensor devices to track depressive symbols has added a new dimension. Scientists are working with different sensors and IoT devices to track depression [54, 55, 58–60].

Wireless body area network is another important area where the work is going on. In a review performed by Raffaele Gravina and team (2016), clear discrimination of multi-sensor data fusion has been discussed [76].

Scientists have performed their study on different IoT-based devices [27] and wireless sensor network (WSN) [44] and wireless body area network (WBAN) for detection and treatment of depression by cognitive and motor rehabilitation [45, 46]. Several research works have been undertaken previously in this domain. Chatbots are being widely used for stress and exhaustion identification and recovery irrespective of gender, age group, education, and employment status [15] for improving the quality of life. Brainwave parameters like alpha, beta, and delta help detect the mental state, and concentration, attention, and breathing index can be judged also along with the stress level [38]. Sahu et al. introduced a promising method for reducing complexities and creating a normal e-health device that may be further enhanced by Internet of Things (IoT) integration. So, the conclusion can be presented as the system is capable of making electronic health more compatible with utility and cost. Having an aim of improving quality of life of people suffering from mental disorder, de la Torrez et al. have shown that 60% of the total research works regarding e-health and m-health applications in our daily life have achieved their goal using sensors and networked devices [16]. For delivering health facilities, various aspects are considered for various situations [19, 31].

Whereas most of the research works of e-health and m-health have focused on the physical health [18, 20–24, 26], some have enlightened the mental health and cognitive science also for better understanding of psychology and mood swing due to various situations in our life. Being the fifth cause of worldwide death since 2016 [28], dementia has been the area of concern of Vitabile et al. in [25] where detection and treatment of abnormal behavior and psychological symptoms have been the main objective. A group of Raspberry Pi's has been fitted in the residing places of the persons to be monitored; the data recorded from those devices has been processed using machine learning algorithms after going through a big data platform to find the anomalies in the concerned person's behavior. Research has also shown that computerized speech and facial recognition can also detect suicidal tendencies. People suffering from anxiety and depression can have reduced acoustic range in their speech, and the sound frequency can differ from the original also [40]. Based on the response to some vignette videos along with body measurements like skin conductance and heart rate, suicidal ideation can be identified where such tendency is not expressed verbally ever.

In [56], with the goal of finding reduction in the disorder when early symptoms of negative mental health state are identified, Ivascu et al. evaluated four disorders among the most popular psychological diseases and found out which type of sensors are able to identify exact symptoms for generating an advanced cautioning system. By following their proposed system, one may forecast probable disease to happen by matching some exact symptoms of that particular one. In [67], Cosma et al. introduced the application of wearable technologies and smart textile as an essential portion of IoT ecosystems, as well as those executed for mental health facility surroundings. The protocol for talking loudly and creating a data analytics system for semantic analysis of the transcripts identify worried and not so worried members. The study exposed important differences between the vocabulary used by worried and not worried and stressed members. This method delivers a better performance in the application of smart textiles to connect to the member's responses toward environments and circumstances as portion of a person-centered method in smart build and growth of textile project and services provided for psychological health.

Almotiri et al. have described the fundamentals of mobile health monitoring suitable for home rehabilitation [26]. They have basically worked on measuring physical conditions like blood pressure, sugar, ECG, etc., but those are the indirect indicators of disturbed mental health condition. Android devices enable concerned physicians to continuously monitor different measures like ECG signal, heart rate, respiration rate, body temperature, and SpO2 and treat the patient with the use of real-time waveform and data monitoring of Java-based application on the mobile phone [32]. Hassanalieragh et al. reviewed the present status of the research works integrating remote health monitoring devices into smart Internet of Things apparatus for clinical practices and found out the probable future directions by identifying the challenges in terms of visualization, analytics, and sensing [33]. Advanced pervasive healthcare systems have been the area of focus in Firouzi et al.'s work [34] where different research hurdles like interoperability, scalability, and security have been addressed of existing applications of Internet of Things paradigm in healthcare. As a solution to the challenges and issues, they have suggested a stronger collaboration between hardware and software technologies, and in the area of big data, pattern recognition, and cloud computing, different breakthroughs can bring the required advancements [35].

Our subconscious mind gets strengthened when it gets instruction to change its behavior by neuro-feedback [47]. Auditory and visual reinforcements are received for this strengthening of the subconscious tracked by computers. Our everyday activities and mental practices can be tracked by external stimuli because stressful events and negative emotions can be controlled accordingly [48–51]. Though detection of signs for mental illness is not so easy with sensors, now IoT has made it possible to estimate this area. A recent study performed by Frank Kruisdijk and team has shown that physical exercise can help reduce mental illness, and they have proposed accelerometer-based sedimentary behavior analysis [70]. In this study they have chosen schizophrenia, multiple personality disorder, and social anxiety disorder patients. Table 12.1 presents a comparative study between different existing works where mental health is the main area of concern and performance in terms of loopholes or drawbacks found in them has been attempted to identify for finding out the future direction of research in this domain.

12.3   Sensors and Devices Used in IoT-Based Applications for Depression Analysis

Sensors play a vital role in different application areas of the Internet of Everything (IoE). IoE includes sensing, computation, data extraction, and exchange as well as interactions together in a device. Wireless body area network (WBAN) has shown its efficiency in different aspects like cognitive and motor rehabilitation where the mental as well as physical health recovery is concerned. The types of probable psychiatric biomarkers are proteins, genetics, neuroimaging findings, or other molecules. With the speedy appearance and acceptance of digital skills, substitute procedures of identifying mental condition and behavior are being established to detect, diagnose, and monitor. In another work, automatic method for accelerating the cardiac arrest response has been developed using ECG signal and sensor devices, where the cardiac defense response can be tracked [77]. In this work, the basic psycho-physiological work has been performed.

The sensors which have been widely used in the existing literature for mind reading and mood detection [54] are described below.

12.3.1   Temperature Sensors

The DS18B20 sensor residing in a thermometer [37] provides 9–12 bit (according to user requirement) Celsius temperature measurement and is widely used in industrial systems and consumer products (Table 12.2).

The pin diagram has been shown in Fig. 12.5 where there exist mainly three pins: voltage supply (VDD), ground (GND), and data in/out current (DQ).

Table 12.1 Comparative study of existing literature

Ref. no.	Methodology used	Dataset with source	Depression type covered (if available)	Performance
[12]	Neural feedback-based system, electroencephalogram	Brain sensing headband	How to cure mental illness	This can tune brain to a relaxed state
[13]	Proximity-based positioning methodology	RFID, IOT	NA	Security context
[14]	User-driven design methodology, decision tree, KNN	Accelerometer, heart rate monitor	NA	98% effectiveness
[17]	Decision tree, neural network	Brainwave reading headset	Not specific type	Measurement through brain wavelength after music therapy
[19]	Flow-based model based on IoT	Wireless sensor network	Anxiety	Future focus on emotional intelligence
[30]	Gesture recognition, decision theory	Pulse sensor	Geriatric depression scale (GDS)	Low cost and use of limited resources
[38]	Digital signal process	Electrooculography sensor. NeuroSky hardware	Depression and anxiety	The importance has been given on hardware-based development based on brainwaves and eye movement
[39]	Short-term depression detector framework	Accelerometers and heart rate monitor sensors	Short-term depression	The study has been done with 5 factors of depression, but sample size was limited to 20 participants only
[52]	Telehealth	AMSTAR tool, no specific sensor	Post-traumatic stress disorder (PTSD)	Female patient was generalized
[70]	Accelerometer-based detection of impact of physical activity on mental illness	Accelerometer/ actigraph	Schizophrenia, personality disorder	They performed t-test and chi square test to analyze the data
[71]	Human stress monitoring patch to detect stress	Skin temperature sensor, pulse wave sensor	Detecting stress by multimodal biosignal	Capable to detect multimodal biosignal
[73]	Tracking anxiety disorder using wearable devices	ECG signal	Post-traumatic stress disorder, social anxiety disorder	It collects multiple biosignals; they extracted features from ECG

Table 12.2 Technical specification of DS18B20 sensor [72]

Supply voltage	3–5.5 V
Pull-up supply voltage	3–5.5 V
Storage temperature range	−55 to +125 °C
Operating temperature range	−55 to +125 °C
Data in/out (DQ) current	5 μA

Fig. 12.5 Pin diagram of DS18B20 sensor

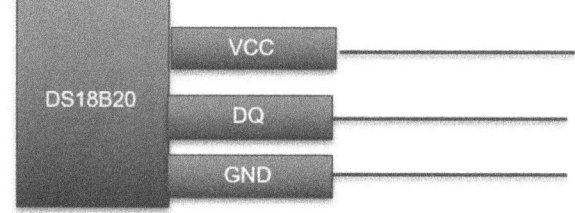

12.3.2 Humidity Sensor

The DHT11 sensor [36] is a widely used humidity and temperature measuring sensor which is able to measure temperature ranging from 0 to 50 °C and humidity from 20% to 90% having an accuracy up to ±1 °C. A sudden drastic change in body temperature can be due to depression, and instant detection of this change can notify the family or the concerned physicians of depressed people so that action can be taken accordingly. Body temperature tracking has been an area of major concern in different research works [12] to predict depression and various mental disorders. The specifications of DHT11 are shown in Table 12.3.

The sensors equivalent to DHT11 include DHT22, SHT71, and AM2302. The pin diagram has been shown in Fig. 12.6.

12.3.3 Proximity Sensors

A proximity sensor senses the presence of closely located objects without any bodily contact [29]. It creates an electromagnetic field around it and finds out if there is any change in the field or if there is any return signal existing. The demands of different proximity sensors vary according to their target, like an inductive proximity sensor always targets some metallic object whereas photoelectric or capacitive proximity sensor always targets some plastic material for sensing. Smart devices containing proximity sensors are widely being used in mental healthcare for different movement and action detection purpose of the concerned people. There are different types of proximity sensors used – inductive sensor, capacitive sensor, etc. The types of proximity sensors have been shown in the following Fig. 12.7.

Table 12.3 Technical specification of DHT11 sensor

Operating voltage	3.5–5 V
Operating current	0.3 mA (measuring) 60 uA (standby)
Resolution	16 bits for both humidity & temperature
Output	Serial data

Fig. 12.6 Pin diagram of DHT11 sensor

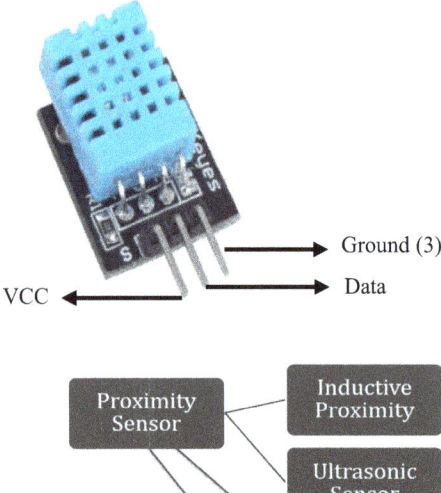

VCC ← | → Ground (3)

→ Data

Fig. 12.7 Types of proximity sensor

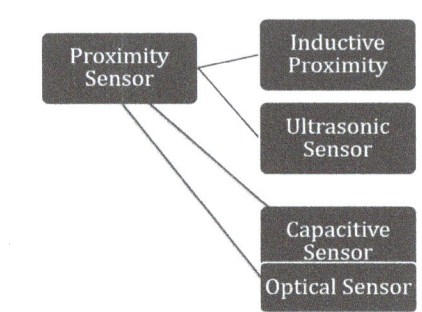

12.3.4 Image Sensors

An image sensor or imager detects and carries information used to create some image. The variable attenuation of light or other electromagnetic waves is converted into signals which are basically small spurts of current carrying information. The image sensors are used basically in analog and digital devices like digital cameras, smartphones, medical imaging instruments, and various others. The tracking of one's movement can be performed by cameras containing image sensors, and any unusual behavior leading to depression can be identified by it. So different researchers have applied textual and image content identified by sensor as one of their mental illness predicting and detecting tools [58]. Serious mental sicknesses most of the times don't have life-long therapies; nevertheless, suitable interference and handling of the issue may ensure long-lasting well-being.

Facial expressions are a vital part in the identification of someone's expressive or sensitive conditions. In reality, facial actions and reactions can be beneficial to diagnose mental diseases also. As an example, we can observe a patient suffering from

Fig. 12.8 Pictorial representation of image sensor components [58]

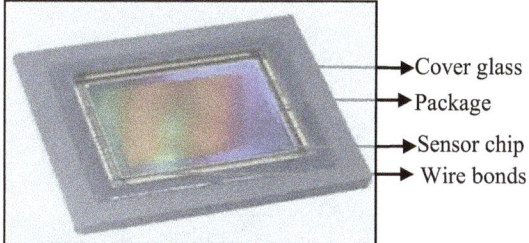

Cover glass
Package
Sensor chip
Wire bonds

schizophrenia often results in decreased facial expression which is also known as flat affect [62]. A number of recent research works have created platforms to categorize different psychological health conditions acquired from facial structures. For example, Tron et al. applied light cameras having 3D structure to detect several facial action units (AUs) of depressed people having schizophrenia [63]. With the use of those features, the proposed classification method attained a great accuracy while distinguishing depression sufferers from normal applicants. Laksana et al. too have utilized facial appearance for identifying suicidal tendency [64]. For the upcoming generation, the authors extracted AUs from facial reactions along with smile data including strength and occurrence, frowning reaction, eyebrow movements, and several head activities. Valstar et al. have used facial structures along with audio signals to identify the intensity of probable symptoms in persons having misery and stress [65]. Most of the studies collected data from different monitored lab surroundings. Nevertheless, the current rise of pervasive equipment containing cameras has been observed and concluded that facial reactions play an important role in identification and treatment of mental sickness. Rui et al. established a scheme where opportunistic capturing of the concerned person's facial languages during the whole day takes place by using a smartphone's front camera [66]. When the smartphones is available to the user, such a system gets able to identify and control psychological problems on a worldwide basis (Fig. 12.8).

12.3.5 Motion Detection Sensors

Passive infrared (PIR) motion sensor which is small, simple, low power, and inexpensive senses movement within a certain range. Pyroelectric sensor containing BISS0001 chip in a PIR sensor is able to detect infrared radiation where resistors and capacitors help it to complete the circuitry as shown in Fig. 12.9. The technical specification is shown in Table 12.4. Level of physical action can be revealing psychological health position. For example, a person suffering from bipolar disorder, mania often shows overactivity, whereas activity level expressively decreases in depression [59]. Decreased level of physical activity is also an identifier of growing symptom severity in patients having schizophrenia [60]. To measure levels of activity, most of the research works applied actigraph—a wrist-worn device which acquires data from accelerometer for gathering duration, strength, and frequency of

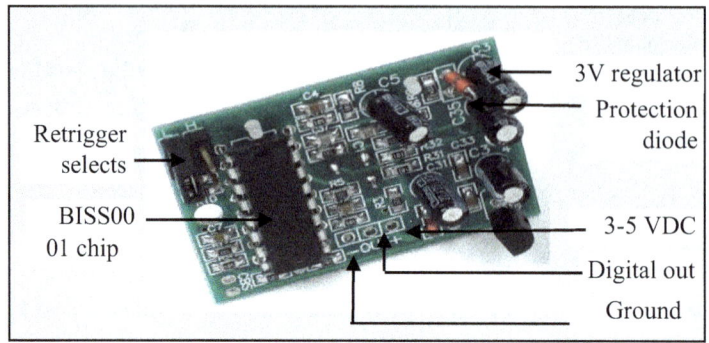

Fig. 12.9 Pictorial representation of PIR motion sensor

Table 12.4 Technical specification of PIR motion sensor

Output	Digital pulse high (3 V) when motion detected and low when idle
Sensitivity range	Up to 20 feet (20 meters)
Power supply	5–12 V input voltage for most modules

physical actions [61]. Motion sensors residing in a smartphone can monitor the movement of a patient and analyzing the number and types of steps taken by him to classify the current mood he possess [39]. Social activity is negatively correlated with the depression level [55], so by tracking the number of text messages and calls one performs and receives, depressive symptoms can be identified also as depression and anxiety lead to isolating nature.

12.3.6   Color Sensors

TCS230 RGB color sensor detects colors using 8×8 array of photodiodes. The reading obtained from photodiodes is converted to a square wave having frequency proportional to light intensity using current to frequency converter. The chronic and relapsing mental abnormalities need long-term follow-up and evaluation process for speedy recovery. Different standard questionnaire formats like PHQ-9 are being used to diagnose and assess one's mental condition, restrained characteristics, and source of the stress. But self-assessing survey sometimes can lead to unreliable outcomes as memory constraint and recall issues may exist there for normal persons anytime. According to psychologists, color therapy can be a tool for boosting up our well-being and confidence as it affects how someone thinks, feels and behaves. The environment and circumstances have a great impact on human mood, and color therapy can treat issues like insomnia and physical pain which sometimes occur due to some negative mental state. It has been observed that colored light generally has a small impact on blood pressure and

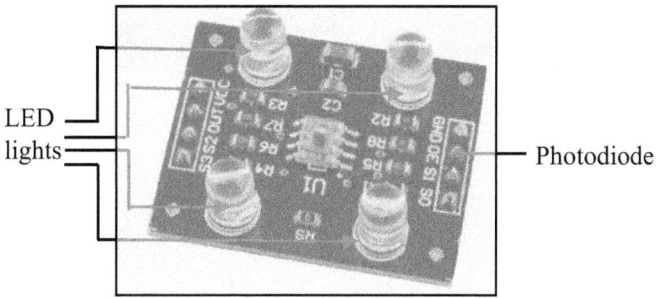

LED
lights

Photodiode

Fig. 12.10 Pictorial representation of TCS230 sensor [57]

heart rate as red light sometimes becomes the reason behind the rise of heart beat and blue light gets able to decrease it. Pink and red colors are connected to the blood circulation in our body and the breathing process. These colors can be applied to increase our pulse, blood pressure, and the speed of breathing, as well as support our veins. Yellow is connected to our tissues and skin, mostly our nervous, metabolism, and digestive system. It can brace our body, handle bronchitis and asthma-type problems, and assist in different skin problems also. Greenish shades have a pleasant-sounding and calming impact, so it can be applied in fighting with infection and as an antiseptic [57]. Blue also inspires us to relax, that is why it sometimes gets applied in treatment of all kinds of pain including muscle pain and stomach as well as heal from tension and stress, colds, and headaches. Indigo is useful for different eye, nose, and ear issues, while violet shades of purple having a pinkish shade can be useful to relax our nervous system and body muscles. Violet colors are also useful when meditating for concentration power and overall well-being (Fig. 12.10).

12.3.7   Pulse Sensors

It is a well-known heart rate sensor which is often used to detect unusual behavior due to mood swing of people having anxiety for automatic cognitive behavioral therapy [40]. Heart rate variability, called HRV in short, gets used to evaluate cardiac autonomic regulation, and it increases with depression intensity [53]. Pictorial view of a heart rate pulse sensor along with different components has been shown in Fig. 12.11. HRV is normally measured by acquiring data from electrocardiogram (ECG). Conventional ECG system can be rather large and, as such, sometimes not suitable in case of nonstop measurement. Nevertheless, the competences of smartwatches may decrease the issue in the forthcoming. As an example, we can see that Apple Watch now can unceasingly monitor the user's heartbeat. Applying that particular dataset, detection of anomalies in HRV patterns is not at all a tough job which is able to identify and notify different symptoms of patients having mental sicknesses.

Fig. 12.11 Pictorial view
of heart rate pulse sensor

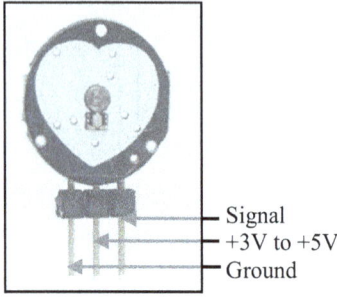

Signal
+3V to +5V
Ground

12.3.8   Skin Sweat Sensor

Wearable sweat sensors are being used for health monitoring for a long time as sweating or perspiration as a form of thermoregulation of human body is an indicator of physiological condition as well as mental disturbance in someone [41]. Various biomedical sensors and biomarkers are getting applied to measure the sweat [42] for diagnosis of chronic and acute stress by healthcare specialists. Figure 12.12 demonstrates one of them which acts as an indicator of anxiety since human beings are prone to sweat more during anxiety.

12.3.9   GPS Sensor

Global Positioning System (GPS) sensors are receivers having antennas which apply a navigation system depending on a system consisting of 24 satellites in orbit around the earth to deliver location, timing information, and velocity [68]. Figure 12.13 shows a pictorial view of GPS module which is to be connected to microcontroller board Arduino for tracking the exact location of some object or person as per the requirement. It uses four pins, VCC, GND, RX, and TX, as it communicates via a simple serial RS232 connection, the same protocol Arduino uses when Serial.begin is written [69].

12.3.10   Accelerometer

Among the three mostly used motion sensors, namely, accelerometer, magnetometer, and gyroscope, the first one gets applied mainly in identifying updates of the device location and movement and tilt about three axes by calculating acceleration forces. Its functionality hinges on the value updates of capacitance, while a portable mass freely passes between the fixed plates in the MEMS. The entire voltage variations from every plate may be noted and used. Figure 12.14 presents the simple 2D structure of the accelerometer. Accelerometer is often used to track the movement

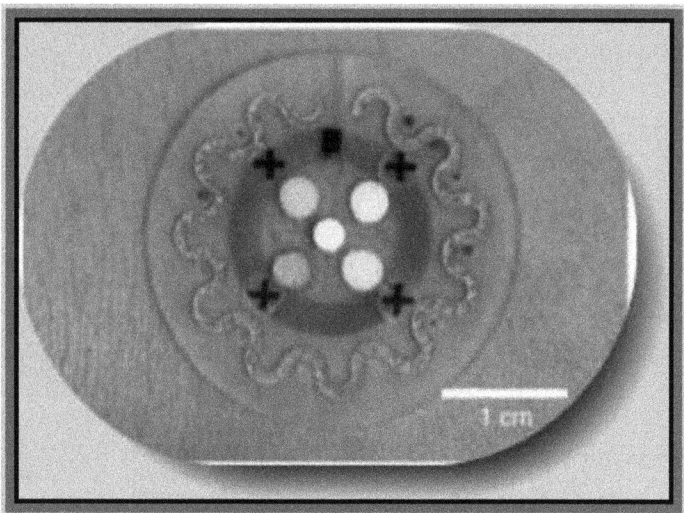

Fig. 12.12 Pictorial representation of wearable sweat sensor [43]

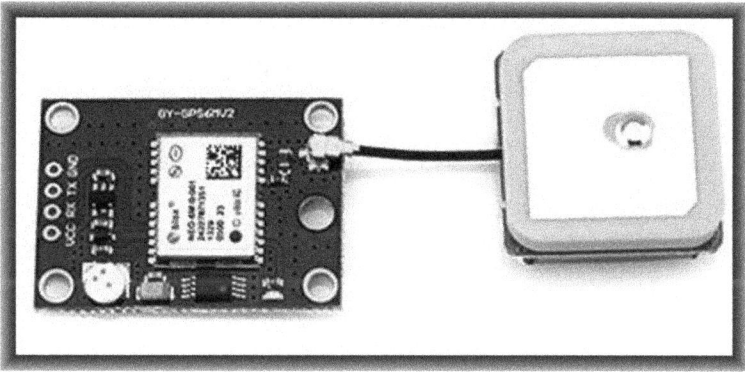

Fig. 12.13 Pictorial view of GPS module

of psychological patients [70], and the difference between the present state and normal behavioral state is analyzed for detecting mental disorder, and proper actions are taken accordingly.

12.3.11 Raspberry Pi

Raspberry Pi is a widely used device in different application domains of Internet of Things (IoT) which is basically a collection of small single-board computers. Research projects like home automation and weather monitoring get benefitted a lot by the device for its low cost and easy portability [31]. The device has been

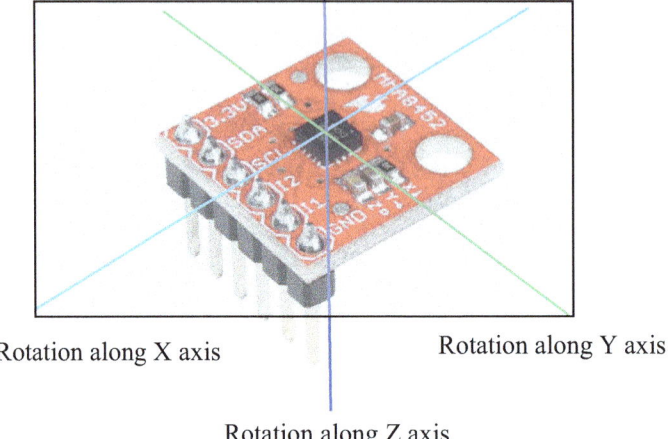

Rotation along X axis   Rotation along Y axis

Rotation along Z axis

Fig. 12.14 Pictorial view of different components of accelerometer

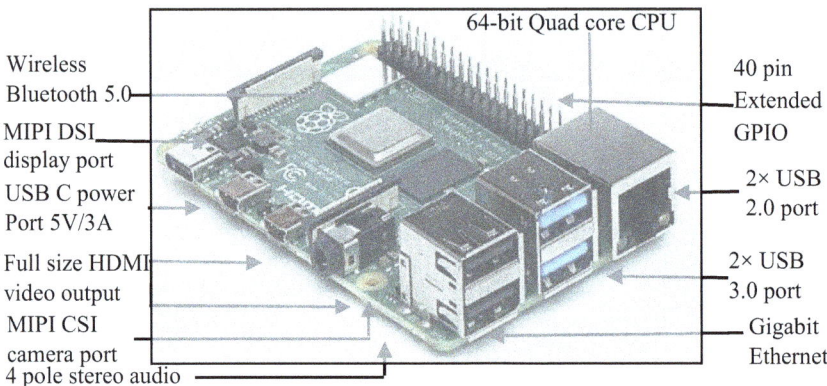

Fig. 12.15 Pictorial view of different components of Raspberry Pi 4 Model B

evolving through different versions in terms of features of its different components like central processing input, network support, memory capacity, and support from peripheral device. Various components of Raspberry Pi 4 Model B has been shown in Fig. 12.15.

12.3.12 Arduino Board

Arduino is a programmable microcontroller board combined with an open-source software (basically IDE) which is an electronic prototyping platform allowing users to make the connected electronic objects interactive in the system. The boards

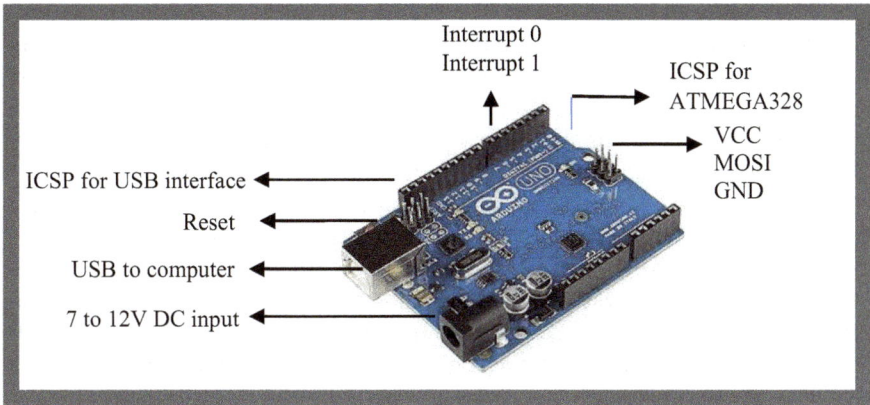

Fig. 12.16 Arduino Uno SMD R3

consist of sets of analog and digital input/output pins which is able to be connected to other circuits via different external boards or shield like breadboard according to the requirement. The language used to program the board is very similar to C/C++ using a standard API and is called as Arduino language. Different Arduino boards based on its features include Arduino RS232, Arduino Diecimila, Arduino Duemilanove, Arduino Micro (AtMega32U4), Arduino Pro Micro (AtMega32U4), Arduino Uno R2, Arduino Uno SMD, Arduino MEGA, Arduino Nano (DIP-30 footprint), Arduino Robot, Arduino Ethernet (AVR + W5100), Arduino Yún (AVR + AR9331), and Arduino Due (ARM Cortex-M3 core). The pictorial representation of different components of the simplest board, i.e., Arduino Uno SMD R3, is shown in Fig. 12.16.

12.4   Sensor Data Formats

The sensor data formats for mental health monitoring can be analyzed based on different factors like mood, sleep, food intake, social activity, physical activity, etc. Physical activity can be defined by accelerometer having three axes which is capable of detecting step and significant motion. Features in terms of mean, standard deviation, skewness, kurtosis, root mean square, and energy can be extracted from the accelerometer data of smartphone and smartwatch and can be further processed to analyze physical activity and the heartbeat rate for mood level detection. Depending on the circumstances being comparatively dark and when the smartphone and watch are providing static data, the potential sleeping hours can be tracked. Seven hours being the daily sleeping duration baseline helps to determine the mental condition by judging the deviation of actual sleeping duration from itself. The amount of interaction with the world can be determined in terms of the number of incoming and outgoing calls and messages, social media communication, and call duration. The food intake has been analyzed from self-reports in most of the studies as obtrusiveness minimization was one of the main concerns in the mental healthcare domain. Category and severity of depression can be measured using all of the mentioned factors, and depression classes can be defined as normal, mildly depressed, moderately depressed, and severely depressed according to PHQ-9.

When the Arduino board is attached to Arduino MKR IMU shield, the MKRIMU library provides an interface to read the registers of IMU sensor. Three axes (X, Y, Z) data for each of the three sensors (accelerometer, gyroscope, magnetometer) provide us nine axes data which is primarily stored in JSON format, and ArduinoJSON library gets applied to write the sensor readings in serial monitor. Later the data can be communicated to Wi-Fi or Bluetooth modules for a greater range transmission.

12.5   Major Challenges of Data Acquisition

The challenges we face during data acquisition [74] can be described as follows which should be addressed in future works in the concerned domain for improved outcome of research.

12.5.1   Study Quality and Reproducibility

A lot of research works replicate the existing studies [75]. As computer science and engineering prefers novelty of research works over generalization, usually the studies analyzing the same behavioral aspects use different features, sensors, and research methods in terms of experimental setup, duration, location, etc. Moreover, the availability of simple techniques and tools is increasing rather than expertise and good quality. Somewhere it has been indicated that in some research, half of the actual result has been removed to obtain greater level of accuracy, so the studies have only indicated that they are feasible under smaller set of conditions, but reliability required for clinical investigation has not been demonstrated at all.

12.5.2   Invisibility and Inaccuracy

A common goal of collecting data is to make the data and the marker as invisible and unobtrusive to the user as possible. Users who provide smaller set of data are more prone to deliver greater accuracy of the models. Customized, active learning data requiring user labeling leads to improved result than static models, and it also removes the shelf-life problem allowing recalibration over time.

12.5.3   Privacy and Ethics

Passively gathered digital data sometimes suffer from privacy and security issues when different researchers possess different opinions and there is a lack of proper guideline regarding the data acquisition method. The privacy rule is to ensure people having control and preference over their personal data used for mental health monitoring. Trust and value of appropriate use of data are the two basic concepts which are needed for people's agreement for sharing their data. What can some data reveal about them, the people should be well informed about it, as the data collected by various sensing devices may result to an identification risk.

12.5.4   Unknown Expiry

Customized sensing algorithms often have shorter period of lives as sensors and actuators get updated frequently, and based on that, the raw data formats get modified over time. The way of applying different platforms and sensing devices can change with time; also like in the last decade, use of smartphone has increased drastically. We prefer to communicate with each other using social media rather than traditional phone calling; we use smartphone for our entertainment also like movie watching, music listening, etc. So, the expirations of the methods used to process the data collected from sensors are unknown totally; thus, decision-making for adapting new methods gets difficult eventually.

12.5.5   Variability

Different characteristics of people and environment result in variation of data source and type. Features of smartphone sensors vary based on the designer. The pattern of social contact can be analyzed, for example, an older person can be more comfortable in calling rather than text messaging like younger people. The body part associated with carrying the smartphone can affect the sensor data a lot like pocket/hand associated with handbag/backpack, etc. The personal sensing field for mental healthcare is still at the beginning and small enough to reach to some uniform agreement for a broad range of sensor data changing over time and purpose.

12.6   Conclusion and Future Scope

When compared with physical health, a smaller number of research works has been conducted on smartphone applications for mental health monitoring and depression detection. The real-time emotional state of a person and suicidal risk can be identified using different technologies like data analytics, cloud computing, and Internet of Things integrated with artificial intelligence for preventing anxiety in people belonging to different societies and motivating them in advance. The treatment plan can be modified accordingly; confidentiality and privacy concerns are essential while developing such systems as the collected data generally becomes sensitive in nature. The present analytical survey will be able to guide the researchers of this domain. The loopholes have been attempted to identify for future enhancement where a direction for future research and innovation has been explored also. None of the review works have described the sensors used in mental health monitoring; they have only focused on the methods. The functionalities and specifications of the concerned sensors have been presented in this chapter; the novelty lies here. The chapter has discussed different mental disorders like depression, anxiety, stress, bipolar disorder, etc., but exhaustive study has not been included for each of them. In future, our target will be to focus on these specific use cases for mental health monitoring and treatment which will be of great benefit in in the healthcare domain.

References

1. WHO Depression Factsheet [Online] (1997). Available: https://www.who.int/news-room/fact-sheets/detail/depression. Accessed on 04 Aug 2020
2. Depression Statistics Everyone Should Know [Online] (2019). Available: https://www.very-wellmind.com/depression-statistics-everyone-should-know-4159056. Accessed on 04 Aug 2020
3. E.Y. Kim, S.H. Kim, H.J. Lee, N.Y. Lee, H.Y. Kim, C.H.K. Park, Y.M. Ahn, A randomized, double-blind, 6-week prospective pilot study on the efficacy and safety of dose escalation in non-remitters in comparison to those of the standard dose of escitalopram for major depressive disorder. J. Affect. Disord. **259**, 91–97 (2019)
4. Depression: Facts, Statistics, and You [Online] (2018). Available: https://www.healthline.com/health/depression/facts-statistics-infographic. Accessed on 04 Aug 2020
5. US Among the Most Depressed Country (2016). Available: https://www.usnews.com/news/best-countries/articles/2016-09-14/the-10-most-depressed-countries. Accessed on 06 Aug 2020
6. H. Ritchie, M. Roger, Mental health (2018). Available: https://ourworldindata.org/mental-health(Dataset). Accessed on 06 Aug 2020
7. Types of Depression [Online]. Available: https://www.webmd.com/depression/guide/depression-types#1. Accessed on 07 Aug 2020
8. V. Patel, J.K. Burns, M. Dhingra, L. Tarver, B.A. Kohrt, C. Lund, Income inequality and depression: A systematic review and meta-analysis of the association and a scoping review of mechanisms. World Psychiatry **17**(1), 76–89 (2018). https://doi.org/10.1002/wps.20492
9. Persistent Depressive Disorder (Dysthymia) [Online] (2018). Available: https://www.mayoclinic.org/diseases-conditions/persistent-depressive-disorder/symptoms-causes/syc-20350929. Accessed on 05 Aug 2020: 10.30 am
10. Psychotic Depression [Online] (2019). Available: https://www.webmd.com/depression/guide/psychotic-depression#1. Accessed on 05 Aug 2020: 11.00 am
11. M.D. Chowdhury, S.A. Counts, E. J. Horvitz, A. Hoff, Characterizing and predicting postpartum depression from shared Facebook data, social technologies and well-being, Baltimore, MD, USA, February 2014

12. E. Almeida, M. Ferruzca, M.D.P.M. Tlapanco, Design of a system for early detection and treatment of depression in elderly case study, in *International Symposium on Pervasive Computing Paradigms for Mental Health*, (Springer, Cham, 2014, May), pp. 115–124

13. S. Ali, M.G. Kibria, M.A. Jarwar, S. Kumar, I. Chong, Microservices model in WoO based IoT platform for depressive disorder assistance, in *2017 International Conference on Information and Communication Technology Convergence (ICTC)*, (IEEE, 2017, October), pp. 864–866

14. M.P. Deepika, V. Suresh, C. Pradeep, IoT powered wearable to assist individuals facing depression symptoms. Int. Res. J. Eng. Technol. (IRJET) **6**(1), 2019 (2019)

15. A. Vaseem, S. Sharma, Depression: A survey on the Indian scenario and the technological work done. Int. Res. J. Eng. Technol. (IRJET), 221–226

16. I. de la Torre Díez, S.G. Alonso, S. Hamrioui, E.M. Cruz, L.M. Nozaleda, M.A. Franco, IoT-based services and applications for mental health in the literature. J. Med. Syst. **43**(1), 11–16 (2019)

17. B.M. Krishna, V.C. Jhansi, P.S. Shama, A.B. Leelambika, C. Prakash, B.V.V.N. Manikanta, Novel solution to improve mental health by integrating music and IoT with neural feedback

18. C. Chinmay, Chapter 5: Mobile health (m-health) for tele-wound monitoring, in *Mobile Health Applications for Quality Healthcare Delivery*, (IGI, 2019), pp. 98–116, ISBN: 9781522580218. https://doi.org/10.4018/978-1-5225-8021-8.ch005

19. C. Chinmay, B. Amit, H.K. Mahesh, G. Lalit, C. Basabi, *Internet of Things for Healthcare Technologies*, Studies in Big Data, vol 73 (Springer, 2020)., ISBN 978-981-15-4111-7. https://link.springer.com/book/10.1007/978-981-15-4112-4

20. L. Syed, S. Jabeen, S. Manimala, H.A. Elsayed, Data science algorithms and techniques for smart healthcare using IoT and big data analytics, in *Smart Techniques for a Smarter Planet*, (Springer, Cham, 2019), pp. 211–241

21. R.S. Istepanian, A. Sungoor, A. Faisal, N. Philip, Internet of m-health Things 'm-IOT' (2011)

22. O.S. Albahri, A.S. Albahri, A.A. Zaidan, B.B. Zaidan, M.A. Alsalem, A.H. Mohsin, K.I. Mohammed, A.H. Alamoodi, S. Nidhal, O. Enaizan, M.A. Chyad, Fault-tolerant mHealth framework in the context of IoT-based real-time wearable health data sensors. IEEE Access **7**, 50052–50080 (2019)

23. A. Santos, J. Macedo, A. Costa, M.J. Nicolau, Internet of things and smart objects for M-health monitoring and control. Procedia Technol. **16**, 1351–1360 (2014)

24. D. Dziak, B. Jachimczyk, W.J. Kulesza, IoT-based information system for healthcare application: Design methodology approach. Appl. Sci. **7**(6), 596 (2017)

25. S. Vitabile, M. Marks, D. Stojanovic, S. Pllana, J.M. Molina, M. Krzyszton, A. Sikora, A. Jarynowski, F. Hosseinpour, A. Jakobik, A.S. Ilic, Medical data processing and analysis for remote health and activities monitoring, in *In High-Performance Modelling and Simulation for Big Data Applications*, (Springer, Cham, 2019), pp. 186–220

26. S.H. Almotiri, M.A. Khan, M.A. Alghamdi, Mobile health (m-health) system in the context of IoT, in *2016 IEEE 4th International Conference on Future Internet of Things and Cloud Workshops (FiCloudW)*, (IEEE, 2016, August), pp. 39–42

27. E. Welbourne, L. Battle, G. Cole, K. Gould, K. Rector, S. Raymer, M. Balazinska, G. Borriello, Building the internet of things using RFID: The RFID ecosystem experience. IEEE Internet Comput. **13**(3), 48–55 (2009)

28. The Top 10 Causes of Death [Online] (2019). Available: https://www.who.int/news-room/fact-sheets/detail/the-top-10-causes-of-death

29. M. Masoud, Y. Jaradat, A. Manasrah, I. Jannoud, Sensors of smart devices in the internet of everything (IoE) era: Big opportunities and massive doubts. J. Sens. **2019**, 1–26 (2019)

30. Design of E-health monitoring of patient using Internet of Things. Int. J. Latest Technol. Eng. Manag. Appl. Sci. **6**(8), 140–144 (2017)

31. R. Kumar, An IoT based patient monitoring system using Raspberry Pi, in *International Conference on Computing Technologies & Intelligent Data Engineering*, (2016)

32. K. Mathan Kumar, R.S. Venkatesan, A design approach to smart health monitoring using android mobile devices, in *IEEE International Conference on Advanced Communication Control and Computing Technologies (ICACCCT)*, (2014), pp. 1740–1744

33. M. Hassanalieragh et al., Health monitoring and management using Internet-of-Things (IoT) sensing with cloud-based processing: Opportunities and challenges, in *IEEE International Conference on Services Computing*, (2015)
34. F. Firouzi, B. Farahani, M. Ibrahim, K. Chakrabarty, From EDA to IoT eHealth: Promise, challenges, and solutions. IEEE Trans. Comput. Aided Des. Integr. Circuits Syst. **37**(12), 2965–2978 (2018). https://doi.org/10.1109/TCAD.2018.2801227
35. D. O Hara, Wearable technology for mental health [Online] (2019). Available: https://www.apa.org/members/content/wearable-technology
36. W. Gay, DHT11 sensor, in *Advanced Raspberry Pi*, (Apress, Berkeley, 2018), pp. 399–418
37. G. Li, Y. Zhao, Principle and application of 1Wire bus digital thermometer DS18B20 [J]. Mod. Electron. Tech. **21** (2005)
38. S. Sahu, A. Sharma, Detecting brainwaves to evaluate mental health using LabVIEW and applications, in *2016 International Conference on Emerging Technological Trends (ICETT)*, (IEEE, 2016, October), pp. 1–4
39. N. Narziev, H. Goh, K. Toshnazarov, S.A. Lee, K.M. Chung, Y. Noh, STDD: Short-term depression detection with passive sensing. Sensors **20**(5), 1396 (2020)
40. A. Vahabzadeh, N. Sahin, A. Kalali, Digital suicide prevention: Can technology become a game-changer? Innov. Clin. Neurosci. **13**(5–6), 16 (2016)
41. M. Chung, G. Fortunato, N. Radacsi, Wearable flexible sweat sensors for healthcare monitoring: A review. J. R. Soc. Interface **16**(159), 20190217 (2019)
42. Can IoT and AI help fundamentally redesign Indias broken mental health system [Online]. Available: https://medium.com/@sukantkhurana/can-iot-and-ai-help-fundamentally-redesign-indias-broken-mental-health-system-4bfaebed2947
43. M. Bariya, H.Y.Y. Nyein, A. Javey, Wearable sweat sensors. Nat. Electron. **1**(3), 160–171 (2018)
44. A. Ghosh, C.C. Ho, R. Bestak, Secured energy-efficient routing in wireless sensor networks using machine learning algorithm: Fundamentals and applications, in *Deep Learning Strategies for Security Enhancement in Wireless Sensor Networks*, (IGI Global, Hershey, 2020), pp. 23–41
45. S. Saha, A. Ghosh, Rehabilitation using neighbor-cluster based matching inducing artificial bee colony optimization, in *2019 IEEE 16th India Council International Conference (INDICON)*, (IEEE, 2019, December), pp. 1–4
46. H. Heinrich, H. Gevensleven, U. Strehl, Neurofeedback -train your brain to train behavior. J. Child Psychol. Psychiatry, 3–16 (2007)
47. M. Balconi, G. Fronda, I. Venturella, D. Crivelli, Conscious, pre-conscious and unconscious mechanisms in emotional behaviour. Some applications to the mindfulness approach with wearable devices. Appl. Sci **7**(12), 1280 (2017)
48. A. Sau, I. Bhakta, Screening of anxiety and depression among the seafarers using machine learning technology. Inform. Med. Unlocked, 1–7 (2018)
49. M. Al Jazaery, G. Guo, Video-based depression level analysis by encoding deep spatiotemporal features. IEEE Trans. Affect. Comput., 1–8 (2018)
50. J.M. Girard, J.F. Cohn, M.H. Mahoor, S. Mavadati, D.P. Rosenwald, Social risk and depression: Evidence from manual and automatic facial expression analysis, in *Automatic Face and Gesture Recognition (FG), 2013 10th IEEE International Conference and Workshops on IEEE*, (2013), pp. 1–8
51. E. Palylyk, C. Argaez, *Telehealth for the Assessment and Treatment of Depression, Post-Traumatic Stress Disorder, and Anxiety: Clinical Evidence* (CADTH, Ottawa, 2018)
52. S. Byun, A.Y. Kim, E.H. Jang, S. Kim, K.W. Choi, H.Y. Yu, H.J. Jeon, Detection of major depressive disorder from linear and nonlinear heart rate variability features during mental task protocol. Comput. Biol. Med. **112**, 103381 (2019)
53. E. Garcia-Ceja, M. Riegler, T. Nordgreen, P. Jakobsen, K.J. Oedegaard, J. Tørresen, Mental health monitoring with multimodal sensing and machine learning: A survey. Pervasive Mob. Comput. **51**, 1–26 (2018)

54. F. Wahle, T. Kowatsch, E. Fleisch, M. Rufer, S. Weidt, Mobile sensing and support for people with depression: A pilot trial in the wild. JMIR mHealth uHealth **4**(3), e111 (2016)
55. T. Ivascu, B. Manate, V. Negru, A multi-agent architecture for ontology-based diagnosis of mental disorders, in *Proc. 17th Int. Symp. Symb. Numer. Algorithms Sci. Comput. SYNASC*, (2015), pp. 423–430
56. How to use colour therapy to boost your wellbeing [Online] (2020). Available: https://www.calmmoment.com/wellbeing/colour-therapy-boost-wellbeing/. Accessed on 06 Aug, 09.00 am, India
57. S. Abdullah, T. Choudhury, Sensing technologies for monitoring serious mental illnesses. IEEE MultiMedia **25**(1), 61–75 (2018)
58. E.A. Wolff, F.W. Putnam, R.M. Post, Motor activity and affective illness: The relationship of amplitude and temporal distribution to changes in affective state. Arch. Gen. Psychiatry **42**(3), 288–294 (1985). psycnet.apa.org/record/1985-20373-001
59. S. Walther et al., Physical activity in schizophrenia is higher in the first episode than in subsequent ones. Front. Psychiatry (2015). ncbi.nlm.nih.gov/pmc/articles/PMC4283447/
60. D. John, P. Freedson, ActiGraph and Actical physical activity monitors: A peek under the hood. Med. Sci. Sports Exerc. (2012). ncbi.nlm.nih.gov/pubmed/22157779
61. R.E. Gur et al., Flat affect in schizophrenia: Relation to emotion processing and neurocognitive measures. Schizophr. Bull. **32**(2), 279–287 (2006). ncbi.nlm.nih.gov/pmc/articles/PMC2632232/
62. T. Tron et al., Automated facial expressions analysis in schizophrenia: A continuous dynamic approach, in *MindCare 2015: Pervasive Computing Paradigms for Mental Health*, (Springer, 2016). link.springer.com/chapter/10.1007/978-3-319-32270-4_8
63. E. Laksana et al., Investigating facial behavior indicators of suicidal ideation, in *12th IEEE International Conference on Automatic Face & Gesture Recognition (FG)*, (2017). ieeexplore.ieee.org/document/7961819/
64. M. Valstar et al., AVEC 2014: 3D dimensional affect and depression recognition challenge, in *4th International Workshop on Audio/Visual Emotion Challenge*, (2014), pp. 3–10. dl.acm.org/citation.cfm?id=2661806.2661807
65. R. Wang, A.T. Campbell, X. Zhou, Using opportunistic face logging from smartphone to infer mental health: Challenges and future directions, in *ACM International Joint Conference on Pervasive and Ubiquitous Computing and ACM International Symposium on Wearable Computers (UbiComp/ISWC'15 Adjunct)*, (2015). dl.acm.org/citation.cfm?id=2804391
66. G. Cosma, D. Brown, S. Battersby, S. Kettley, R. Kettley, Analysis of multimodal data obtained from users of smart textiles designed for mental wellbeing, in *International Conference on Internet of Things for the Global Community (IoTGC)*, (2017), pp. 1–6
67. N. Chadil, A. Russameesawang, P. Keeratiwintakorn, Real-time tracking management system using GPS, GPRS and Google earth, in *2008 5th International Conference on Electrical Engineering/Electronics, Computer, Telecommunications and Information Technology*, vol. 1, (IEEE, 2008, May), pp. 393–396
68. T.W. Boonstra, J. Nicholas, Q.J. Wong, F. Shaw, S. Townsend, H. Christensen, Using mobile phone sensor technology for mental health research: Integrated analysis to identify hidden challenges and potential solutions. J. Med. Internet Res. **20**(7), e10131 (2018)
69. F. Kruisdijk, J. Deenik, D. Tenback, et al., Accelerometer-measured sedentary behaviour and physical activity of inpatients with severe mental illness. Psychiatry Res. **254**, 67–74 (2017). https://doi.org/10.1016/j.psychres.2017.04.035
70. S. Yoon, J.K. Sim, Y.H. Cho, A flexible and wearable human stress monitoring patch. Sci. Rep. Nature **6**, 23468 (2016). https://doi.org/10.1038/srep23468
71. I. Diez et al., IoT-based services and applications for mental health in the literature. J. Med. Syst. **43**, 11 (2019). https://doi.org/10.1007/s10916-018-1130-3
72. M. Elgendi, C. Menon, Assessing anxiety disorders using wearable devices: Challenges and future directions. Brain Sci. MDPI **9**(50), 2–12 (2019). https://doi.org/10.3390/brainsci9030050

73. C.J. Peñafort-Asturiano, N. Santiago, J.P. Núñez-Martínez, H. Ponce, L. Martínez-Villaseñor, Challenges in data acquisition systems: Lessons learned from fall detection to nanosensors, in *2018 Nanotechnology for Instrumentation and Measurement (NANOfIM)*, (IEEE, 2018, November), pp. 1–8
74. U. Bilal, F.H. Khan, An analysis of depression detection techniques from online social networks, in *International Conference on Intelligent Technologies and Applications*, (Springer, Singapore, 2019, November), pp. 296–308
75. R. Gravania et al., Multi-sensor fusion in body sensor networks: State-of-the-art and research challenges. Inform. Fusion **35**, 68–80 (2017)

Chapter 13
Role of Sensors, Devices and Technology for Detection of COVID-19 Virus

Monoj Kumar Singha, Priyanka Dwivedi, Gaurav Sankhe, Aniket Patra, and Vineet Rojwal

13.1   Introduction

Many people in Hubei Province of China with symptoms like cough, fever, and shortness of breaths were first admitted into local hospitals in December 2019 [1, 2]. Initial screening by doctors using CT (computed tomography) scan suggested that patients have symptoms like pneumonia. But RT-PCR (real-time polymerase chain reaction) results suggested that the disease was not related to pneumonia. It has different origins. Later in January month it was discovered that the virus has similarity to SARS-CoV, Middle East respiratory syndrome coronavirus (MERS-CoV) and bat coronavirus of RaTG13 with ~80%, 50% and 96% similarity, respectively [3]. This virus was named SARS-CoV-2 (severe acute respiratory syndrome coronavirus 2) and the resultant pandemic is known as COVID-19. The world is caught off guard by the SARS-CoV-2 which has infected a total of over 27.5 million people and caused ~900,000 deaths worldwide (WHO, 2020) as of 9 September 2020 [4]. After two localized outbreaks, viz. SARS coronavirus (SARS-CoV) in 2002 and

M. K. Singha · V. Rojwal
Department of Instrumentation and Applied Physics, Indian Institute of Science, Bangalore, India

P. Dwivedi (✉)
Department of Electronics and Communication Engineering, Indian Institute of Information Technology (IIIT), Sri City, Chittoor, India
e-mail: priyanka.dwivedi@iiits.in

G. Sankhe
Centre for Biosystems Science and Engineering, Indian Institute of Science, Bangalore, India

Division of Infectious Diseases, MSKCC, New York, NY, USA

A. Patra
Dipartimento di Fisica, Universitàdella Calabria, Rende, Italy

© The Author(s), under exclusive license to Springer Nature Switzerland AG 2021   293
C. Chakraborty et al. (eds.), *Efficient Data Handling for Massive Internet of Medical Things*, Internet of Things,
https://doi.org/10.1007/978-3-030-66633-0_13

Middle East Respiratory syndrome coronavirus (MERS-CoV) in 2012, SARS-CoV-2 is the third severe pandemic of this century caused by coronavirus. Immunocompromised and those on active therapy have higher vulnerability to COVID-19 [5, 6]. Mainly the lungs, heart, kidneys, genitals and liver are affected due to COVID-19 [7]. Acute symptoms like acute kidney injury, abnormal hepatic function, cardiac injury and acute respiratory distress syndrome (ARDS) have been found in patients having acute COVID-19 symptoms [8–11]. Most people who are 60+ years or having health problems like heart and lung disease, diabetics or those who have poor immune systems are easily affected and vulnerable to COVID-19 [12]. Initially, most of the infected individuals were showing some disease symptoms for the virus infection, but presently many cases have arisen without any symptoms, thereby emphasizing its asymptomatic nature. These asymptomatic individuals further spread the virus in their community. Mostly human beings are spreading the virus knowingly or unknowingly through their communities. This virus quickly spread throughout the world and halted daily activity. The rapid transmissivity guided by asymptomatic infectivity and quick spreading of this virus demand rapid detection tools along with urgent strategies of interventions [13].

As of now no medicines are available to cure it. Therefore, there are enormous challenges for us to solve the problem globally with the help of government, citizens and common people. To solve this problem, we have to use the available techniques, precaution and safety. To understand the spectrum of techniques which can be employed for rapid and robust detection of the pathogen, we have to understand its biological properties. The existing knowledge of the biological characteristics of the virus can be exploited for evolving the existing diagnostic tools. The key biological attributes central to the virus can be briefly presented as its genomic organisation, replication timespan and mutation rate which are important for sensitivity of nucleic acid-based diagnostic technique and the features of viral entry and disease pathogenesis. Therefore, in this chapter we have discussed the biological property of COVID-19, followed by transmission of the disease to human being. Finally we have discussed the available techniques, sensors, devices, future techniques and technologies that can be used to detect the virus rapidly.

13.2 Biological Characteristics of COVID-19

The biological characteristics of SARS-CoV-2 are described briefly as follows:

13.2.1 Genome

SARS-CoV-2, a beta-coronavirus, has a single-stranded positive-sense ribonucleic acid (RNA) genome. The specialty of a positive-sense RNA genome is the ability to be directly used for translating the nucleic acid molecule to generate multiple copies

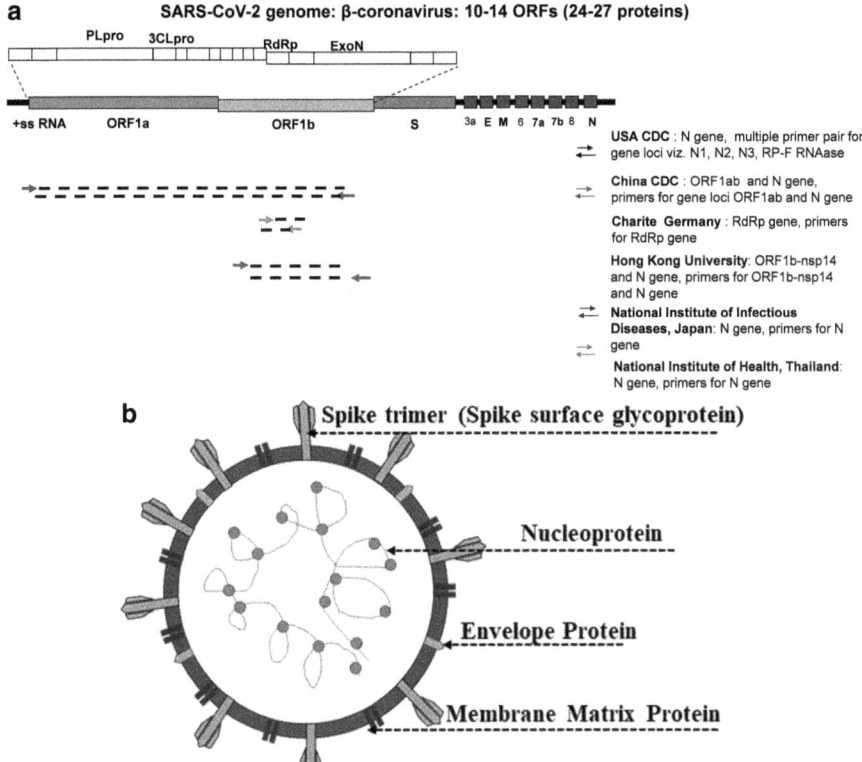

Fig. 13.1 (**a**) Genomic organization of SARS-CoV-2 virus and utilization of various genes by different infectious disease organizations across the world. The genome encodes for 2 large open reading frames (ORF1a and ORF1b) and 8–12 other genes translating to 24–27 proteins. The colour-coded arrows define the directionality of amplification in RT-PCR technique used as a COVID-19 diagnostic tool followed by the information of genes and primer pairs utilized by the organization to detect SARS-CoV-2 in the patient sample using RT-PCR. (**b**) Structural organization of SARS-CoV-2 virus

of protein molecules. This RNA genome has ten genes which are utilized to synthesize proteins. Usually one gene codes for one protein, but in this unique design, one gene is involved in coding different proteins. Such a unique design is possible due to one long gene *orf1ab* which leads to the formation of a polyprotein that is cleaved into 16 proteins by proteases (Fig. 13.1a). The genome has nucleotide identity of about 50%–96% nucleotide identity with other viruses of the coronavirus family [14]. Apart from proteases, RNA polymerase (RNA-dependent RNA polymerase which generates a RNA molecule from another template RNA molecule) and a proofreading exonuclease essential for error-proof replication, the genome predominantly encodes for four structural proteins, namely, (I) spike surface glycoprotein, (II) small envelope protein, (III) two membrane-bound matrix proteins and (IV) nucleoprotein or nucleocapsid (Fig. 13.1b) [15].

13.2.2   Replication Timespan and Mutation Rates

In comparative analysis with other coronavirus family of viruses, SARS-CoV-2 virion is estimated to enter the nasal epithelial cell within 10 minutes of adherence, multiplies to generate intracellular virions in approximately 10 hours and bursts open from the infected cells with a burst size of 1000 virions [16]. The mutation rate defined as the number of substitutions per nucleotide site per replication cycle is a key parameter governing viral evolution. Having an error correction mechanism, it is estimated that SARS-CoV-2 accumulates 10^6 mutations per replication cycle which implies about 1000 mutations getting fixated per year in the viral genome. Overall, replication timespan of the virus is considered as 10 hours with a burst size of 1000 virions. These estimations are crucial in designing diagnostic tools, mathematically modelling viral spread and strategies of intervention against the virus [14].

13.2.3   Viral Entry and Pathogenesis

Using colocalization fluorescence experiments, Zhou et al. [2] demonstrated the interaction of angiotensin-converting enzyme 2 (ACE2) receptor with SARS-CoV-2. The viral entry requires binding of spike protein (S) to receptor ACE2 present almost ubiquitously in all types of host cell [17, 18]. Patients, who become critical post-infection, develop acute respiratory distress syndrome (ARDS) [19]. ARDS is marked by collapse of lung function due to maladaptive immune response. One of the leading causes of such immune response is activation of lung-resident immune cells activating complement system driving the release of pro-inflammatory cytokines, thus accounting for the damage of vascular endothelial cells of blood vessels supplying lung alveoli [20].

13.3   Transmission and Risk Factors

It was reported that initially consumption of wild animals/seafoods in Hubei Province is the source of COVID-19 [21]. Later it was transmitted from human to human in a market and became widespread [22, 23]. Due to the attributes of the infection, some people are showing symptoms, whereas others are asymptomatic. These asymptomatic and symptomatic individuals touching uninfected people or coughing in crowded areas are the reasons for fast spread in heavily populated areas [24–26]. It was reported that aerosols (droplets) having dimension less than 5 μm can live for at least 3 hours. Researchers also showed that COVID-19 can be alive on metal or plastic surfaces or on the clothes also [27]. If the proper environment is found, then COVID-19 can be alive for a few days even in wastewater also. From China, COVID-19 spread into Asian countries like South Korea, Japan and Thailand in January 2020 [28]. By the end of January, the USA has the first case of coronavirus. In Europe the first COVID-19 patients were found in Italy (Milan region). Similarly in India, the first case was reported in Kerala State. These persons had a flight history from China [29, 30]. Sudden increase of patients was found in India when the "Shramik special" train was introduced in India at the end of May. Many migrant labourers are travelling on these trains to reach their native places. Suddenly an increase of positive cases was found in India. In the present situation, there are many positive reported cases per day (>30,000) in Brazil, the USA and India. These trends prove that transmission of this virus is due to human interaction, touching and gathering in small occluded places.

13.4 Methods to Collect the Samples

Before diagnosis, sample collection is the first step, and it is as per the demand of the diagnosis test. The predominantly used diagnostic tool for rapid detection of infection with high sensitivity involves employing reverse transcriptase polymerase chain reaction (RT-PCR). The sample used to extract viral RNA is obtained from the upper respiratory tract samples like nasopharyngeal and oropharyngeal swabs or washes and aspirates (interim guidelines by Centers for Disease Control and Prevention). Serological tests used to probe antibodies generated in response to viral proteins involve harvesting blood plasma from patients after a minimum of 5 days post-infection [31].

13.5 Diagnostic Tools

Initially the symptoms of the patients were fever, shortness of breath and coughing. These symptoms are similar to pneumonia, influenza or normal cold. So, doctors have difficulties in determining the exact cause of the disease. Later nucleic acids tests were performed to confirm the virus. Due to its new biological structure and properties, RT-PCR was first used to diagnose the virus followed by CT scan of the chest. There are also different techniques available which can be used to determine COVID-19. They are discussed below.

13.5.1 RT-PCR

RT-PCR is the routine diagnostic tool employed to detect RNA virus infections [32]. RT-PCR forms the primary method to detect SARS-CoV-2 and diagnose COVID-19. RT-PCR, in brief, involves exponential amplification of a template RNA to cDNA (complementary DNA) using gene-specific primers (short DNA probes) by using RNA-dependent DNA polymerase called reverse transcriptase. For strain specificity and sensitivity in detection of viral genome in patient samples, primer design should be furnished with utmost precision [33]. The process flow of generating RT-PCR-based diagnostic kit comprises two steps: (a) sequence alignment and primer design for viral strain-specific gene and (b) assay optimization for amplification, sample preparation and testing. The target genes used by various existing diagnostic kits have been displayed in diagrammatic representation of viral genome for better visualization of RT-PCR diagnostic tool (Fig. 13.1a). Positive controls for setting up reaction standards are generated by using in vitro transcription kits for transcribing the template viral gene of interest already inserted in a plasmid [34]. Since RNA has relatively low stability and ribonuclease (RNAse) from various sources is a robust and abundant enzyme omnipresent on any lab bench setup, isolating viral RNA from patient samples emerges as the biggest bottleneck. Use of standard RNA isolation kits, therefore, is a prerequisite for using this diagnostic tool. To alleviate this requirement, efforts are ongoing to generate an agile RNA preparation method for COVID-19 detection [35].

13.5.2 Chest CT Scan

Chest computed tomography (CT) scan is an alternative and confirmation technique for the detection of COVID-19. A group of doctors led by Dr. T. Ai in the department of radiology at Tongji Medical College in Wuhan, China, had conducted chest CT and RT-PCR for 1014 patients between 6 January and 6 February 2020 [36]. They have used RT-PCR as a reference and performed the chest CT for confirmation of the virus. Similarly dynamic conversion of RT-PCR results of a patient, i.e. positive to negative or negative to positive results of RT-PCR, are analysed with serial chest CT scan results for more than 4 days. They revealed that chest CT scan is a better diagnostic tool for COVID-19 with higher sensitivity. Positive results of 88% was found when chest CT scan was conducted compared to 59% positive RT-PCR. Among the negative RT-PCR results, chest CT scan showed 75% positive results. Chest CT scan showed 97% sensitivity, 25% specificity and 68% accuracy for the detection of COVID-19.

In Rome, Italy, tests were conducted for chest CT scan along with RT-PCR between 4 March 2020 and 19 March 2020 [37]. A total of 158 cases were studied. After taking swab for RT-PCR studies from the patients, they went for chest CT image acquisition. Images were captured while the patients were in supine position without any contrast medium injection. Patients having both positive RT-PCR and chest CT scan ground glass opacities, bilateral pneumonia and sub-segmental vessel enlargement (>3 mm) were confirmed for 100%, 91% and 89%, respectively, compared to RT-PCR cases. Their results are also similar to the results published by Chinese researchers. Sensitivity, specificity and accuracy from the study were found to be 97%, 25% and 68%, respectively. Though chest CT scan shows high accuracy to predict the infected individuals, it has several limitations. First of all, the chest CT scan is a bulky system. It needs specialized technicians to operate, and finally to conclude the results, we need specialists in those areas. These are the main disadvantages for chest CT scan.

13.5.3   Optical Plasmonic-Based Detection

Optical methods can be used to determine COVID-19. There are several techniques in optical-based detections among which SERS (surface-enhanced Raman spectroscopy) and localized surface plasmon resonance (LSPR) methods are the most reliable and trusted ones. SERS is an optical technique used to determine the biological (single molecule) and chemical samples. A report has been published on single-molecule SERS (SM-SERS) where bovine serum albumin (BSA) was the protein sample and Traut's reagent (TR) was chosen as a protein linker [38]. The binding between BSA and TR on the gold surface changes the spectral response of SERS, which detects the presence of targeted virus protein. As we discussed earlier COVID-19 consists of a protein; therefore, SM SERS method with suitable plasmonic materials can be used in the future to detect COVID-19.

Localized surface plasmon resonance (LSPR) is another promising alternative detection technique for sensing analytes for biosensing application. LSPR is a collective oscillation of free surface electrons of materials (generally metal or highly doped semiconductors) in the presence of light. Combining thermoplasmonics (localized heating in nanostructure) and LSPR effect, G. Qiu et al. have published a work on SARS-CoV-2 detection [39]. Thermoplasmonic effects are used to generate heat for hybridization methods of complementary strands of DNA like the methods used for RT-PCR techniques, and these hybridization methods can be detected simultaneously using LSPR method. According to G. Qiu et al.'s device design, AuNI nanostructures was able to generate thermoplasmonic heat (532 nm wavelength as laser source), and then the hybridization of nucleic acid of SARS-CoV-2 virus was transduced using LSPR. LSPR was generated at the interface between glass and the liquid environment using a wide-spectrum LED. The response of the LSPR was retrieved using the windowed Fourier transform phase extraction method. By using the 532 nm-centred wavelength excitation laser with 32 mW power, they were able to generate ~41.08 °C.

For real-time sensing, they used artificially synthesized DNA sequences of SARS-CoV-2. They functionalized the surface of sensors by forming Au−S bond between the synthesized thiol cDNA of RdRp-COVID and AuNIs. When they injected the analytes with different molar concentrations (0.1 pM–50 μM), the RdRp-COVID sequence was hybridized with the surface-functionalized thiol cDNA of RdRp-COVID in the presence of heating. Thus the refractive index near the AuNI surface changed; therefore, there is a change of LSPR response. From the change of LSPR response, they have detected the presence of SARS-CoV-2. According to their studies without the presence of thermoplasmonic can show false-positive response which is not reliable. By using thermoplasmonics, they were able to sense

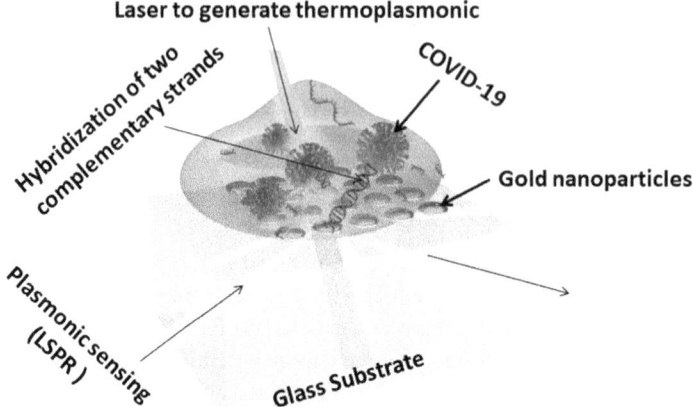

Fig. 13.2 Schematic illustration of the device. Two complementary strands of RNA are hybridized on the gold surface in the presence of green lasers. LSPR responses were recorded from the bottom of the device using a white light

0.22 ± 0.08 pM concentrated RdRp-COVID sequence which is very promising for real-time application. Figure 13.2 depicts the working principle of thermoplasmonic effect to detect COVID-19.

13.5.4 FET-Based Biosensor

FET (field effect transistor)-based biosensors are used in many cases to detect the biological samples [40]. Fast detection with less quantity of samples and high sensitivity makes it popular biosensors and point-of-care applications. Mainly oxide materials, 2D materials are used for FET-based biosensor applications. FET-based biosensors can be an alternative to detect COVID-19 viruses. Recently one journal paper and one patent were published/filed for detecting the COVID-19 virus using graphene and diamond nanocarbon as a sensing layer. Graphene was earlier used to detect RNA [41]. G. Seo et al. have used graphene as a sensing layer of FET for detection of COVID-19 [42]. They have discussed thoroughly how to prepare the sample and detect the virus. In their study, specific antibodies against COVID-19 spike proteins were used to bind it, and the concentrations of 1 fg/mL in phosphate-buffered saline and 100 fg/mL clinical transport medium were detected.

Among all the proteins, spike protein has distinct characteristics like it is predominantly a transmembrane and highly immunogenic protein of the virus with highly specific amino acid sequence. These features were used in their study to bind this protein with antibodies. Antibody-coated COVID-19 samples were placed on the FET through 1-pyrenebutyric acid N-hydroxysuccinimide ester (PBASE) as a medium. This medium acts as an interface coupling to be a probe linker for gate terminal. Measurement was performed at constant gate voltage, and by measuring

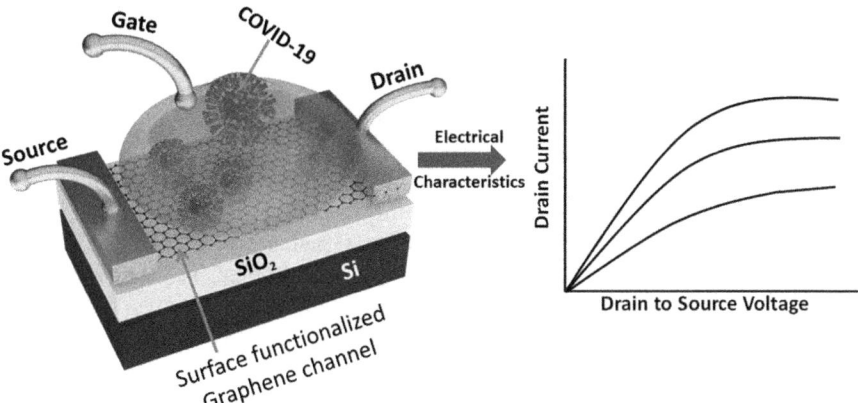

Fig. 13.3 Schematic of FET-based biosensor with electrical characteristic representation

the change of slope due to presence of antibody, they have detected the virus. They have found the limit of detection (LOD) of graphene-based FET sensor to 1 fg/ml of target SARS-CoV-2 with antigen protein.

Another group in China (X. Zhang et al.) has also used graphene-based FET to develop a coronavirus immunosensor. In their study they have shown that their device can capture the spike protein S1 in COVID-19 within 2 minutes with a detection limit of 0.2 pM [43]. Figure 13.3 shows the schematic diagram of FET-based biosensors and their electrical characteristic representation. Instead of graphene, any other oxide materials and 2D transition metal dichalcogenides can be also used as a channel material (sensing). AKHAN Semiconductor, a prominent diamond semiconductor technology, has applied for a patent in US Patent and Trademarks Office (USPTO) to detect COVID-19 using Miraj Diamond nanocarbon materials technology for biosensing field-effect transistors (bio-FET) [44].

13.5.5 Electrochemical-Based Sensors

Electrochemical-based approach can be useful to determine COVID-19. Many researchers have used electrochemical techniques to determine protein [45]. SARS-Cov-2 has some protein structures. If it is able to bind with sensing materials, then there is a change of current. By measuring the changing of current, COVID-19 can be determined. Mostly metal oxides, nanowires, CNTs and graphene are used for electrochemical detection of proteins. Due to high surface-to-volume ratio, nanostructures are preferred in determining the proteins and other biosensor applications. A.T. EzhilViliana et al. have fabricated the sensing layer on polycarbonate substrate where gold wire acts as a working electrode and 1-ethyl-3-(3-dimethylaminopropyl)carbodiimide hydrochloride/N-hydroxysuccinimide-activated 3-mercaptopropionic acid (MPA) was used as a self-assembled monolayer agent and bovine serum albumin (BSA) acted as a blocking agent before immobilizing the C-reactive protein (CRP) [46]. They have measured trace amount of CRP, a biomarker for real-time monitoring of cardiovascular disease and inflammation, using electrochemical techniques. A highly selective electrochemical platform was developed for detection of protein kinase activity in normal human serum [47]. S.K. Arya et al. have used electrochemical ELISA method to detect bladder cancer protein markers, nuclear mitotic apparatus protein 1 (NUMA1) and complement factor H-related 1 (CFHR1) in urine [48]. Similarly screen-printed gold electrode with modified rGO and CNTs was used as electrochemical ELISA-like immunosensor [49]. These sensors were used to detect two miRNAs, viz. miR-141 (a prostate biomarker) and miR-29b-1 (a lung cancer biomarker).

13.5.6   Enzyme-Based Detection

Onset of any infection is characterized by protective response generated by the immune system in the form of antibodies against a specific protein or a short peptide sequence of protein called antigen from the infectious agent [50]. Enzyme-based assays rely on strong and specific antigen-antibody interaction. Enzyme-linked immunosorbent assay (ELISA) has been effectively developed for a reliable diagnosis of COVID-19. Based on the recombinant nucleocapsid protein of SARS-CoV-2, antibodies against the coronavirus were detected in patients with confirmed or even suspected COVID-19 at about 40 days post-onset of symptoms. This serodiagnostic ability of the test was investigated for sensitivity, specificity, consistency rate, positive predictive value (PPV) and negative predictive value (NPV) [51].

13.5.7   Micro-PCR

In order to reduce the processing time per patient sample for this test, loop-mediated isothermal amplification (LAMP) enables nucleic acid amplification in short time by utilization of 4–6 specially primers and a DNA polymerase with chain displacement activity under constant temperature. Combined with reverse transcription, RT-LAMP allows rapid and direct detection of RNA. Named as iLACO (isothermal LAMP-based method for COVID-19), such coupling of RT-LAMP along with pH-driven, colorimetric detection technique has been recently developed [52].

13.5.8   Paper-Based COVID-19 Detection

Due to rise of asymptomatic individuals, there is a challenge to rapidly detect the virus and keep them quarantined for preventing the further spreading of the virus in the community. Recent research shows that COVID-19 can be alive in wastewater for several days and viruses can be isolated from the faeces and urine of infected people. It is a problem for the locality where asymptomatic people live. Therefore there is a challenge to determine the virus in those areas. Recently researchers have shown the ability of paper-based sensors to detect different pathogens like malaria. Paper-based sensors are inexpensive, use-and-throw and rapid detection techniques. Paper-based sensors are easy to fabricate in large scales. Due to its small size, lots of sensors can be easily transported, thus allowing easy diagnoses in large residential areas. Recently K. Mao group has shown that paper-based sensors and devices can be used to detect COVID-19 in wastewater [53]. Recently B.S. Batule et al. have developed paper-based RNA detection from mosquito-borne disease [54]. They have selectively detected RNAs of Zika from the serum samples.

13.6 Use of Technology: About Technology/Electronics Tools

Existing methods like RT-PCR, chest CT scan and enzyme-linked immunosorbent assay (ELISA) can be used to detect the virus. But these processes are time-consuming. So there is a gap between detection of infected people and spreading the virus in the locality as human beings are primarily a source for spreading COVID-19 in masses. But the spreading of viruses is done by human beings. It is easy to find the COVID-19-affected person. By quarantining him/her, we can stop the spread of the virus. But the problem is the asymptotic person. If he/she is not tested for the virus, there is a high chance that the affected asymptotic person can spread the virus in large areas. In this scenario existing technology like artificial intelligence (AI), machine learning (ML), Internet of Things (IoT), computer vision, big data analysis and image processing can be used to stop the spreading of the virus. Deep learning can be developed as an automatic, accurate, cost-effective, time-efficient and easily performed system for screening COVID-19. Many institutes such as the Allen Institute and leading research groups are collaborating and providing weekly updates of open research dataset regarding COVID-19 [55]. These data become scholar articles which help to conduct further research projects and improvisation. In this pandemic situation, it is mandatory to integrate and analyse the COVID-19 patients' data at the large scale using advanced machine learning algorithms, understanding pattern of spread, improvement in diagnostic accuracy and speed and identifying the sensitive cases based on genetics and physiology of the person.

Since the worldwide COVID-19 outbreak, advanced machine learning methods are already being used in CRISPR-based detection assay, taxonomic classification of genomes, survival prediction of severe patients and searching for potential drugs to treat COVID-19 [56–58]. Certainly, any experimental hypothesis must be tested further for improvement with fine experimental designs and tools to make the system more reliable.

Machine learning, a subset of artificial intelligence, is presently used by researchers and technologists to combat COVID-19 pandemic. Many researchers' ongoing efforts have developed few diagnostic and testing approaches through machine learning algorithms. High-sensitivity and fast CRISPR-based system for screening of SARS-CoV-2 virus has started using machine learning. Using past patterns of distinct respiratory images of COVID-19 patients, a neural network classifier was developed for large-scale screening. Moreover, time-efficient automated monitoring system of COVID-19 patients uses deep learning analysis of thoracic CT data [57, 59, 60]. Hosting, modelling and sharing of integrated computational data whether it is scientific, clinical or biomedical are critical to accelerate the operationalization of AI protocol to respond to COVID-19 pandemic worldwide.

Artificial intelligence and machine learning not only play an important role in rapid and accurate testing for diagnosis but also make a protected protocol to stop spread by eliminating contacts with infected people which might help the hospital arrangement and patients to operate COVID-19 pandemic. Google DeepMind has developed a deep learning system which recently released protein structures of COVID-19. This will become valuable information in making vaccine cocktails against it in a short span [56, 61].

To get reliable results on predictions, past records could be exchanged and shared to a framework. Figures 13.4 and 13.5 show the application of AI, machine learning, big data analysis and smartphones to tackle COVID-19. Such processes help to grow transfer learning and framework dataset to construct large datasets using multiple smartphone onboard sensors.

Nowadays, smartphones are not simple instruments but embedded with many sensors and computational capabilities. Therefore, smartphones are able to sense several parameters or visual data simultaneously about daily activities. Capability to capture, collect and store large volume data can be useful to make artificial intelligence systems either suspect or affirm infected cases of COVID-19 [62]. More importantly, if smartphone cameras are able to capture CT scan images of infected patients then comparative analysis with the recorded data to diagnose or detect the level of lung inflammation. Research suggests some well-known symptoms of

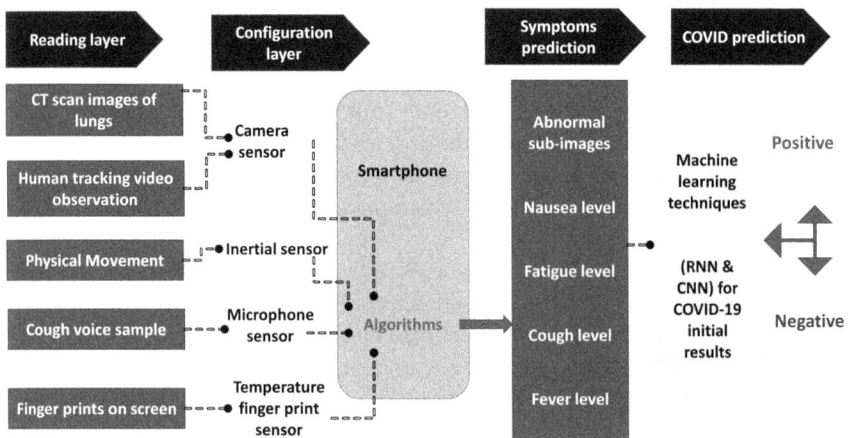

Fig. 13.4 Application of artificial intelligence and machine learning in the fight against COVID-19

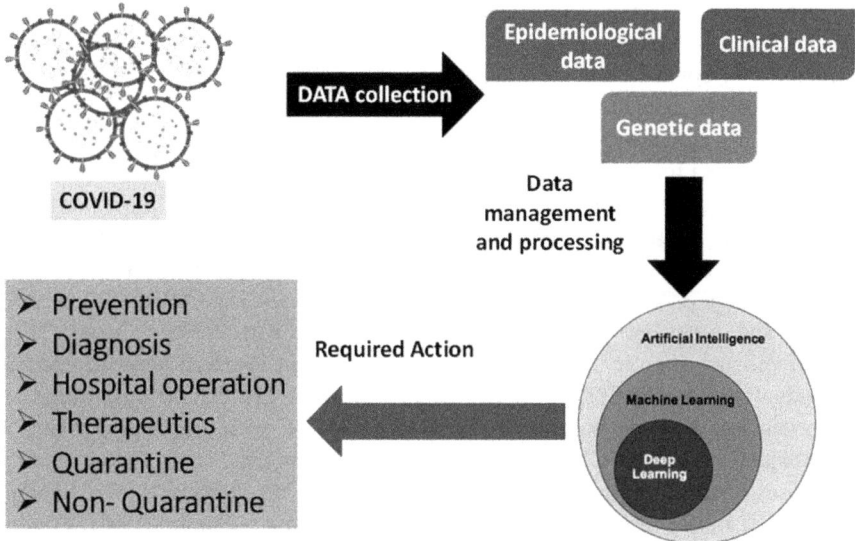

Fig. 13.5 Cloud computing and big data analysis for COVID-19 detection

infected cases such as headache, dry cough, fever, fatigue and interruption in breathing. These symptoms will become important parameters to differentiate COVID-19 from other infections like flu, cold or hay fever.

An important task is to make a framework using each level of every symptom monitored by onboard embedded sensors in smartphones. These main sensors are cameras, microphone, temperature sensor, inertial sensors etc. Existing COVID-19 symptoms would be used to read, detect, monitor and confirm infection by smart sensors of phones. Machine learning algorithms are separately applied to these sensors, most importantly detecting the level of symptoms, for example, camera-captured images or activity videos, to measure human fatigue in different circumstances. Temperature fingerprint sensor is to detect fever level through the touchscreen. Apart from this onboard inertial camera (accelerometer sensor) can also be optimised to measure fatigue level. Camera and inertial sensors in smartphone can be used to measure and monitor the neck posture and level of human headache. Similarly nausea prediction can be accomplished through video-observation using smartphones. In addition, using microphone chipset in comprehensive studies has been done to indicate the type of cough [63–67].

Smartphone-based apps were implemented in the USA and the UK. A total of 2,450,569 UK and 168,293 US citizens used the app to report the symptoms for COVID-19 between 24 March and 21 April 2020. Among all, 18,401 individuals have undergone COVID-19 tests, and 65.03% individuals tested positive when they have reported losing smell, whereas 21.71% tested positive who do not have symptoms like losing of smell. Then a mathematical model was implemented, and using all the app data, it was predicted that 140,312 individuals will have COVID-19 [68]. Singaporean government has introduced "Trace Together app" on 20 March 2020 to find COVID-19-infected people nearby [69, 70]. Similarly the Government of India also introduced "Aarogya Setu" App to find the individuals who have SARS-Cov-2 symptoms by contact tracking on 22 April 2020 [71]. If any individual is affected with COVID-19, then any person, who has contact history with the affected person, can be easily recognized by using these apps, and so medical check-up and testing will be arranged for them. Many other countries have also introduced similar types of app. A. Imran et al. have developed an app "AICOVID-19"which uses artificial intelligence to predict COVID-19 by analysing the cough sample. Cloud-based AI engine was used to diagnose or predict the affected person by analysing the cough samples within 2 minutes. This AI engine can differentiate the COVID-19-infected person and other non-affected COVID-19 coughs with 90% accuracy [72]. Therefore, such mobile apps based on AI are excellent alternate ways to find the individual who needs COVID-19 testing immediately. Big data analysis plays an important role in analysing the pandemic like SARS-Cov-2. The National Health Command Center (NHCC) of Taiwan uses big data to stop and control the spreading of viruses. The NHCC has used immigration and customs database with the health insurance database for making big data analysis. After the declaration of COVID-19 by the WHO, the NHCC used these databases along with new technology like QR code scanning, travel history and health symptoms to identify the persons with travel history to infected areas. Then they were quarantined at home and were monitored through their phone. Using big data analysis along with other modern technologies, Taiwan has stopped spreading the virus and prevented the epidemic in their country [73].

13.7 Plasma Therapy and Vaccine for Treatment of COVID-19

At present no particular vaccines are available to cure this disease. Many virologists, pharmaceutical companies and research institutes are now trying to develop the drugs or vaccine for COVID-19. But it is too early. It will take time to develop the final version of drugs as it requires many trials. Presently alternative ways to cure the patients were found by using plasma therapy. Here plasma is collected from the patients who have recovered from COVID-19, and then these plasmas are used as vaccines and applied to other infected patients who have symptoms like COVID-19. Favourable results were found using plasma therapy [74, 75] (Table 13.1).

13.8 Technology Challenges

There is a challenge for any government, research institutes and hospitals and the human race when a pandemic condition like COVID-19 breaks out. Due to the enormous population, it is very tough for the organization to control and prevent the

Table 13.1 Emerging techniques for SARS-CoV-2 diagnostics

Platform used	Type of detection	Working principle	Type of clinical sample	Biomarker	Ref.
CRISPR	CIA	CRISPR-/Cas12-based lateral flow biosensor	Serum	Nucleic acid	[76]
Electro-chemical	ELISA	Binding of biomolecules with electrochemical signal collection	Urine	Protein	[48]
LAMP	LAMP	Isothermal DNA synthesis using self-recurring strand displacement reactions; positive detection leads to increased sample turbidity	Throat swabs	Nucleic acid	[77]
FET-based sensor	Electrical	Graphene layer is used as a channel of FET and characterized drain voltage and current	Throat swabs	Spike protein	[42, 43]
Paper based	RT-LAMP	Two-step advanced paper systems for simultaneous extraction, amplification and detection of viral RNAs	Serum	Nucleic acid	[54]
Antibody test	ELISA	Antibody response with COVID-19 and evaluation of serodiagnostic value	Nasopharyngeal and/or oropharyngeal swabs	Protein	[51]
Smartphone app	App	App is used for checking the cough and others	Cough, sound	NA	[66–68]
RT-lamp	LAMP	Reverse transcriptase LAMP reaction for RNA targets	Nasopharyngeal aspirates	Nucleic acid	[78]
RT-PCR	Real-time fluorescence	Detection of the white blood cell	Throat swabs	Nucleic acid	[79]
Artificial intelligence	Machine learning recorded data	Detection of many parameters such as CT scan, X-ray, posture, fatigue level, fever level etc. and compare with past positive data	–	–	[62, 72]
Thermo-plasmonic	Optical	Localized heating at plasmonic resonance starts in situ hybridization	–	Nucleic acid	[39]

pandemic. Therefore, the need for advancements in the medical field gained more attention. People are also very cautious about their daily routine and health conditions. In order to check COVID-19 symptoms like cough, fever, fatigue etc., there are several android app-based solutions proposed by several information technology (IT) researchers. In order to satisfy the needs of the people in the medical field, a cost-efficient and effective healthcare system that can monitor continuously the person is needed. In case of an emergency situation, the patient's condition is not notified to anyone where he cannot receive any help. In this type of scenario, this may even lead to death. So, in order to reduce such a situation, there is a need for systems that monitor the patient's condition 24/7 and notifies when there is a sudden change in the patient's condition. There are many researchers working in the area of healthcare monitoring systems, where most of the time they do not have storage of any continuous monitoring data that will help for future predictions; that is one of the challenges of using technology for COVID-19.

Real-time patient prediction can be a technological solution using the Internet of Things (IoT) and machine learning (ML) that can continuously monitor the patient/user and calculate or measure his/her vital sign information and make predictions using the user's data stored in the cloud. After successful ML algorithm implementation, it can be used for prediction of COVID-19 symptoms; also, people can have real data of affected patients.

References

1. *Report of the WHO-China Joint Mission on Coronavirus Disease 2019 (COVID-19)* (WHO, Geneva, 2020)
2. P. Zhou et al., A pneumonia outbreak associated with a new coronavirus of probable bat origin. Nature **579**, 270–273 (2020). https://doi.org/10.1038/s41586-020-2012-7
3. R. Lu et al., Genomic characterisation and epidemiology of 2019 novel coronavirus: Implications for virus origins and receptor binding. Lancet **395**, 565–574 (2020). https://doi.org/10.1016/S0140-6736(20)30251-8
4. *WHO Coronavirus Disease (COVID-19) Dashboard* (WHO, Geneva, 2020). https://covid19.who.int/. Accesses on 9th Sept
5. E.D. Wit, N.V. Doremalen, D. Falzarano, V.J. Munster, SARS and MERS: Recent insights into emerging coronaviruses. Nat. Rev. Microbiol. **14**, 523–534 (2016). https://doi.org/10.1038/nrmicro.2016.81
6. M. Dai et al., Patients with cancer appear more vulnerable to SARS-COV-2: A multicenter study during the COVID-19 outbreak. Cancer Discov. (2020). https://doi.org/10.1158/2159-8290.CD-20-0422
7. Z. Varga, A.J. Flammer, P. Steiger, M. Haberecker, R. Andermatt, A.S. Zinkernagel, M.R. Mehra, R.A. Schuepbach, F. Ruschitzka, H. Moch, Endothelial cell infection and endotheliitis in COVID-19. Lancet **395**, 1417–1418 (2020). https://doi.org/10.1016/S0140-6736(20)30937-5
8. L. Ma, W. Xie, D. Li, L. Shi, Y. Mao, Y. Xiong, Y. Zhang, M. Zhang, Effect of SARS-CoV-2 infection upon male gonadal function: A single center-based study. medRxiv (2020). https://doi.org/10.1101/2020.03.21.20037267
9. X. Yang et al., Clinical course and outcomes of critically ill patients with SARS-CoV-2 pneumonia in Wuhan, China: A singlecentered, retrospective, observational study. Lancet **8**, 475–481 (2020). https://doi.org/10.1016/S2213-2600(20)30079-5
10. Z. Fan, L. Chen, J. Li, C. Tian, Y. Zhang, S. Huang, Z. Liu, J. Cheng, Clinical features of COVID-19 related liver damage. Clin. Gastroenterol. Hepatol. **18**, 1561–1566 (2020). https://doi.org/10.1016/j.cgh.2020.04.002
11. X. Li, L. Wang, S. Yan, F. Yang, L. Xiang, J. Zhu, B. Shen, Z. Gong, Clinical characteristics of 25 death cases with COVID-19: A retrospective review of medical records in a single medical center, Wuhan, China. Int. J. Infect. Dis. **94**, 128–132 (2020). https://doi.org/10.1016/j.ijid.2020.03.053
12. COVID-19: Vulnerable and high risk groups, WHO Western Pacific (2020). https://tinyurl.com/ybqhfnx4

13. B. Rockx et al., Comparative pathogenesis of COVID-19, MERS, and SARS in a nonhuman primate model. Science **368**, 1012–1015 (2020). https://doi.org/10.1126/science.abb7314
14. Y.M. Bar-On, A. Flamholz, R. Phillips, R. Milo, SARS-CoV-2 (COVID-19) by the numbers. eLife **9**, e57309 (2020). https://doi.org/10.7554/eLife.57309
15. B. Udugama et al., Diagnosing COVID-19: The disease and tools for detection. ACS Nano **14**, 3822–3835 (2020). https://doi.org/10.1021/acsnano.0c02624
16. W. Sungnak et al., SARS-CoV-2 entry factors are highly expressed in nasal epithelial cells together with innate immune genes. Nat. Med. **26**, 681–687 (2020)
17. M. Hoffmann et al., SARS-CoV-2 cell entry depends on ACE2 and TMPRSS2 and is blocked by a clinically proven protease inhibitor. Cell **181**, 271–280 (2020). https://doi.org/10.1016/j.cell.2020.02.052
18. A.C. Walls et al., Structure, function, and antigenicity of the SARS-CoV-2 spike glycoprotein. Cell **181**, 281–292 e286 (2020). https://doi.org/10.1016/j.cell.2020.02.058
19. W.J. Guan et al., Clinical characteristics of coronavirus disease 2019 in China. N. Engl. J. Med. **382**, 1708–1720 (2020). https://doi.org/10.1056/NEJMoa2002032
20. A.M. Risitano et al., Complement as a target in COVID-19? Nature reviews. Immunology (2020). https://doi.org/10.1038/s41577-020-0320-7
21. C. Wang, P.W. Horby, F.G. Hayden, G.F. Gao, A novel coronavirus outbreak of global health concern. Lancet **395**, 470–473 (2020). https://doi.org/10.1016/S0140-6736(20)30185-9
22. J.F.W. Chan et al., A familial cluster of pneumonia associated with the 2019 novel coronavirus indicating person-to-person transmission: A study of a family cluster. Lancet **395**, 514–523 (2020). https://doi.org/10.1016/S0140-6736(20)30154-9
23. W.B. Yu, G.D. Tang, L. Zhang, R.T. Corlett, Decoding the evolution and transmissions of the novel pneumonia coronavirus (SARS-CoV-2/HCoV-19) using whole genomic data. Zool. Res. **41**, 247–257 (2020). https://doi.org/10.24272/j.issn.2095-8137.2020.022
24. X. Pan, D. Chen, Y. Xia, X. Wu, T. Li, X. Ou, L. Zhou, J. Liu, Asymptomatic cases in a family cluster with SARS-CoV-2 infection. Lancet Infect. Dis. **20**, 410–411 (2020). https://doi.org/10.1016/S1473-3099(20)30114-6
25. A. Kimball et al., Asymptomatic and presymptomatic SARS-CoV-2 infections in residents of a long-term care skilled nursing facility —King County, Washington. MMWR **69**, 377–381 (2020)
26. C. Rothe et al., Transmission of 2019-nCoV infection from an asymptomatic contact in Germany. N. Engl. J. Med. **3682**, 970–971 (2020). https://doi.org/10.1056/NEJMc2001468
27. N.V. Doremalen et al., Aerosol and surface stability of SARS-CoV-2 as compared with SARS-CoV-1. N. Engl. J. Med. **382**, 1564–1567 (2020). https://doi.org/10.1056/NEJMc2004973
28. Novel Coronavirus (2019-nCoV) Situation Report-12, WHO, 1 February (2020).
29. G. Lalit, C. Emeka, N. Nasser, C. Chinmay, G. Garg, Anonymity preserving IoT-based COVID-19 and other infectious disease contact tracing model. IEEE Access **8**, 159402–159414 (2020. ISSN: 2169-3536). https://doi.org/10.1109/ACCESS.2020.3020513
30. A. Miani, E. Burgio, P. Piscitelli, R. Lauro, A. Colao, The Italian war-like measures to fight coronavirus spreading: Re-open closed hospitals now. EClinicalMedicine **21**, 100320 (2020). https://doi.org/10.1016/j.eclinm.2020.100320
31. W. Zhang et al., Molecular and serological investigation of 2019-nCoV infected patients: Implication of multiple shedding routes. Emerg. Microbes Infect. **9**, 386–389 (2020). https://doi.org/10.1080/22221751.2020.1729071
32. V.M. Corman et al., Assays for laboratory confirmation of novel human coronavirus (hCoV-EMC) infections. Eurosurveillance **17**, 20334 (2012). https://doi.org/10.2807/ese.17.49.20334-en
33. C. Drosten et al., Identification of a novel coronavirus in patients with severe acute respiratory syndrome. N. Engl. J. Med. **348**, 1967–1976 (2003). https://doi.org/10.1056/NEJMoa030747
34. J.F. Chan et al., Improved molecular diagnosis of COVID-19 by the novel, highly sensitive and specific COVID-19-RdRp/Hel real-time reverse transcription-PCR assay validated in vitro and with clinical specimens. J. Clin. Microbiol. **58** (2020). https://doi.org/10.1128/JCM.00310-20

35. A. Ladha, J. Joung, O. Abudayyeh, J. Gootenberg, F. Zhang, A 5-min RNA preparation method for COVID-19 detection with RT-qPCR. medRxiv, 2020.2005.2007.20055947 (2020). https://doi.org/10.1101/2020.05.07.20055947

36. T. Ai, Z. Yang, H. Hou, C. Zhan, C. Chen, W. Lv, Q. Tao, Z. Sun, L. Xia, Correlation of chest CT and RT-PCR testing in coronavirus disease 2019 (COVID-19) in China: A report of 1014 cases. Radiology, online publication 26 Feb, 2020. https://doi.org/10.1148/radiol.2020200642

37. D. Caruso, M. Zerunian, M. Polici, F. Pucciarelli, T. Polidori, C. Rucci, G. Guido, B. Bracci, C. Dominicis, A. Laghi, Chest CT features of COVID-19 in Rome, Italy. Radiology (2020). https://doi.org/10.1148/radiol.2020201237

38. L.M. Almehmadi, S.M. Curley, N.A. Tokranova, et al., Surface enhanced Raman spectroscopy for single molecule protein detection. Sci. Rep. **9**, 12356 (2019). https://doi.org/10.1038/s41598-019-48650-y

39. G. Qiu, Z. Gai, Y. Tao, J. Schmitt, G.A. Kullak-Ublick, J. Wang, Dual-functional plasmonic photothermal biosensors for highly accurate severe acute respiratory syndrome coronavirus 2 detection. ACS Nano **14**, 5268–5277 (2020). https://doi.org/10.1021/acsnano.0c02439

40. Y.C. Syu, W.E. Hsu, C.T. Lin, Review—field-effect transistor biosensing: Devices and clinical applications. ECS J. Solid State Sci. Technol. **7**, Q3196 (2018). https://doi.org/10.1149/2.0291807jss

41. M. Tian, S. Xu, J. Zhang, X. Wang, Z. Li, H. Liu, R. Song, Z. Yu, J. Wang, RNA detection based on graphene field-effect transistor biosensor. Adv. Condens. Matter Phys. **2018**, 8146765 (2018). https://doi.org/10.1155/2018/8146765

42. G. Seo et al., Rapid detection of COVID-19 causative virus(SARS-CoV-2) in human nasopharyngeal swab specimens using field-effect transistor-based biosensor. ACS Nano **14**, 5135–5142 (2020). https://doi.org/10.1021/acsnano.0c02823

43. X. Zhang et al., Electrical probing of COVID-19 spike protein receptor binding domain via a graphene field-effect transistor. arXiv:2003.12529 (2020)

44. https://tinyurl.com/yaprylgs

45. F. Islam, M. Haque, S. Yadav, M.N. Islam, V. Gopalan, N.T. Nguyen, A.K. Lam, M.J.A. Shiddiky, An electrochemical method for sensitive and rapid detection of FAM134B protein in colon cancer samples. Sci. Rep. **7**, 133 (2017). https://doi.org/10.1038/s41598-017-00206-8

46. A.T.E. Viliana et al., Efficient electron-mediated electrochemical biosensor of gold wire for the rapid detection of C-reactive protein: A predictive strategy for heart failure. Biosens. Bioelectron. **142**, 111549 (2019). https://doi.org/10.1016/j.bios.2019.111549

47. Q. Hua, Q. Wang, C. Jiang, J. Zhang, J. Kong, X. iZhang, Electrochemically mediated polymerization for highly sensitive detection of protein kinase activity. Biosens. Bioelectron. **110**, 52–57 (2018). https://doi.org/10.1016/j.bios.2018.03.030

48. S.K. Arya, P. Estrela, Electrochemical ELISA-based platform for bladder cancer protein biomarker detection in urine. Biosens. Bioelectron. **117**, 620–627 (2018). https://doi.org/10.1016/j.bios.2018.07.003

49. H.V. Tran, B. Piro, S. Reisberg, L.H. Nguyen, T.D. Nguyen, H.T. Duc, M.C. Pham, An electrochemical ELISA-like immunosensor for miRNAs detection based on screen-printed gold electrodes modified with reduced graphene oxide and carbon nanotubes. Biosens. Bioelectron. **62**, 25–30 (2014)

50. D. Jacofsky, E.M. Jacofsky, M. Jacofsky, Understanding antibody testing for COVID-19. J. Arthroplasty (2020). https://doi.org/10.1016/j.arth.2020.04.055

51. F. Xiang et al., Antibody detection and dynamic characteristics in patients with COVID-19. Clin. Infect. Dis. (2020). https://doi.org/10.1093/cid/ciaa461

52. L. Yu et al., Rapid detection of COVID-19 coronavirus using a reverse transcriptional loop-mediated isothermal amplification (RT-LAMP) diagnostic platform. Clin. Chem. (2020). https://doi.org/10.1093/clinchem/hvaa102

53. K. Mao, H. Zhang, Z. Yang, Can a paper-based device trace COVID-19 sources with wastewater-based epidemiology? Environ. Sci. Technol. **54**, 3733–3735 (2020). https://doi.org/10.1021/acs.est.0c01174

54. B.S. Batule, Y. Seok, M.G. Kim, Paper-based nucleic acid testing system for simple and early diagnosis of mosquito-borne RNA viruses from human serum. Biosens. Bioelectron. **151**, 111998 (2020). https://doi.org/10.1016/j.bios.2019.111998
55. L.L. Wang et al., CORD-19: The Covid-19 open research dataset. arXivPrepr. arXiv2004.10706 (2020)
56. Y. Ge et al., A data-driven drug repositioning framework discovered a potential therapeutic agent targeting COVID-19. bioRxiv (2020)
57. H.C. Metsky, C.A. Freije, T.-S.F. Kosoko-Thoroddsen, P.C. Sabeti, C. Myhrvold, CRISPR-based COVID-19 surveillance using a genomically-comprehensive machine learning approach. bioRxiv (2020)
58. G.S. Randhawa, M.P.M. Soltysiak, H. El Roz, C.P.E. de Souza, K.A. Hill, L. Kari, Machine learning using intrinsic genomic signatures for rapid classification of novel pathogens: COVID-19 case study. PLoS One **15**(4), e0232391 (2020)
59. O. Gozes et al., Rapid development cycle for the coronavirus (covid-19) pandemic: Initial results for automated detection & patient monitoring using deep learning ct image analysis. arXivPrepr. arXiv2003.05037 (2020)
60. Y. Wang, M. Hu, Q. Li, X.-P. Zhang, G. Zhai, N. Yao, Abnormal respiratory patterns classifier may contribute to large-scale screening of people infected with COVID-19 in an accurate and unobtrusive manner. arXivPrepr. arXiv2002.05534 (2020).
61. A.W. Senior et al., Improved protein structure prediction using potentials from deep learning. Nature, 1–5 (2020)
62. H.S. Maghdid, K.Z. Ghafoor, A.S. Sadiq, K. Curran, K. Rabie, A novel ai-enabled framework to diagnose coronavirus covid 19 using smartphone embedded sensors: Design study. arXivPrepr. arXiv2003.07434 (2020).
63. E. Maddah, B. Beigzadeh, Use of a smartphone thermometer to monitor thermal conductivity changes in diabetic foot ulcers: A pilot study. J. Wound Care **29**(1), 61–66 (2020)
64. S.B. Karvekar, *Smartphone-Based Human Fatigue Detection in an Industrial Environment Using Gait Analysis* (Rochester Institute of Technology, Rochester, 2019)
65. W. Lawanont, M. Inoue, P. Mongkolnam, C. Nukoolkit, Neck posture monitoring system based on image detection and smartphone sensors using the prolonged usage classification concept. IEEJ Trans. Electr. Electron. Eng. **13**(10), 1501–1510 (2018)
66. L. Kvapilova et al., Continuous sound collection using smartphones and machine learning to measure cough. Digit. Biomarkers **3**, 166–175 (2019). https://doi.org/10.1159/000504666
67. M. Sterling, H. Rhee, and M. Bocko, Automated cough assessment on a mobile platform. J. Med. Eng. Article ID 951621, 9 pages (2014). https://doi.org/10.1155/2014/951621
68. C. Menni et al., Real-time tracking of self-reported symptomsto predict potential COVID-19. Nat Med (2020). https://doi.org/10.1038/s41591-020-0916-2.
69. Help speed up contact tracing with TraceTogether, Singapore Government Blog, March (2020). https://www.gov.sg/article/help-speed-up-contact-tracing-with-tracetogether
70. H. Cho, D. Ippolito, Y.W. Yu, Contact tracing mobile apps for COVID-19: Privacy considerations and related trade-offs. arXiv:2003.11511.
71. Aarogyasetu App, Govt. of India. https://www.aarogyasetu.gov.in/
72. A. Imran et al., AI4COVID-19: AI enabled preliminary diagnosis for COVID-19 from cough samples via an app. arXiv:2004.01275v5.
73. C.J. Wang, C.Y. Ng, R.H. Brook, Response to COVID-19 in Taiwan big data analytics, new technology, and proactive testing. JAMA **323**, 1341–1342 (2020)
74. M. Ye, D. Fu, Y. Ren, F. Wang, D. Wang, F. Zhang, X. Xia, T. Lv, Treatment with convalescent plasma for COVID-19 patients in Wuhan, China. J. Med. Virol. (2020). https://doi.org/10.1002/jmv.25882
75. M. Rojas et al., Convalescent plasma in Covid-19: Possible mechanisms of action. Autoimmun. Rev. **19**, 102554 (2020). https://doi.org/10.1016/j.autrev.2020.102554
76. O. Mukama et al., An ultrasensitive and specific point-of-care CRISPR/Cas12 based lateral flow biosensor for the rapid detection of nucleic acids. Biosens. Bioelectron. **159**, 112143 (2020). https://doi.org/10.1016/j.bios.2020.112143

77. M. Imai et al., Rapid diagnosis of H5N1 avian influenza virus infection by newly developed influenza H5 hemagglutinin gene-specific loop-mediated isothermal amplification method. J. Virol. Methods **141**(2), 173–180 (2007)
78. K. Shirato et al., Diagnosis of human respiratory syncytial virus infection using reverse transcription loop-mediated isothermal amplification. J. Virol. Methods **139**(1), 78–84 (2007)
79. G. Lippi, A.-M. Simundic, M. Plebani, Potential preanalytical and analytical vulnerabilities in the laboratory diagnosis of coronavirus disease 2019 (COVID-19). Clin. Chem. Lab. Med. **1**, ahead-of-print (2020)

Chapter 14
Implementation of the Internet of Medical Things (IoMT): Clinical and Policy Implications

Rohan D'Souza

14.1 Introduction

There has never been a better time to scale the IoMT than the present. The COVID-19 pandemic led to a four-time increase in telehealth usage among consumers, from 11% to 46% coupled. As per a McKinsey report, virtual care could replace 24% of outpatient consultations, 20% of emergency visits, and 35% of home-based care. Telehealth is just the first step in increasing the democratization in healthcare [1]. As access to clinicians and other healthcare professionals increases, so also will the increase to health data to supplement these consultations and help the individual take health into their own hands. The key gaps at the moment can be divided based on the stakeholder. At the patient level, addressing access to wearable technology, conversion of data to actionable insights, and reimbursement is going to be critical. For the physician, integration of big data into standard of care, assimilation of big data and healthcare analytics, and translation of this data into actionable prescriptive advice will be essential. At payor and provider levels, a transformation is occurring across the industry with new reimbursement strategies and user experience tactics being central to adapting to the new normal. At the policy level, it is critical to drive the creation of infrastructure to safely and accurately collect, store, secure, and manage health data. The key is end-to-end regulations to ensure not only the accuracy of devices and quality of data but also the equitability of access to improve healthcare outcomes at an individual, community, and country levels.

Contribution Although IoMT has an often spoken about topics, this chapter seeks to give the reader a holistic view of the landscape from the clinical perspective in an

R. D'Souza (✉)
University of California, Berkeley, Berkeley, CA, USA
e-mail: rohan.dsouza@berkeley.edu

© The Author(s), under exclusive license to Springer Nature Switzerland AG 2021
C. Chakraborty et al. (eds.), *Efficient Data Handling for Massive Internet of Medical Things*, Internet of Things,
https://doi.org/10.1007/978-3-030-66633-0_14

attempt to address the obstacles in going from research lab to patient. The aim of this chapter is to assess the adoption of IoMT in healthcare as a surrogate to estimate the current maturity of the industry, identify the key gaps in its implementation, and call out specific areas of focus for the future.

Structure The chapter is structured around these key stakeholders, the patient, the clinician, the provider, the payor, and the policy makers. Each subsection covers the various drivers and obstacles to adoption and scaling of IoMT as well as some real-world use cases currently in practice.

Nancy was woken up by her sleep monitoring device playing soft meditative music. Her device told her she had not slept well, and she could feel it. Her REM cycles were clearly not as per her regular patterns. It was the stress; she knew it was the big presentation and did not need the stress monitor in her watch to tell her that her stress levels were up. She went into the bathroom and began brushing her teeth. The smart mirror she saw her reflection in scanned her face and told her she had a mole on her right cheek that needed to be monitored. She ignored it and slipped into her bathtub. She started the jets which conducted a full body scan and reminded her again about the uterine mass that needed her gynecologist's attention. She got out of the bathroom and hit the send button, when asked if she wanted to set up a tele-consultation the next day. As soon as she gave her approval for the consultation, the data was sent to the doctor's office via the blockchain network. "Thank goodness I don't have to go into the hospital anymore," she thought.

This anecdote is fictional, but these IoT devices and capabilities are closer than you think [2–4].

14.2   What Healthcare Stakeholders Want: Defining the Status Quo and Drivers Toward IoMT

Contrast this with the current patient journey, in which the individual controls none of their data, is subjected to long lines and waiting times in the healthcare settings, and where it is close to impossible to see a consolidated view of one's health. This chapter will go over the three key stakeholders critical for the implementation of the Internet of Medical Things: the patient, the doctor, and the hospital. It also touches on supporting players like the government, payors, and regulators.

14.2.1   Patient

14.2.1.1   Shift of Power

When patients enter the traditional healthcare setting, they are exceedingly frustrated with their care providers. The frustration is attributed to factors such as long waiting times, inconvenient clinic timings, insufficient communication, the persistence of disease and symptoms, inadequate understanding of the disease, and treatment [5]. Paternalism in healthcare, where the doctor is king, is slowly ebbing away [6]. Doctor shopping is now a regular new phenomenon, much like selecting among consumer options in e-commerce. Physicians are subjected to similar market forces with platforms such as Vitals, Healthgrades, and RateMDs used to rate clinicians [7]. Hospitals too are exceedingly being rated by patient safety measures, patient experience, outcomes, process measures, and cost measures over and above pressures to comply with industry standards such as HEDIS and Joint Commission International. [8, 9] The Healthcare Effectiveness Data and Information Set, or HEDIS, is a used performance enhancement tool that includes the effectiveness of care, access, experience, and utilization [10].

Other initiatives target health records, such as Patients Know Best, and allow patients to control their own medical records in the UK, including all clinician notes and lab results [11]. GoodRx allows consumers to track prescription drug prices and provides coupons to avail discounts on medications across over 75,000 pharmacies in the USA [12]. Even medical innovation has been disrupted by patient and caregiver drive like the "We Are Not Waiting" movement to facilitate innovation for type I diabetes [13].

14.2.1.2 $N = 1$: The Move Toward True Patient Centricity

Randomized controlled trials are considered the clinical standard to verify an intervention's efficacy and safety. However, with the move toward individualized medicine, the focus needs to go from larger sample sizes to an n or sample size of one. For individualized medicine, the use of an individual's genomics, transcriptomics, epigenomics, metabolomics, and other "omics" is more important than larger sample sizes of a population [14]. This opens the doors to wearables, 'omics,' and a host of other sources of healthcare data to create personalized health plans.

14.2.1.3 The Democratization of Genomics

Rather than a scientist, Angelina Jolie changed the landscape of genome mapping. "The Angelina Effect" was the headline used by Time magazine to report the rise in Internet searches related to breast cancer genetics and an increase in genetic testing after her BRCA testing and mastectomy [15]. The cost of sequencing a human genome has reduced from $2.7B to $1000 since The Human Genome Project [16]. Companies such as 23andMe, Foundation Medicine, and Guardant Health have increased access to genomic testing and genome mapping. However, physicians lack an understanding of genomic test results, and hence individuals either need to receive reports from the genomic companies or access to genetic counselors to break down the complex evolving science. Genomic data is also set to significantly increase the volume of healthcare data [17]. The future Internet of Medical Things will have to build recommendations taking the genetic and epigenetic risks into consideration.

14.2.1.4 The Wearables' Wave for Health and Disease

The evolution of wearable dates back to seventeenth century with abacus ring, a smart ring to perform calculations. With the gradual evolution from the 1970s with cassette players, digital audio hearing aids (1987), smart clothes, GoPro wearable action camera (2004), fitbit tracker (2009), and Google glass (2013), technology has been evolving in health wearable areas. Current AR/VR headsets, immersive spectacles, bioprinted surface electrodes, and smart sensors will continue to evolve [151]. As access to wearable in the consumer market surges with marketplaces such as the Amazon Wearable Technology Marketplace, the parameters that can be tracked by individuals are expanding as well [18]. These currently include basic heart rate, temperature, blood pressure, and oxygen saturation; posture, physical activities' electrocardiogram (ECG), sleep pattern, fall identification among the elderly, mental status monitoring, and obesity and weight control are commonplace. However, the types of wearables and their indications have been expanding as well [19]. Medical technology companies are now giving patients the power to manage their disease. Some examples in various therapy areas include:

Pulmonology Spire Health (digital biomarkers for patients with severe chronic obstructive pulmonary disease, COPD, to predict exacerbations), [20] Propeller Health (smart inhaler for asthmatic patients) [21].

Mental Health PIP (a tiny device designed to give immediate feedback about stress levels) [22], Muse (EEG-based neuro-feedback headband) [23], Takeda Pharmaceuticals, Cognition Kit, and Apple Watch to monitor major depressive disorder [24].

Cardiology AliveCor's KardiaMobile (an FDA-approved, medical-grade ECG recorder) [25].

Women's Health Ava (helps track menstrual cycles to understand more about fertility, pregnancy, and menstrual health) [26], Yono (an in-ear ovulation predictor) [27].

Dermatology My Skin Track UV (made by a subsidiary of L'Oréal; tracks exposure to UV, pollen, humidity, and pollution) [28].

Pediatrics Owlet (develops wearables for infants that track heart rate, oxygen levels, and sleep) [29], TempTraq (temperature monitoring) [30].

Neurology Embrace2 (epilepsy monitoring) [31], Apple Movement Disorder API (Parkinson's monitoring) [32].

Nephrology Awak (wearable peritoneal dialysis device with FDA Breakthrough designation) [33].

Gastroenterology Proteus (digital pill) [34].

Diabetes Eversense, FreeStyle Libre (a smart continuous glucose monitoring device); Gocap, InPen, and Esysta (smart insulin pen caps); OpenAPS (a closed-loop automated artificial pancreas system) [35].

Oncology Intravascular cancer cell detection device [36].

14.2.1.5 Beyond the Traditional Biomarkers: Non-clinical Data Sources for the Internet of Medical Things

IoMT should extend beyond wearables and traditional diagnostics. In the age of social determinants of health and personalized medicine, there have been several non-traditional markers used to predict the health of an individual.

Social Determinants of Health

Factors influencing an individual's health include social and economic background of their parents and grandparents, location, culture, tradition, education, employment, income, wealth, lifestyle, and genetic disposition. These are factors that are currently not integrated into the management of a patient or used in the risk determination process as per the current clinical guidelines. However, on the Internet of medical and healthcare things, these parameters will probably be on par with traditional clinical parameters collected by wearables and in EHRs [37]. These are gradually finding their way into mainstream medicine. Social determinants are even the focus of ICD-10 codes, which providers use to classify diagnoses for reimbursement claims [38].

Social Media

Social media has been used in some studies to diagnose mental disorders. Facebook and Twitter have both been used to predict depression, suicidality, post-traumatic stress disorder, and postpartum depression [39–45]. Other studies have used a comparison of medical records and the statuses from their Facebook timelines to diagnose depression using International Classification of Diseases (ICD) codes and have demonstrated moderate accuracy [46, 47].

The empowered patient is an essential cog of the healthcare system that is currently ignored. Next, the physician, the traditional stalwart of the medical system.

14.2.2   The Physician

14.2.2.1   The Twenty-First-Century Physician

The fact that medicine is changing is not a modern phenomenon. In his 1989 essay, Karl Jaspers spoke of the technological convergence and its implication on the clinician's role [48]. Healthcare is a slow-moving industry that does not undergo dramatic changes very often, but the past few decades have witnessed "tech-tonic" shifts for clinicians with more paradigm shifts to come [49].

14.2.2.2   A Day in the Life

Today's practice of medicine is significantly different compared to 20 years ago and even more than that of 40 years ago. Sir Theodore Fox, an erstwhile famous editor of The Lancet, once wrote that "lack of time made us all bad doctors." [50]. Much like the hours in the day, the lack of time among medical professionals has never changed. However, the usage of time has seen dramatic changes over the decades [51]. One needs only to look at the break-up of a typical resident's day in an inpatient setting as per a JAMA study [52]. 80 residents were included in the study and observed over 194 shifts (2173 hours) The number of hours and percentages exceeded 24 hours and 100%, respectively, since some activities extend across multiple buckets:

- Three hours, or 13%, spent on face-to-face patient interaction, down from 25% a few decades ago.
- Five hours spent rounding, wherein clinical teams move from patient-to-patient, updated care plans, information handovers at the end of a shift.
- 1.8 hours on education, or 7%
- 15.9 hours, or 66%, on indirect care with 10.3 hours spent updating electronic medical records and other documentation

This will not come as a surprise, and electronic health record (EHR) woes are well-known to anyone remotely associated with healthcare. However, the promises of EHR, including interoperability and clinically actionable insights, are yet to come to fruition [53].

An intended consequence of technology integrated into the care pathway and in process management is "documentation overload." Burnout cost the US healthcare system $4.6 billion, as per an American Medical Association study, which accounted to approximately $7600 per physician, annually [54]. Several initiatives attempted to address this, including personalized user interfaces, natural language processing, and digital assistants [55]. The AMA and Nuance's collaboration in ambient clinical intelligence (ACI) to transform patient-physician interactions into reliable medical chart notes was one notable initiative in 2020 [56].

There have been numerous predictions made about the physician of the future. Some notable publications include the essay "A glimpse into the future: a typical day in the NHS in the year 2050" complete with genome clinics, brain-enhancing puzzles, and telesurgery [57]. The reality of the situation is we need to learn to manage a doctor's interaction with technology rather than inundate them with new makeshift solutions.

14.2.2.3 The "Dataism" Overload

Information overload, much like technology convergence, has also been written about since the 1990s. Hunt and Newman in 1997, in a study titled "Medical knowledge overload: a disturbing trend for physicians," documented the woes of 500 physicians regarding both the lack of time to read journal articles and the difficulty in retrieving information [58]. Back then, an electronic knowledge management system was considered the answer [59].

This rate of increase in clinical literature is exemplified in the current COVID-19 pandemic. As of 19 July 2020, the WHO global literature on coronavirus disease database had 45,938 publications [60]. As a practitioner, it is impossible to stay up to date with the current rate of generation of clinical information.

The Internet of Medical Things will further increase the health informatics volume. Within healthcare centers alone, organizations have seen a data growth rate of 878% since 2016, reaching 8.41 petabytes (PB) on average in 2018 [61]. Genomics and neuroimaging alone generated over 30 petabytes of data annually between 2015 and 2019 [62]. Healthcare IoT devices will constitute 30.7% of IoT device market by volume and generate 507.5 zettabytes of data from 50 billion connected devices [63, 64]. Developing user interfaces and delivering actionable insights are as essential as collecting server's worth of data.

How do we prevent collecting data for the sake of data? A study by Univadis of 550 physicians across specialties reported that less than 50% of the publications they reviewed translated to an impact in practice [65]. Perhaps, a model similar to Cochrane Reviews, which utilize high-quality systematic reviews and meta-analysis to provide specific insights directly to physicians, may be the answer [66].

Besides journal publications, clinical guidelines are another key component of a physician's "continuous medical education." Hibble, in a 1998 study, referred to the ever-changing UK-based primary care clinical guidelines as "the Tower of Babel" and found that there were 855 guidelines that year, weighing 28 kilograms and stood 68 cm high [67]. How do we update clinical guidelines in the face of ever-changing insights, and how often? The process of gathering senior clinicians, or key opinion leaders, along with accessing clinical trial evidence every few years is possibly a practice that warrants reconfiguration as we attempt to amalgamate decades of clinical experience with data-driven insights.

Making IoMT data translatable and relevant to a clinician is critical to its usability in the clinical setting.

14.2.2.4   From Art to Science to Art Again?

The twenty-first-century physician is no longer the hallowed "gatekeeper" of medical information as they once were. The locus of knowledge is shifting from the mind of the physician to search engines. There lies the importance of transforming medical education and physician-patient engagement to focus on how a patient feels rather than what diagnostic and therapeutic interventions the physician prescribed [68].

Medical education needs an overhaul from its current state. The AMA released its "Five competencies of the 21st-century physician" in 2014: inquiry and improvement, interdependency, information management, interest and insight, and involvement [69]. A number of elite medical education establishments have proactively begun embracing these competencies in their curricula.

Inquiry and Improvement Exploring the unknowns and being curious. Examples: Stanford Discovery Curriculum (focused on students discovering career passions and pursuing research) [70], Inquiry Curriculum, UCSF (designed to help students recognize the limits of current knowledge, engage in scientific discovery) [71].

Interdependency Working across teams beyond the customary clinical team. Examples: University of Toronto, Centre for Interprofessional Education for physician competency training.

Information Management Managing the intersection of technology and healthcare. Example: Harvard-MIT Health Sciences and Technology (HST) program for MDs [72].

Interest and Insight Cutting through the data to deliver key insights to patients. Examples: Genes to Society curriculum, Johns Hopkins University (centered around human variability, risk, and the ability to modulate disease presentation and outcomes.) [73].

Involvement Empathy and relationship building. Examples: COMPASS Curriculum, McMaster University (based on principles of learning drawn from cognitive psychology), Narrative Medicine, Columbia Medical School (teaching students to design care plan around patients' unique plights) [74, 75].

The physicians of tomorrow will likely be digital natives, better trained in dealing with data and technology, empathizing with patients, and working across multifunctional teams.

14.2.2.5   Will the Algorithm See You Now: Sensitivity or Sensitivity?

Framing the right question is critical in the age of big data. So far, this has largely centered around "AI versus doctor." Several studies have demonstrated the potential of machine learning across radiology, dermatology, pathology, and other image-based specializations [76]. A Google algorithm when compared with six certified radiologists had 11% less false positives and detected 5% more cancers than the clinicians [77]. Studies found algorithms to be comparable if not better than their human counterparts: This extends to breast cancer screening, skin cancer screening, Alzheimer's disease, and rare congenital diseases [78–83]. This is just the beginning, with technology companies partnering the providers and health systems to use the data science prowess of the former to tap into the vast stores of healthcare information with the latter: These include household names like Google, Amazon, IBM Watson, Facebook, and Apple [84].

Where the issue arises is trust. We have access to journals, risk calculators, disease information, and diagnostic and lab test, yet patients still appeared to resist medical AI as per a perception study by Longoni et al. [85]. The study found that the key reason was that participants felt that the algorithm ignored their "uniqueness" and not the fear that AI provided inferior care, cost more, or was inconvenient. Augmented intelligence is a well-rehearsed topic at medical conferences, but personalization of AI and the patient experience is an essential element for both clinicians and providers to consider [86]. Patients clearly still yearn for empathy as much as accuracy.

The role of the physician and the medical education itself will need a "reboot" with the entry of the Internet of Medical Things [87].

14.2.3   The Provider

Physicians aside, another key stakeholder that will have to transform with the onset of IoMT is hospitals and healthcare providers.

Hospitals already struggle with their EBITDA and profit margins, and the onset of COVID-19 worsened their financial health [88]. However, the digital technology wave will further pressure the system into embracing change to adapt to this new paradigm [89]. A key component of this revolution includes revamping the patient journey, right from making primary care more navigable and accessible to focusing on the patient experience rather than outcome alone. Clinicians are already dealing with exceedingly proactive patients keen to be involved in their care plan rather than silent spectators who follow instructions.

Based on a study by Vahdet et al., the factors influencing patient participation in the care pathway include the relationship with their clinician, their disease knowledge, the time allocated to the patient as well their past experience with the healthcare system and emotional connection [90]. These require a transformational change compared to the transactional relationship that patients currently have with their healthcare provider.

14.2.3.1   Financial Health as a Driver for Change

Kaufman Hall's analysis, from November 2018 to November 2019, covering close to 800 hospitals, reported a 21.3% decline in operating margins and a 14.5% decrease in EBITDA operating margins. This decline in operating EBITDA margins was across hospital categories regardless of the number of beds, and larger hospitals fared the worst with five consecutive months of reported decrease in profitability. Furthermore, there were also significant reductions in volumes. Traditional revenue generators like operating rooms had a 9.4% reduction in operating minutes, and adjusted patient days reduced by 7.6% [91]. The need to be leaner has increased with the introduction of bundled payments and value-based payments. This financial pressure has also driven the need to develop the brand of the health center to be more innovative and improve member satisfaction.

14.2.3.2   Every Penny Counts: The Changing Reimbursement Landscape

Value-based care reimbursement ties payment to quality of care and outcomes. The Health and Human Services (HHS) and Centers for Medicare and Medicaid (CMS) in the USA set a goal of converting 30% of fee-for-service payments to value-based payment models by 2016 and 50% by 2018 [92].

The shift to bundled payment (payments based on predetermined expected costs of a group of related healthcare services) from fee-for-service has seen changes in the practices within the healthcare system. This switch was associated with a 10% decline in spending and a 5–15% reduction in the utilization of healthcare services included within a bundle. Hospitals were increasingly under pressure to ensure that the entire cost of care is controlled rather than over-investigating and readmitting patients [93].

The healthcare IT ecosystem has moved toward the quality-based realm of MACRA, the Medicare Access and CHIP Reauthorization Act of 2015. The measures include outcome measures outside of typical clinical outcomes such as patient-reported outcomes and functional status measures, patient experience, care coordination measures, and appropriate use of services. The Merit-Based Incentive Payment System and Alternative Payment Model frameworks are expected to help providers develop the technical and management competencies to meet these requirements [94].

The argument for IoMT adoption is made stronger by studies such as that by Accenture in 2017, which found that 73% of healthcare professionals reported cost savings with the adoption of IoMT. The issue seems to lie in adoption, as the same report also mentioned that half of all healthcare executives interviewed believed that their leadership did not understand the impact of IoMT to the organization. The key barriers included data security, budgetary constraints, integration with legacy systems, lack of human capital like data scientists, and uncertain return on investment [95].

14.2.3.3   Re-Examining the Care Pathway and Patient Journey

As mentioned in the anecdote in the beginning of this chapter, the patient journey is set to change. The patient journey is currently defined as the series of steps a patient passes through from admission to discharge. However, this definition appears to be an outdated method of defining this journey. Process mapping allows providers to understand the patient's experience. Improvements in this process involve multidisciplinary coordination that extends beyond just the realm of current clinical care. This is beneficial not only in achieving clinical outcomes but also in improving efficiency, eliminating wastage, reducing costs, and increasing stickiness among consumers. Creating IoMT solutions that clearly address an unmet need in these new care pathways will be critical to adoptions and reimbursement [96].

As this expansion of the journey occurs outside the clinical setting, digital journeys are all the more important. Digital journeys toward a health solution are similar to those in other industries wherein the key is understanding all touchpoints and consumer preferences. Consumer adoption of digital health has steadily increased, and a study by the EU Digital Transformation Monitor in 2017 reported that 83% of patients are more willing to share health data for their treatment [97].

Patients are ready, but are the hospitals?

14.2.3.4   The COVID-19 Effect

The COVID-19 pandemic has led to a paradigm shift in the adoption of telehealth among providers, payors, and physicians. Consumer adoption in the USA rose from 11% to 46% as outpatient departments across the country shut their doors and 70% of in-person visits were cancelled. Providers were agile and the adoption of telehealth services increased 50 to 175 fold in the post-COVID period. The Centers for Medicare and Medicaid approved more than 80 telehealth services during this period. McKinsey estimated that $250B of the current healthcare spend could be turned virtual [98]. The decline in in-person visits was the largest in surgical specialties and in pediatrics, traditionally strong revenue generators in the hospital income statement [99, 150]. This may have been the nudge that the telehealth industry needed.

14.2.3.5   Case Studies of Hospitals Adopting IoT

Boston Children's Hospital   The Boston Children's Hospital adopted IoT to address wayfinding, a key contributor to the underwhelming patient experience. Patients struggle to maneuver their way through the care setting leading to stress and struggling to assimilate the complex nature of the healthcare system. The hospital admits 25,000 inpatients and caters to 500,000 through its outpatient department annually. It stretches across 300,000 square feet over 12 buildings and 5 floors, and hence anxious parents with their children struggled to find their way around the facility. The hospital developed MyWay, a GPS-based app to sense patient or visitors' location and guide them in the right direction as well as map the fastest route to facilities like parking lots and information desks. In the first 6 months, the app was downloaded over 4500 times and was reported to improve patient experience among 65% of users [100].

MD Anderson The state-of-the-art oncology center uses a smart monitoring system, known as CYCORE, for oncology patients. Patients randomized to CYCORE experienced less severe symptoms and drug-related side effects compared to patients who went in for weekly physician visits and no additional monitoring. MD Anderson also uses CYCORE for clinical research to wirelessly send data from the patient's home to the research center [101].

Mt. Sinai The Mt. Sinai Medical Center in New York City partnered with GE Healthcare to develop Autobed – an IoT-based software to track bed occupancy and utilization. The software helped reduce waiting times by one hour for 50% of patients admitted through the Emergency Department. This software helped maximize resources and track occupancy among its 1200 units along with other metrics to assess the individual patient's needs [102].

University of Missouri Health System University Hospital It ranks among the most technologically advanced hospitals in the USA. The electronic medical record system has received the top-level HIMSS recognition, Stage 7, and allows barcode-based scanning of every medication and integration with medical equipment to improve patient safety and monitoring. The "smart rooms" allow vital parameters, like blood pressure and heart rate, to be recorded automatically for review by the care team [103].

Smart hospitals utilize healthcare technology to increase patient-centricity and improve patient experience and clinical outcomes. [104]

14.2.4 Payors

Payors, too, are increasingly adopting IoT into their processes to increase their efficiency. Technology implementation use cases include medical underwriting, real-world monitoring, care optimization, curbing fraud, and payment management [105]. Some notable use cases include:

Jon Hancock, Vitality Platform Vitality Active Rewards is an incentivization strategy in which members receive an Apple Watch and a set of personalized activity goals. The goals are structured to help recipients pay off the watch through goal compliance. A healthier patient theoretically translates to less claims and lower payouts for the insurer [106].

Medical Underwriting Using IoT Medical underwriting utilizes health records to determine the risk of an individual to apply for a medical claim in the future and hence dictates the person's healthcare premium. IoT is now beginning to be discussed to increase the robustness of this process so as to improve prediction and reduce the insurers medical loss ratio [107].

Humana and Fitbit Humana partnered with Fitbit to release a virtual care platform. Fitbit's acquisition of fitness training platform Twine Health helped participants achieve better wellness outcomes combining fitness tracking and coaching. Humana did not publish details regarding insurance discounts or additional incentives, but the objective was largely expected to center around helping members manage chronic diseases, guide them toward healthier lifestyles, and build stronger data around participants [108].

14.2.5   Regulatory Bodies

The Internet of Healthcare Things is the amalgamation of data from different sources. It has the potential to aggregate data from patient records, wearable, laboratories, diet, social services, environment, and social networking. This data is currently neither standardized nor interoperable, and a policy intervention can nudge the ecosystem in this direction with a top-down approach [109].

14.2.5.1   Regulating Without Suffocating

The medical device and pharmaceutical regulations have been in the eye of the storm for several years, with numerous books and documentaries highlighting these fallacies [110]. The FDA is already overwhelmed; it oversees $2.5 trillion worth of products and accounts for 25 cents of every dollar spent covering over 19,000 prescription drugs, 6000 medical devices, 12% of imported goods, and 85,000 tobacco products [111].

The regulation of software as a medical device, telehealth, digital health is a relatively new advance in the regulatory landscape and is in an ongoing process. "Software as medical device" is defined by the International Medical Device Regulators Forum (IMDRF) as "software intended to be used for one or more medical purposes that perform these purposes without being part of a hardware medical device." [112]. The Digital Health Innovation Action Plan delineates the FDA's efforts to ensure the quality, safety, and efficacy of these products. The Center for Devices and Radiological Health (CDRH), within the FDA, established the Digital Health program, to foster collaborations within the ecosystem and develop regulatory strategies for the new wave of healthcare solutions [113]. This new center will overlook solutions in artificial intelligence and machine learning, software as a medical device, cybersecurity, health IT, medical device data systems, mobile applications, telemedicine, and wireless medical devices. Some key steps in the right direction include hiring of digital health experts to the FDA and the development of the Digital Health Software Precertification Pilot Program [114].

Pear Therapeutics was the forerunner and received approval for reset, the first prescription digital therapeutic proven to improve patient outcomes of patients with substance abuse disorders [115]. The Apple Watch Series 4 approval as a medical device began a wave of approvals among wearables and other digital health solutions [116]. Since then, the sheer range in the types of products going through the approval pathway is staggering, and this adds pressure onto an already burdened FDA.

Some of the wearables approved by the FDA in 2019 include the IB-Stim (battery-powered electrical nerve stimulator that emits low-frequency electrical pulses to treat abdominal pain associated with irritable bowel syndrome), the VivaQuant's RX-1 (a continuous ECG monitor) and KardiaMobile (a touchpad-based ECG monitoring device tethered to a smartphone), monitoring platform by Current Health (device attached to the arm that tracks vital parameters and predicts health declines), and the Monarch eTNS which is the first FDA-approved digital health solution for ADHD [117]. In 2020, Akili announced that its solution for children with attention-deficit/hyperactivity disorder (ADHD), EndeavorRxTM (AKL-T01), was approved by the FDA. This was the first prescription treatment which is delivered through a video game experience [118].

14.2.5.2 From Patient-Owned to Patient-Generated Data

The least utilized resource in the care pathway is the patient. The HITECH Act encouraged healthcare providers to adopt electronic health records across the USA and achieved this adoption through financial incentivization. The USA spent $27B on EHR, and adoption went from 9% in 2008 to 84% in 2015, and, in 2017, 96% of hospitals had a certified EHR [119]. However, data from sensors, tablets, smartphones, and other data sources mentioned in section one of this chapter are not captured in health records. A similar movement is necessary to adopt the Internet of Medical Things into the formal healthcare ecosystem.

14.2.5.3 Government Infrastructure

For-profit and not-for-profit organizations have all contributed toward setting up infrastructure toward IoMT. Below are significant examples in this direction.

Building "Omics" Databases

Genome sequencing is already on the uptick as discussed earlier in the chapter with the Angelina Effect. The volume and the sensitivity of this data have nudged some governments to implement regulatory policies and frameworks to safeguard the data and attempt to implement evidence-based policy. England announced plans to sequence 100,000 genomes among its citizens, and Saudi Arabia also followed suit [120]. The USA announced the All of Us research project, which will map one million genomes and the Human Microbiome Project to map human microbiomes for research [121, 122]. China has multiple initiatives related to genome sequencing. In 2018 the Beijing Genomic Institute (BGI) published an analysis of 141,431 expectant mothers from across China who had their genome mapped, one of the largest genetic analyses ever conducted [123]. In India, the Southern state of Andhra Pradesh announced in 2018 that it would secure the DNA data of 50 million citizens using blockchain. The Government partnered with a precision medicine company called Shivom to run a pilot in an attempt to make this a reality [124].

Estonia: The Digital Nation

The ultimate goal for any healthcare system is to be able to integrate all the sources of health-related data around a single individual, be it genomic, health records, wearables, social services, etc. The country whose model seems to be closest to that healthcare singularity is Estonia. The European nations began a digital journey over two decades ago and are now reaping the rewards of digital transformation. A key part of this transformation has been the fact that healthcare was merely one of the many facets that were digitized. The X-Road platform allows citizens to access all services on one digital platform, from healthcare and education to banking, taxes, and voting. 78% of the country's bureaucracy is digitized [125].

The vision for 2025 for the e-health system is "better information, better health." The digital health ecosystem was built in piecemeal with a national EHR in 2008, followed by digital prescriptions, e-consultations 2 years later, e-ambulances in 2015, and in 2017 a drug interaction decision support system [126].

Estonia has also built a blockchain-based network to facilitate interoperability and data sharing. The Government developed a data security framework and partnered with Guardtime in 2017 to develop KSI blockchain technology to ensure the security of medical records [127].

However, it is not just infrastructure, but its utilization as well. Over a quarter of the population have had their genome mapped and risk profiled, and there is a political nudge from the highest offices for all citizens over 18 years of age to have their genome mapped for various risk factors. In 2018, the Estonian Genome Center offered free genetic testing to over 100,000 Estonians [128]. The country even enacted the Human Genes Research Act to regulate privacy and research based on genomes [129].

Cancer Biomedical Informatics Grid (caBIG) [130]

The National Cancer Institute (NCI) developed an informatics program to improve patient care and accelerate scientific discoveries. Large volumes of data are collected, analyzed, and harmonized to promote collaboration among researches and affiliated organizations. The NCI aimed to address the key unmet need associated with the inability to collect, process, share, and archive biospecimen data across the entire oncology network. Since 2004, over 700 organizations are involved in this initiative. These include researchers, patients, oncologists, physicians, data scientists, bioinformatics specialists, executives, academics from community cancer centers, academic centers, medical centers, government, and pharmaceutical and biotechnology companies from across the globe.

The four key principles of the project are:

- Open access.
- Open development (the infrastructure on the platform are open to the entire oncology community, both from a utilization and contribution perspective to increase the breadth of data and the possibility of solutions).
- Open source (the software code is freely available for use and modification by any organization).
- Federation (data is controlled locally or integrated across sites. The decentralized approach obviates the need for a central authority).

eVIN (Electronic Vaccine Intelligence Network) [131]

Electronic Vaccine Intelligence Network was developed in India to address the issues associated with the country's massive vaccination effort. Inventory management and cold chain are critical to the success of this program, and this solution was developed indigenously and implemented by the United Nations Development Program (UNDP) to address these issues using a smartphone-based application. The network currently extends across 12 states in India and supports the effort of the government to implement India's Universal Immunization Program. It provides real-time updates on vaccine inventory, product flow, and temperature across each point in the cold chain. eVIN has aided data-driven policy making around vaccination programs, streamlined planning of vaccine drives, and improved procurement cycles. At the moment, teams of additional human resources are critical for the network to run seamlessly including temperature loggers, cold-chain handlers, cold-chain managers, and cold-chain technicians in every district across the participating states.

China's COVID-19 Response

China has invested heavily in IoT in the past, but the true depth of IoT penetration and adoption was seen with the COVID-19 outbreak. Skynet, Alibaba, and mobile operators during the early days of the pandemic mobilized to contribute toward disease control. Alibaba implemented a Skynet across over 100 cities by leveraging smartphone apps and the power of mobile IoT. The Alipay Health Code enabled large-scale, real-time monitoring across the country in an effort to control the outbreak. An AI company, SenseTime, deployed contactless temperature detection technology in stations, schools, and other locations across various regions in China that used a combination of temperature screening and facial recognition to identify infected individuals. The company Tencent launched a QR-code-based tracking feature to address contact tracing within the country. Although there were privacy issues reported, the scale of the IoT initiative was unparalleled in healthcare [132].

The Rare Diseases Registry Program (RaDaR)

For rare diseases registries are critically important to build advocacy groups, share best practices, and generate evidence-based care recommendations. The Rare Diseases Registry Program (RaDaR) was initiated by the National Center for Advancing Translational Sciences to provide guidance and offer recommendations and data standards for rare disease registries. The program offers stepwise overviews to set up and manage these disease registries and ensure the efficient and secure collections and management of data. It also creates frameworks to protect patient data and ensure standardization to facilitate the sharing of data between patients and providers as well as researchers and the industry [133].

Rhode Island: Increasing Interoperability

Rhode Island partnered with InterSystems to use its analytics tool to consolidate and analyze data for patients across the state. The Rhode Island Quality Institute (RIQI) used a grant to care to build analytics capabilities for its diabetic population. The objective was to reduce readmissions, emergency visits, and length of stay among inpatients. The system used metrics such as key diabetes clinic parameters, admission trends across facilities, and providers. The initiative found that about 10% of lab tests performed in over 25% of the state's population were medically unnecessary and helped improve the efficiency and the cost-effectiveness of diabetic care [134].

New England Healthcare Exchange Network (NEHEN)

The New England Healthcare Exchange Network, established in 1998, is a consortium of payers and providers. The working group designed and implemented a secure health information exchange platform. The key objective being the improvement of patient care and safety while reducing administrative costs. The network boasts of 40-member organizations consisting 8 health insurance plans, over 50 hospitals, and thousands of healthcare practitioners. The network currently generates over eight million transactions a month [135].

14.3 The Way Forward

14.3.1 Accountability

Checks and balances are critical in healthcare. Currently, in cases of negligence or medical error, healthcare professionals and providers face lawsuits and litigation [136]. However, with the increase in the volume of data and the decision-making coming down to an algorithm, where does accountability lie? With the clinicians? With the manufacturer/developer?

Additionally, in cases of data breaches, who bears the legal burden? These are questions that have larger social implications but could become stumbling blocks in the IoMT future. Accountability is centered around checks and balances to power, but in the world of algorithms, the concept of accountability remains murky [137].

14.3.2 Accuracy

97,000 health and fitness apps and 52% of users collect health data from their smartphones [138]. Twenty-one percent of Americans use a health tracker or a smart watch [139].

While wearables, fitness trackers, and digital apps encourage users to be more active, eat more consciously, and live healthier, they are not necessarily accurate. The vast majority of these direct-to-consumer solutions currently do not go through a stringent regulatory process. Companies such as Fitbit have faced lawsuits due to inaccuracy in the past, and, although not large scale, some studies have suggested that these devices are not entirely accurate [140].

Genome testing has had a thorny relationship with the FDA in the past, and other sources of health data on which an intervention is to be based should fall under a regulatory umbrella to ensure efficacy, reliability, accuracy, and data security [141].

Once the data is collected, the analysis and insights pose the next hurdle. For the cognitive technologies that drive the analysis of IoMT data, robust peerreviewed evaluation is difficult for machine learning algorithms. The inability to look "under the hood" coupled with the impracticality of constant reapproval of algorithms makes it all the more complicated. When any change whatsoever is made to a drug or a device, the FDA is sent an update by the manufacturer. This format will lead to redundancies for self-learning algorithms constantly updating themselves [142].

14.3.3 Equity

Universal access to healthcare services has been a thorn in the side of healthcare. With IoMT this is true as well. With regard to wearables, according to a Pew study,

31% of Americans in households with annual earnings over $75,000 extensively used a smart watch or fitness tracker. Compare that with 12% in households with annual incomes below $30,000. There were also differences reported based on education level, gender, race, and ethnicity [143].

AI algorithms have already shown to be biased on the basis of gender, ethnicity, and age [144, 145]. There are several reasons behind these biases including judgmental data sets, ingrained social injustices, unconscious clinical biases, clinical trial homogeneity with primarily white males, etc. [146] While it's important to ensure that everyone has access to resources, both human and technological, it is critical that we address these deeper fallacies to avoid further deepening the healthcare access divide [147].

14.3.4 Patient and Patient Data Safety

The Department of Health and Human Services in the USA passed The Common Rule of 1991 and was updated in 2018. The Common Rule regulations focus on the ethics and safety of patients in clinical trials and research and at the same time attempt to confer for flexibility for low-risk studies to increase participation. The Act covers collection, storage, transmission, and secondary use of the data by healthcare entities [148]. However, the Act does not focus sufficiently on the individual, and a new set of regulations are essential to address the increasing democratization of IoMT. Data protection is covered elsewhere in this book.

Regulators and policy makers aside, despite an increase willingness from patients to share data, there is an increasing concern over data security when it comes to sensitive healthcare data. Thus, any strategy must cover not only the specifics of increasing security but also increasing public awareness on measures taken to safeguard healthcare data [149].

14.4 Conclusions and Final Thoughts

The Internet of Medical Things can profoundly change the face of healthcare as we know it and take us from sick care to health care. To truly make a difference at scale, adoption of this technology needs to cut across all the stakeholders mentioned in this chapter: patients, physicians, providers, payors, policy makers, regulatory bodies, and authorities. The one key gap is the lack of interoperability in healthcare. Health data will be the center of everything, and beyond collection and storage, sharing of data across the value chain is essential. As technologists, creating breakthrough IoT technology and infrastructure alone will mean nothing if it isn't integrated into the current care and reimbursement pathways.

For the industry, looking ahead and preparing for the healthcare of tomorrow requires focusing on the next big IoMT breakthroughs. The key will be to work with researchers, innovators, technologists, and others to go beyond the science and focus on acceptability, adaptability, and affordability. There have been multiple interventions in the past that created hype and never saw the light of day given healthcare's paternalism and bureaucracy. For inventors and founders, understanding the highly nuanced healthcare system, its stakeholders, its incentives, the flow of money, and, of course, the patient is crucial.

References

1. Telehealth: a quarter-trillion-dollar post-COVID-19 reality? McKinsey May 29, 2020. https://www.mckinsey.com/industries/healthcare-systems-and-services/our-insights/telehealth-a-quarter-trillion-dollar-post-covid-19-reality. Accessed 8/8/2020
2. United States Patent and Trademark Office, Patent Number US020160206244A120160721 Link. Accessed 7/10/2020
3. Oura Sleep tracking Ring https://ouraring.com/. Accessed 8/8/2020
4. Blockchain: A Superhighway for Health Data Exchange – HIMSS March 21, 2019. https://www.himss.org/resources/blockchain-superhighway-health-data-exchange. Accessed 7/10/2020
5. R.A. Sansone, L.A. Sansone, Doctor shopping: a phenomenon of many themes. Innov. Clin. Neurosci. **9**(11–12), 42–46 (2012)
6. S.M. Gallagher, Paternalism in healthcare decision making. Ostomy Wound Manage **44**(4), 22–25 (1998)
7. Rating Doctors: What you need to know. US News Feb. 15, 2018. https://health.usnews.com/health-care/patient-advice/articles/rating-doctors-what-you-need-to-know. Accessed 7/10/2020
8. How to Use Online Ratings for a Hospital. WebMD https://www.webmd.com/health-insurance/how-use-online-ratings-hospital#. Accessed 7/25/2020
9. JCI – Joint Commission International, http://www.jointcommissioninternational.org/jci-accreditation-standards-for-hospitals-6th-edition/?ref=PATHWAY. Accessed 7/10/2020
10. HEDIS, https://www.ncqa.org/hedis/. Accessed 7/10/2020
11. Patients Know Best, https://patientsknowbest.com/. Accessed 7/25/2020
12. GoodRx, https://www.goodrx.com/. Accessed 7/10/2020
13. The #WeAreNotWaiting Diabetes DIY Movement – Healthline May 5, 2019, https://www.healthline.com/health/diabetesmine/innovation/we-are-not-waiting#1. Accessed 7/10/2020
14. E.O. Lillie, B. Patay, J. Diamant, B. Issell, E.J. Topol, N.J. Schork, The n-of-1 clinical trial: the ultimate strategy for individualizing medicine? Per Med. **8**(2), 161–173 (2011). https://doi.org/10.2217/pme.11.7
15. A. Liede, M. Cai, T.F. Crouter, D. Niepel, F. Callaghan, D.G. Evans, Risk-reducing mastectomy rates in the US: a closer examination of the Angelina Jolie effect. Breast Cancer Res. Treat. **171**(2), 435–442 (2018). https://doi.org/10.1007/s10549-018-4824-9
16. The Cost of Sequencing a Human Genome National Human Genome Research Institute, https://www.genome.gov/about-genomics/fact-sheets/Sequencing-Human-Genome-cost. Accessed 7/24/2020
17. C.M. Weipert, K.A. Ryan, J.N. Everett, et al., Physician experiences and understanding of genomic sequencing in oncology. J. Genet. Couns. **27**(1), 187–196 (2018). https://doi.org/10.1007/s10897-017-0134-3
18. Amazon Wearable Technology, https://www.amazon.com/Wearable-Technology/b?ie=UTF8&node=10048700011. Accessed 7/24/2020
19. M. Wu, J. Luo, Wearable technology applications in healthcare: as literature review. Online J. Nurs. Inform. **23**, 3 (2019)

20. Spire, https://spirehealth.com/pages/about-us. Accessed 7/24/2020
21. Propeller Health, https://www.propellerhealth.com/. Accessed 7/24/2020
22. PIP, https://thepip.com/en-eu/. Accessed 7/24/2020
23. Muse, https://choosemuse.com/. Accessed 7/24/2020
24. Takeda and Cognition Kit Present Results from Digital Wearable Technology Study in patients with Major Depressive Disorder (MDD), https://www.takeda.com/en-us/newsroom/news-releases/2017/takeda-and-cognition-kit-present-results-from-digital-wearable-technology-study-in-patients-with-major-depressive-disorder-mdd/. Accessed 7/24/2020
25. AliveCor, https://www.alivecor.com/. Accessed 7/24/2020
26. Ava, https://www.avawomen.com/. Accessed 7/24/2020
27. Yono, https://www.yonolabs.com/. Accessed 7/24/2020
28. My Skin Track UV, https://www.laroche-posay.us/my-skin-track-uv-3606000530485.html. Accessed 7/24/2020
29. Owlet, https://owletcare.com/. Accessed 7/24/2020
30. Temptraq, https://www.temptraq.com/Home. Accessed 7/24/2020
31. Empatica, https://www.empatica.com/en-gb/embrace2/. Accessed 7/24/2020
32. Movement Disorder API, https://developer.apple.com/documentation/coremotion/monitoring_movement_disorders. Accessed 7/24/2020
33. Awak, https://awak.com/. Accessed 7/24/2020
34. Proteus, https://www.proteus.com/. Accessed 7/10/2020
35. 10 examples of the Internet of Things in healthcare E-consultancy 2019, https://econsultancy.com/internet-of-things-healthcare/. Accessed 7/24/2020
36. T.H. Kim, Y. Wang, C.R. Oliver, et al., A temporary indwelling intravascular aphaeretic system for in vivo enrichment of circulating tumor cells. Nat. Commun. **10**, 1478 (2019)
37. M. Marmot et al., WHO European review of social determinants of health and the health divide. Lancet **380**(9846), 1011–1029 (2012)
38. ICD10 CDC, https://www.cdc.gov/nchs/icd/icd10cm.htm. Accessed 7/24/2020
39. J.C. Eichstaedt et al., Facebook language predicts depression in medical records. Proc. Natl. Acad. Sci. **115**(44), 11203–11208 (2018)
40. M. De Choudhury, M. Gamon, S. Counts, E. Horvitz, Predicting depression via social media. ICWSM **13**, 1–10 (2013)
41. A.G. Reece et al., Forecasting the onset and course of mental illness with Twitter data. Sci. Rep. **7**, 13006 (2016)
42. H.A. Schwartz et al., Towards assessing changes in degree of depression through Facebook, in *Proceedings of the Workshop on Computational Linguistics and Clinical Psychology: From Linguistic Signal to Clinical Reality*, (Association for Computational Linguistics, Stroudsburg, 2014), pp. 118–125
43. M. De Choudhury, S. Counts, E.J. Horvitz, A. Hoff, Characterizing and predicting postpartum depression from shared Facebook data, in *Proceedings of the 17th ACM Conference on Computer Supported Cooperative Work & Social Computing*, (Association for Computational Linguistics, Stroudsburg, 2014), pp. 626–638
44. C.M. Homan et al., *Toward Macro-Insights for Suicide Prevention: Analyzing Fine-Grained Distress at Scale* (Association for Computational Linguistics, Stroudsburg, 2014)
45. G. Coppersmith, M. Dredze, C. Harman, Quantifying mental health signals in twitter, in *Proceedings of the Workshop on Computational Linguistics and Clinical Psychology: From Linguistic Signal to Clinical Reality*, (Association for Computational Linguistics, Stroudsburg, 2014), pp. 51–60
46. K.A. Padrez et al., Linking social media and medical record data: a study of adults presenting to an academic, urban emergency department. BMJ Qual. Saf. **25**, 414–423 (2015)
47. N.H.T. Trinh et al., Using electronic medical records to determine the diagnosis of clinical depression. Int. J. Med. Inform. **80**, 533–540 (2011)
48. K. Jaspers, The physician in the technological age. Theor. Med. **10**(3), 251–267 (1989)
49. Medtech and the Internet of Medical Things – Deloitte Center for Health Solutions

50. A.J. Dunning, Status of the doctor—present and future. Lancet **354**, SIV18 (1999)
51. C.P. West, L.N. Dyrbye, T.D. Shanafelt, Physician burnout: contributors, consequences and solutions. J. Intern. Med. **283**(6), 516–529 (2018)
52. K.H. Chaiyachati, J.A. Shea, D.A. Asch, et al., Assessment of inpatient time allocation among first-year internal medicine residents using time-motion observations. JAMA Intern. Med. **179**(6), 760–767 (2019)
53. N. Menachemi, T.H. Collum, Benefits and drawbacks of electronic health record systems. Risk Manag. Healthc. Policy **4**, 47–55 (2011). https://doi.org/10.2147/RMHP.S12985
54. S. Han, T.D. Shanafelt, C.A. Sinsky, K.M. Awad, L.N. Dyrbye, L.C. Fiscus, et al., Estimating the attributable cost of physician burnout in the United States. Ann. Intern. Med. **170**(11), 784–790 (2019)
55. B. Furlow, Information overload and unsustainable workloads in the era of electronic health records. Lancet Respir. Med. **8**(3), 243–244 (2020)
56. AMA, Nuance partner to pilot innovations to prevent physician burnout. AMA, https://www.ama-assn.org/press-center/press-releases/ama-nuance-partner-pilot-innovations-prevent-physician-burnout. Accessed 7/10/2020
57. H. Wilson, A glimpse into the future: a typical day in the NHS in the year 2050. BMJ **349**, g6881 (2014)
58. R.E. Hunt, R.G. Newman, Medical knowledge overload: a disturbing trend for physicians. Health Care Manag. Rev. **22**(1), 70–75 (1997)
59. A. Hall, G. Walton, Information overload within the health care system: a literature review. Health Inform. Libr. J. **21**(2), 102–108 (2004)
60. WHO Global literature on coronavirus disease, https://search.bvsalud.org/global-literature-on-novel-coronavirus-2019-ncov/. Accessed 7/19/2020
61. Dell Technologies Global Data Protection Index, https://www.delltechnologies.com/en-us/data-protection/gdpi/index.htm. Accessed 7/10/2020
62. I.D. Dinov, Volume and value of big healthcare data. J. Med. Stat. Inform. **4**, 3 (2016)
63. S. Shukla, M.F. Hassan, M.K. Khan, L.T. Jung, A. Awang, An analytical model to minimize the latency in healthcare internet-of-things in fog computing environment. PLoS One **14**(11), e0224934 (2019) Published 2019 Nov 13
64. R.K. Naha, S. Garg, D. Georgakopoulos, P.P. Jayaraman, L. Gao, Y. Xiang, et al., Fog computing: survey of trends, architectures, requirements, and research directions. IEEE Access **6**, 47980–48009 (2018)
65. The Doctor's Dilemma, http://t.go.univadis.com/webApp/APP167#7. Accessed 7/12/2020
66. Cochrane Library, https://www.cochranelibrary.com/about/about-cochrane-reviews. Accessed 7/7/2020
67. H. Arthur, K. David, P. David, P. Fiona, Guidelines in general practice: the new tower of babel? BMJ **317**, 862 (1998)
68. The Art of Medicine in the Age of Technology Mark Kaufmann – Practical Dermatology. Accessed 7/19/2020
69. 5 competencies of the 21st-century physician – Accelerating Change in Medical Education AMA APR 11, 2014
70. 2020 Health Trends Report Stanford, http://med.stanford.edu/dean/healthtrends.html
71. UCSF – Inquiry Curriculum, https://meded.ucsf.edu/inquiry-curriculum. Accessed 7/10/2020
72. Harvard Medical School, https://hms.harvard.edu/. Accessed 7/10/2020
73. John Hopkins Curriculum, https://www.hopkinsmedicine.org/som/curriculum/genes_to_society/year-one/index.html. Accessed 7/10/2020
74. Our Curriculum – McMaster University, https://mdprogram.mcmaster.ca/md-program/our-curriculum/what-is-compass
75. Columbia University, Narrative Medicine, https://sps.columbia.edu/academics/masters/narrative-medicine. Accessed 6/20/2020

76. Will artificial intelligence replace doctors? Ken Budd. July 2019. Association of American Medical Colleges, https://www.aamc.org/news-insights/will-artificial-intelligence-replace-doctors. Accessed 7/23/2020
77. D. Ardila, A.P. Kiraly, S. Bharadwaj, et al., End-to-end lung cancer screening with three-dimensional deep learning on low-dose chest computed tomography. Nat. Med. **25**, 954–961 (2019)
78. A. Rodriguez-Ruiz et al., Stand-alone artificial intelligence for breast Cancer detection in mammography: Comparison with 101 radiologists. JNCI J. Natl. Cancer Instit. **111**(9), 916–922 (2019)
79. A. Esteva, B. Kuprel, R. Novoa, et al., Dermatologist-level classification of skin cancer with deep neural networks. Nature **542**, 115–118
80. N. Bhagwat et al., Modeling and prediction of clinical symptom trajectories in Alzheimer's disease using longitudinal data. PLoS Comput. Biol. **14**(9), e1006376 (2018)
81. T. Hsieh, M.A. Mensah, J.T. Pantel, et al., PEDIA: prioritization of exome data by image analysis. Genet. Med. **21**, 2807–2814 (2019)
82. J.M. Banda, A. Sarraju, F. Abbasi, et al., Finding missed cases of familial hypercholesterolemia in health systems using machine learning. npj Digit. Med. **2**, 23 (2019). https://doi.org/10.1038/s41746-019-0101-5
83. M. Signaevsky, M. Prastawa, K. Farrell, et al., Artificial intelligence in neuropathology: deep learning-based assessment of tauopathy. Lab. Investig. **99**, 1019–1029 (2019). https://doi.org/10.1038/s41374-019-0202-4
84. 36 hospitals, health systems that partnered with big tech in 2019
85. Andrea Park – Friday, December 27th, 2019, https://www.beckershospitalreview.com/healthcare-information-technology/36-hospitals-health-systems-that-partnered-with-big-tech-in-2019.html. Accessed 7/23/2020
86. C. Longoni, A. Bonezzi, C.K. Morewedge, Resistance to medical artificial intelligence. J. Consum. Res. **46**(4), 629–650 (2019)
87. G.R. Cutter, Y. Liu, Personalized medicine: the return of the house call? Neurol. Clin. Pract. **2**(4), 343–351 (2012). https://doi.org/10.1212/CPJ.0b013e318278c328
88. S.A. Wartman, The physician in the 21st century. Rev. Med. **95**, 11–14 (2016)
89. Kaufmann Hall National Hospital Flash Report May 2020, https://www.kaufmanhall.com/sites/default/files/documents/2020-05/may_2020_national_hospital_flash_report_-_kaufmanhall.pdf. Accessed 7/10/2020
90. National Academies of Sciences, Engineering, and Medicine; Health and Medicine Division; Board on Health Care Services; Board on Global Health; Committee on Improving the Quality of Health Care Globally. Crossing the Global Quality Chasm: Improving Health Care Worldwide. Washington (DC): National Academies Press (US); 2018 Aug 28. 3, Optimizing the Patient Journey by Leveraging Advances in Health Care
91. S. Vahdat, L. Hamzehgardeshi, S. Hessam, Z. Hamzehgardeshi, Patient involvement in health care decision making: a review. Iran Red Crescent Med J **16**(1), e12454 (2014). https://doi.org/10.5812/ircmj.12454
92. National Hospital Flash Report 2019, https://flashreportmember.kaufmanhall.com/national-hospital-report-december-2019. Accessed 7/23/2020
93. Better Care. Smarter Spending. Healthier People: Paying Providers for Value, Not Volume, https://www.cms.gov/newsroom/fact-sheets/better-care-smarter-spending-healthier-people-paying-providers-value-not-volume
94. P.S. Hussey et al., Closing the quality gap: revisiting the state of the science (vol. 1: Bundled payment: effects on health care spending and quality). Evid. Rep. Technol. Assess. **2081**, 1 (2012)
95. MACRA – CMS, https://www.cms.gov/Medicare/Quality-Initiatives-Patient-Assessment-Instruments/Value-Based-Programs/MACRA-MIPS-and-APMs/MACRA-MIPS-and-APMs. Accessed 7/25/2020
96. Accenture 2017 Internet of Health Things Survey

97. Process mapping the patient journey: an introduction
98. European Commission (2017). Digital Transformation Monitor: Update of digital solutions in the healthcare industry
99. Telehealth: a quarter-trillion-dollar post-COVID-19 reality? – McKinsey May 2020, https://www.mckinsey.com/industries/healthcare-systems-and-services/our-insights/telehealth-a-quarter-trillion-dollar-post-covid-19-reality. Accessed 7/10/2020
100. A. Mehrotra, et al., The Impact of the COVID-19 Pandemic on Outpatient Visits: A Rebound Emerges," To the Point (blog), Commonwealth Fund, May 19, 2020. https://doi.org/10.26099/ds9e-jm36
101. Making Sense of IoT: How the Internet of Things Became Humanity's Nervous System' by Kevin Ashton
102. Information Technology Tools Helping With Clinical Trials – MD Anderson, https://www.mdanderson.org/publications/cancer-newsline/information-technology-helping-cancer-clinical-trials.h35-1587468.html
103. Looking to Industry for the Next Digital Disruption New York Times Nov. 23, 2012, https://www.nytimes.com/2012/11/24/technology/internet/ge-looks-to-industry-for-the-next-digital-disruption.html?pagewanted=all&_r=1&. Accessed 7/10/2020
104. MU Healthcare, https://www.muhealth.org/about-us/quality-care-patient-safety. Accessed 7/10/2020
105. Finding the future of care provision: the role of smart hospitals – McKinsey 5/31/2019, https://www.mckinsey.com/industries/healthcare-systems-and-services/our-insights/finding-the-future-of-care-provision-the-role-of-smart-hospitals#:~:text=Smart%20hospitals%20are%20patient%2Dcentric,patient%20satisfaction%20(Exhibit%203). Accessed 7/10/2020
106. Digital ecosystems for insurers: opportunities through the Internet of Things, https://www.mckinsey.com/industries/financial-services/our-insights/digital-ecosystems-for-insurers-opportunities-through-the-internet-of-things#. Accessed 7/10/2020
107. Jon Hancock Vitality Platform, https://www.johnhancockvitality.com/. Accessed 7/10/2020
108. IoT Applications for Healthcare Payors, https://www.iotforall.com/iot-applications-healthcare-payers/. Accessed 7/10/2020
109. Fitbit Press Release 9/19/2018, https://investor.fitbit.com/press/press-releases/press-release-details/2018/Fitbit-and-Humana-Expand-Strategic-Partnership-to-Drive-Healthy-Habits-and-Prevent-and-Manage-Chronic-Disease/default.aspx. Accessed 7/10/2020
110. Big Data at Center of Disruptive Technologies, McKinsey Global Institute (May 2013)
111. http://www.mckinsey.com/insights/business_technology/disruptive_technologies. Accessed 7/10/2020
112. It's Time for a Reckoning on Medical Devices 4/29/2020, https://www.nytimes.com/2019/05/04/opinion/sunday/medical-devices.html. Accessed 7/10/2020
113. R.M. Califf, M. Hamburg, J.E. Henney, et al., Seven former FDA commissioners: the FDA should be an Independent Federal Agency. Health Aff. (Millwood). **38**(1), 84–86 (2019)
114. International Medical Device Regulators Forum (IMDRF), https://www.fda.gov/medical-devices/cdrh-international-programs/international-medical-device-regulators-forum-imdrf. Accessed 7/10/2020
115. Digital Health Innovation Action Plan – US FDA, https://www.fda.gov/media/106331/download. Accessed 7/10/2020
116. Digital Health – FDA, https://www.fda.gov/medical-devices/digital-health. Accessed 7/10/2020
117. Pear Therapeutics September 14, 2017., https://peartherapeutics.com/fda-obtains-fda-clearance-first-prescription-digital-therapeutic-treat-disease/. Accessed 7/10/2020
118. Apple Watch Series 4, https://www.accessdata.fda.gov/cdrh_docs/reviews/DEN180044.pdf. Accessed 7/10/2020
119. Non-federal Acute Care Hospital Electronic Health Record Dashboard. The Office of the National Coordinator for Health Information Technology. https://dashboard.healthit.gov/quickstats/pages/FIG-Hospital-EHR-Adoption.php. Accessed 7/10/2020

120. Akili Announces FDA Clearance of EndeavorRx™ for Children with ADHD, the First Prescription Treatment Delivered Through a Video Game 6/15/2020, https://www.akili-interactive.com/news-collection/akili-announces-endeavortm-attention-treatment-is-now-available-for-children-with-attention-deficit-hyperactivity-disorder-adhd-al3pw. Accessed 7/10/2020

121. Non-federal Acute Care Hospital Electronic Health Record Dashboard, https://dashboard.healthit.gov/quickstats/pages/FIG-Hospital-EHR-Adoption.php. Accessed 7/10/2020

122. Z.D. Stephens et al., Big data: astronomical or genomical? PLoS Biol. **13**(7), e1002195 (2015)

123. All of Us Project, https://allofus.nih.gov/news-events-and-media/news/all-us-research-project-historic-effort-sequence-one-million-genomes. Accessed 7/10/2020

124. Human Microbiome Project, https://www.hmpdacc.org/. Accessed 7/10/2020

125. S. Liu et al., Genomic analyses from non-invasive prenatal testing reveal genetic associations, patterns of viral infections, and Chinese population history. Cell **175**(2), 347–359 (2018)

126. An Indian state is using blockchain to collect DNA data of 50 million citizens Quartz 4/8/2018, https://qz.com/india/1244824/andhra-pradesh-is-using-blockchain-to-collect-dna-data-of-50-million-citizens/. Accessed 7/13/2020

127. Estonia- The Digital Republic. The New Yorker 12/18/2017, https://www.newyorker.com/magazine/2017/12/18/estonia-the-digital-republic. Accessed 7/13/2020

128. Estonia e-Health vision, https://www.sm.ee/sites/default/files/content-editors/sisekomm/e-tervise_strateegia_2020_15_en1.pdf. Accessed 7/13/2020

129. PwC Estonia Prescribes Blockchain for healthcare data security 3/2017, http://pwc.blogs.com/health_matters/2017/03/estonia-prescribes-blockchain-for-healthcare-data-security.html. Accessed 7/13/2020

130. Estonian Genome Center, https://www.geenivaramu.ee/en. Accessed 7/13/2020

131. Human Genes Research Act, https://www.riigiteataja.ee/en/eli/531102013003/consolide. Accessed 7/13/2020

132. Institute of Medicine (US), in *Digital Infrastructure for the Learning Health System: The Foundation for Continuous Improvement in Health and Health Care: Workshop Series Summary*, ed. by C. Grossmann, B. Powers, J. M. McGinnis, (National Academies Press (US), Washington, DC, 2011) B, Case Studies for the Digital Health Infrastructure

133. electronic Vaccine Intelligence Network (eVIN). National Health Mission, Ministry of Health and Family Welfare, Government of India, 2016., https://smartnet.niua.org/content/d9b14fcf-c907-4260-bfd7-3ee9fa94c8d4. Accessed 7/13/2020

134. Coronavirus: China's tech fights back BBC 3/3/2020, https://www.bbc.com/news/technology-51717164

135. RaDaR, https://registries.ncats.nih.gov/about-radar/. Accessed 7/13/2020

136. The Key to Breakthrough Healthcare Leveraging Interoperability to Address Hospital Readmissions, https://www.intersystems.com/wpcontent/uploads/assets/Leveraging_Interoperability_to_Address_Readmissions_WP.pdf. Accessed 7/13/2020

137. NEHEN, http://nehenportal.com/. Accessed 7/13/2020

138. Medical Litigation – Health and Human Services, https://aspe.hhs.gov/terms/medical-litigation. Accessed 7/13/2020

139. A. Rosenblat, T. Kneese, D. Boyd, Algorithmic accountability. The Social, Cultural & Ethical Dimensions of "Big Data," March (2014)

140. Innovative Healthcare Mobile Apps, https://www.ortholive.com/blog/mhealth-healthcare-mobile-app-trends-in-2019#:~:text=There%20are%20more%20than%2097%2C000,to%20mobile%20or%20tablet%20devices. Accessed 7/13/2020

141. About one-in-five Americans use a smart watch or fitness tracker Pew Research Center January 9, 2020, https://www.pewresearch.org/fact-tank/2020/01/09/about-one-in-five-americans-use-a-smart-watch-or-fitness-tracker/. Accessed 7/13/2020

142. H.M. Husted, T.L. Llewellyn, The accuracy of pedometers in measuring walking steps on a treadmill in college students. Int. J. Exerc. Sci. **10**(1), 146–153 (2017) Published 2017 Jan 1

143. The FDA Warns Against the Use of Many Genetic Tests with Unapproved Claims to Predict Patient Response to Specific Medications: FDA Safety Communication, https://www.fda.gov/medical-devices/safety-communications/fda-warns-against-use-many-genetic-tests-unapproved-claims-predict-patient-response-specific. Accessed 7/13/2020

144. C.J. Kelly, A. Karthikesalingam, M. Suleyman, et al., Key challenges for delivering clinical impact with artificial intelligence. BMC Med. **17**, 195 (2019)

145. About one-in-five Americans use a smart watch or fitness tracker Pew Research Center January 9, 2020, https://www.pewresearch.org/fact-tank/2020/01/09/about-one-in-five-americans-use-a-smart-watch-or-fitness-tracker/. Accessed 7/13/2020

146. S. Vartan, Racial bias found in a major health care risk algorithm. Sci. Am. https://www.scientificamerican.com/article/racial-bias-found-in-a-major-health-care-risk-algorithm/

147. M.A. Gianfrancesco, S. Tamang, J. Yazdany, G. Schmajuk, Potential biases in machine learning algorithms using electronic health record data. JAMA Intern. Med. **178**(11), 1544–1547 (2018). https://doi.org/10.1001/jamainternmed.2018.3763

148. Z. Obermeyer et al., Dissecting racial bias in an algorithm used to manage the health of populations. Science **366**(6464), 447–453 (2019)

149. M. Brodie et al., Health information, the internet, and the digital divide: despite recent improvements, Americans' access to the internet—and to the growing body of health information there—remains uneven. Health Aff. **19**(6), 255–265 (2000)

Chapter 15
Applicability of Blockchain Technology in Healthcare Industry: Applications, Challenges, and Solutions

Nikhil Sharma, Bharat Bhushan, Ila Kaushik, and Narayan C. Debnath

15.1 Introduction

In the last few years, the decentralized architecture has gained satisfactory response in many fields because of its demands. IoT also uses this architecture to overcome the problems such as security, autonomic control, and scalability [1]. A bitcoin based on cryptocurrency is a network where each system passes information directly to another without involvement of any central entity, or a digital network through which digital cryptocurrency can be transferred from one user to the other without having any involvement of any intermediaries [2]. It was first introduced by blockchain technology. For authorization, no personal details have to be provided by the user every time. Anyone can perform a transaction after becoming a part of blockchain [3]. The consensus algorithm with a public leader is responsible to solve all the trust and security aspects. The public blockchain, that is, Ethereum and bitcoin utilized the consensus algorithm called Proof of Work (PoW) [4]. Miners is a special node which validates all the transactions. The private or public key pair is distributed among the participants and by using that the transaction gets executed [5]. In public ledger, the rest of the nodes disprove the transaction if any of the record is found tampered because it is an inflexible chain of transactions [6].

N. Sharma
Ambedkar Institute of Advanced Communication Technologies & Research, Delhi, India

B. Bhushan (✉)
School of Engineering and Technology, Sharda University, Greater Noida, Uttar Pradesh, India

I. Kaushik
Krishna Institute of Engineering & Technology, Ghaziabad, Uttar Pradesh, India

N. C. Debnath
Eastern International University, Thủ Dầu Một, Vietnam

© The Author(s), under exclusive license to Springer Nature Switzerland AG 2021
C. Chakraborty et al. (eds.), *Efficient Data Handling for Massive Internet of Medical Things*, Internet of Things,
https://doi.org/10.1007/978-3-030-66633-0_15

Blockchain has the perspective to be acquired by the government organizations, banking sectors as well as by the financial sector for different applications, for example, use of blockchain in e-voting [7]. According to the Survey conducted by IBM, the blockchain technology would successfully implement by 66% of financial institutions and 91% of banking sector as revealed by approximately 200 financial institutes [8]. According to the report given by business consultant institute regarding blockchain technology, there will be investment of 3.160 trillion dollars expected in 2030. The healthcare data management has been transformed using expansive networking technologies, hardware and software. The objective of all these technologies is to upgrade the quality standard of drugs and medical care, pharmaceutical treatment, the detection of diseases and their causes, and to entrench worldwide mitigation schemes for chronic infections. The early medical records on papers are now transformed to Electronic Health Records (EHRs) [9]. To deliver an aggregate view of patient's medical history for providing exact, timely, and precise patient care, EHRs are required to be shared and allocated among patients, various hospitals, medical insurance providers, researchers, pharmacists, government, and medical drug manufacturers [10]. While using traditional client-server healthcare database management system the distribution and allocation of EHRs becomes an expensive and time-consuming process as every hospital or clinic needed to manage their own patient's database medical records. This condition directly effects and delays the patient's treatments when they move or referred to other hospital across various cities or countries, as the preferred hospital repeats several radiology and laboratory tests that were already done in earlier hospital [11]. Sometimes, it is necessary for the patients to have several radiology and laboratory tests again. The medical information of patients is stored in cloud storage so that it can be easily accessed by the patients and healthcare suppliers. Before uploading the patient-related information on the cloud server, all the sensitive information of patient's medical data gets encrypted. The cloud-based data management system requires large memory to store all the patient-related information, which is not appropriate as it increases the cost as well as patients are very much aware of risk that their information can be misused. In 2017, approximately 51 lakhs medical data got breached and in 2018, twice of 2017 medical data, that is, 13,236,569 records breached, as per the statistics report provided by the HIPAA (Health Insurance Portability and Accountability Act) [12].

To overcome the issues such as vulnerability, security, lack of traceability, real time information access, data fragmentations, which currently exist in client server architecture, blockchain technology gets employed as it uses fixed, shared, and transparent ledger which has great potential to solve all these kinds of issues. In blockchain technology, a block of various timestamped transactions is generated where each transaction is timestamped, and by using various cryptographic techniques, every block gets linked to its previous block to serve immutability. In 1991, the concept of timestamping was introduced to build immutability. A mechanism was suggested by researchers at Telcordia Technologies [13] to build a fixed record of linked documents. According to this mechanism for timestamping process, the possessor transmits the hashed document with the possessor identification to a server. With the current timestamp, the document gets digitally signed by the server and then hashes the signed document, sender's identification, along with the preceding document's hash.

Blockchain became popular after the introduction of bitcoin (digital cryptocurrency). In 2008, a white paper was published by Satoshi Nakamoto in which he suggested a direct peer-to-peer online payment without involving any third party such as financial institution or banking sector [14]. This solves the problem of twice spending in digital cryptocurrency by associating every transaction with the previous one in a public ledger for building a fixed record of transactions. It also eliminates the requirement of a central database server which works as an intermediary amid the peers because the whole network will be pretentious, if the server fails. For supporting high volumes of network traffic, the usage of network bandwidth of the server must be high [15]. In a centralized network, all the sensitive data of users are stored in the server; hence, the major concern will be its security. Blockchain is a decentralized network; therefore, it can handle these abovementioned issues as every participant should have equal impact over the network, and in the form of a ledger, it allocates a copy of transaction information. The duplication of information provides local ingress to the data and also assists to upgrade fault tolerance whenever the information on any nodes act maliciously. The information once stored in the blockchain is unchangeable, that is, the information cannot be removed or altered once it gets stored. Any deletion or alteration of the information can be easily detected in the blockchain fundamental mechanism [16]. By using hash of preceding block, every block in the chain gets hashed for creating a fixed chain. All these characteristics of blockchain have activated its espousal for healthcare data management. In the healthcare domain, blockchain mainly focused on bitcoin which suffers from various limitations such as low transactions throughput, poor scalability, and high-power consumption. So, while developing a blockchain technology-based healthcare data management system, all these limitations should be taken into consideration.

The rest of this chapter is organized as follows. Section 15.2 presents the related work. Section 15.3 presents the conceptual background of blockchain technology and highlights its key features, architecture, and related consensus protocols. Section 15.4 elucidates the need and applicability of blockchain technology in healthcare industry. Section 15.5 outlines the major challenges faced by the adoption of blockchain technology in healthcare industry and lists the future research directions in this area. Finally, this chapter concludes itself in Sect. 15.6.

15.2   Related Work

Healthcare data management is an essential process which is used to store all the health-related record of patient and manage it to deliver better care, successfully tracking disease and its causes. The stored data can also be used in the research and development process of any medical drugs. Nowadays, the hospitals are widely using EHRs to manage health records of their patients using a client-server-based architecture [17]. But in these types of healthcare data management system, the data get managed by the hospitals as they are primary curator for that information [18]. It is difficult for the healthcare professionals or researcher to make an accurate disease diagnosis whenever needed. As these records are even not available at different clinics and hospitals; therefore, it is also difficult for the patient to view their medical history. Therefore, to overcome these types of situations, different industries and academia have introduced various healthcare management systems based on cloud technology [19]. This is a centralized database system in which patients can easily store their health records and can be accessed whenever required. But these types of cloud facilities are highly prone to different cyber-attacks. The data cannot be easily exchanged or shared as it will also get accessed by the attacker while sharing the information. The major issues which effect the normal functioning of the medical data management systems based on cloud technology are privacy, data fragmentation, different system vulnerabilities, and security.

Different researchers adopted blockchain technology for the purpose of sharing the data securely. It is the technology where the participants can record the transactions and share that with others connected to the network. This is how the data get immediately shared with the other participants. In most of the work, researchers used blockchain to address security and privacy-related issues of healthcare data by storing hash to the cloud. Because of the cloud server facility, the system is prone to a single point failure. Many researchers also introduce different techniques which blockchain use for the healthcare data such as communication-based mechanisms, digital signature-based schemes, a key generator method, or encryptions and decryptions techniques. In 2016, Azaria et al. [20] introduced MedRec, that is, an information sharing application based on blockchain which enables interoperability by integrating with the current data storage system of the doctors. In the year 2018, Dagher et al. [21] and Li et al. [22] suggested a framework which deploys smart contract network (i.e., Ethereum-based blockchain network) for accessing health data. This network utilizes lot of energy as it is based on PoW consensus mechanism. In the same year 2018, Fan et al. [23] have introduced MedBlock which is a healthcare data sharing system based on blockchain technology that permits the user to efficiently ingress and recover the EHRs. Instead of using PoW, MedBlock uses PBFT (Practical Byzantine Fault Tolerance) consensus mechanism as it consumes low energy as compared to the PoW. But it does not permit the patients to distribute its health records to the blockchain network that would assist the health professionals for improving the diagnosis. Dey et al. [24] and Yue et al. [25] suggested the utilization of blockchain technology to share patient's health records. In this system, the patients can upload the medical records for maintaining the primary attention. This system only permits the health professionals to see the health records of the patients, but it does not permit the health professionals to distribute the patient's health data to the networks. Uddin et al. [26] introduced a blockchain-based health information system through which the medical records of the patients can be shared among the various hospitals and patients. This framework permitted both the hospital and patients to upload their medical records to the distributed ledger, so that history of patient's medical records can be easily accessible whenever required. For generating a block, it consumes high energy as it uses a mining-based consensus mechanism. Ismail et al. [27] suggested a highly scalable architecture in which blockchain network gets divided into clusters. Each cluster is having a Blockchain Manager (BCM) which manages a single copy of the ledger and permits the distribution of patient's personal health and medical record to the network. This network architecture uses canal through which other enable cooperating group can execute the confidential transactions by managing a ledger available to the canal participants. This is an energy-efficient architecture as it uses PBFT consensus mechanism. Table 15.1 shows the hardiness and weakness of proposed mechanism by various researchers in the healthcare Industry.

Table 15.1 Hardiness and weakness of proposed mechanism by various researchers in healthcare industry

Reference	Confidentiality	Scalability	Energy efficient	Distribution of personal medical data	Distribution of personal health data	Outcomes
Azaria et al. [20]	No	No	No	Yes	No	Due to usage of PoW consensus, a large amount of energy is consumed
Dagher et al. [21]	Yes	Yes	No	Yes	No	Due to usage of POW consensus, a large amount of energy is consumed. It can be scaled up as it keeps on records hashes in the backing store area and minimum nodes are required for transaction purposes
Li et al. [22]	No	No	No	Yes	No	System cannot be scaled up as involvement of high amount of energy is required by power consensus mechanism

(continued)

Table 15.1 (continued)

Reference	Confidentiality	Scalability	Energy efficient	Distribution of personal medical data	Distribution of personal health data	Outcomes
Fan et al. [23]	Yes	Yes	Yes	Yes	No	Scalability of system is improved and it consumes least energy. Using signature-based security technique, privacy is achieved
Dey et al. [24]	Not described	Not described	No	No	Yes	Due to usage of POW consensus, a large amount of energy is consumed
Yue et al. [25]	Yes	Not described	Not described	No	Yes	Usage of proposed purpose-centric model, privacy is achieved
Uddin et al. [26]	Yes	No	Yes	Yes	Yes	No scalability is improved as mining-based model is used. Usage of proposed purpose-centric model, privacy is achieved. Privacy can also be achieved using trusted canals for performing secret logic unit of work within group of participants

(continued)

Table 15.1 (continued)

Reference	Confidentiality	Scalability	Energy efficient	Distribution of personal medical data	Distribution of personal health data	Outcomes
Ismail et al. [27]	Yes	Yes	Yes	Yes	Yes	Blockchain network is divided into clusters having a Blockchain Manager (BCM) which manages a single copy of the ledger and permits the distribution of patient's personal health and medical record to the network

15.3 Blockchain Technology

This section presents the background knowledge of blockchain technology and highlights its key inherent features that make it suitable for healthcare applications.

15.3.1 Overview and Architecture

In a corporate world, stakeholders need multiple features for the constancy of the services provider. The very first characteristic required in any transaction is data integrity. It is defined as network security characteristic which ensures that no alteration or updation of message takes place within a network, that is, data or transaction should be received without any alteration or modification at the receiver's end. The implementation of cryptographic schemes helps to achieve the data integrity in any network. Another required characteristic is linking of trust which can be acquired by consensus. Consensus controls inclusion of latest items as it contains the rule for resolving strife, broadcasting, and validating logical unit of work and blocks. The participants depend on authority to carry on transactions in centralized systems. For example, in the banking sector, the customers depend on the banking systems which alter the customer account balance after completion of each transaction [28]. The central authority can modify the whole system by directly updating and altering database at the backend in the central system. As the centralized system is a single service

provider, it does not allow the distribution of authority [29]. The examples of centralized system are government, payment, courts, and cloud system [30]. The working of
these systems is carried out eminently keeping in view the urge for leveraging the
elementary possession of a better system which includes public access, data integrity,
trust, and transparency. But this system is also having some limitations such as if a
single service provider crashes then it will affect the entire system as well as the stakeholders. The approach behind the utilization of decentralized system is to deliver distributed computing system where the distribution of authority could take place without
having trust on single service providers on any centralized system [31]. This system
provides a number of possessions such as data integrity, public access, transparency,
and trust. The popular examples of these systems are implementations of Ethereum
and bitcoin. The call for blockchain is impending to achieve interoperability and also
to provide publicly accessible infrastructure. For untrusted users, it provides distributed software infrastructures and also sanctions building of decentralized applications. As it is a single service provider, the major limitation of centralized system is
that it is highly susceptible to single point failure, that is, if there is any crash in the
service provider, the entire system functioning as well as the stakeholders will be
affected. Hence, the centralized system does not provide data integrity, data immutability, fair access to assets, non-repudiation of transactions accomplished, and transparency. The basic architecture of blockchain is depicted in Fig. 15.1 and explained in
the following subsections.

Blockchain is defined as a network of blocks, data structure, or distributed system that is instructed in the form of list. Every block in a blockchain is associated
using cryptographic schemes. In blockchain, each block of record consists of cryptographic hash of preceding block, transaction information, and timestamp. There
are two types of blockchain, the first one is public blockchain and the second one is
permissioned blockchain. In public blockchain, any user can participate and carryout
transactions or even responsible for modifying the blockchain by becoming part of
consensus process. It is highly susceptible to attacks such as sybil attack in which
the users are unidentified and have different identities to affect the consensus
process. Whereas permissible blockchain is close ended which includes parity,
corda and quorum, BigChainDB, Multichain and Hyperledger Fabric, and
Interplanetary. The block consists of transactions followed by different peers within
networks [32]. In blockchain, the blocks are associated with preceding blocks which
consists of cryptographic hash of it. This chain guarantees integrity of transaction;

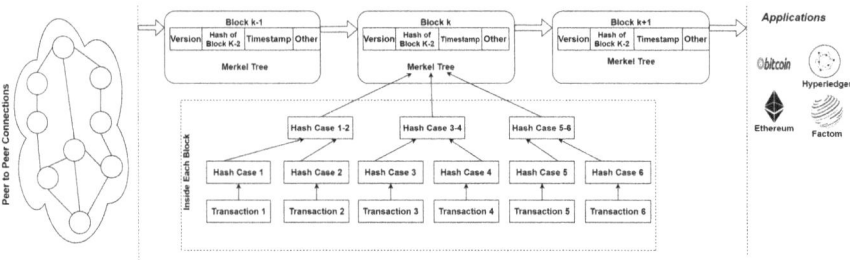

Fig. 15.1 Basic architecture of blockchain

therefore, every transaction is not operated that was made earlier and tries to modify with any of these transactions without PoW results in disproving the chain of hashes. Therefore, in the blockchain technology, trust and transparency are the major components that oblige a number of organizations to accept and implement blockchain in their specific infrastructure. Bitcoin is referred as the first-generation implementation of blockchain which uses public ledger to get secure cryptographically financial transactions, and smart contract is the second-generation implementation. For keeping information of all computational results, it provided a programmable platform. For performing programmable transactions, conditions and business logics are implemented by smart contracts which make it different from other techniques. To keep funds till defined responsibility, a smart contract system is being implemented by Escrow. Ethereum is also a common example of blockchain that uses smart contracts. The aggressor signs transactions in order to make sure that the spending of funds or to design and implement contracts based on smart functioning. The very first aggressor based on logic unit of work is generated to the blockchain nodes which approved the generated transactions to other points in the network till the transaction's details are approved and shared by all systems without involving any central authority in the network. Blockchain depends on the miners for validating logic unit of work after reaching concord on the entire network level. For this purpose, the consensus procedure acquired Proof of Stake (PoS).

15.3.2   Characteristics of Blockchain

The characteristics of blockchain are explained as follows:

15.3.2.1   Improved Security

As compared to traditional technology, blockchain has an improved security as there are no chances of system failure occurring in it. In this technology, the network is made up of nodes which is used to confirm the transactions. Every information is hashed using cryptographically techniques which helps in hiding the true nature of the information on the network. Every block in the ledger has its own unique hash and also contains hash of the preceding block.

15.3.2.2   Immutability

In blockchain, once the information gets stored, it cannot be altered or modified easily. For delivering secured transaction in the network, the information is added to the block after getting the approval from every node. Those who validated the transactions and add that to the block are called miners.

15.3.2.3   Decentralized Storage

As it is a decentralized network, there is no need of any governing bodies or authority. A group of nodes manage the network for storing and sharing the information. Using this technology, we can securely store our important data, documents, or any other digital assets. In blockchain network, every node has a similar copy of the data.

15.3.2.4   No Need of Third-Party Authorization

As it is a decentralized network, there is no need of any third party's involvement for the transactions. It only permitted the transactions between two parties, that is, sender and receiver. It eliminates the need of third-party authorization because in the network everyone can authorize the transactions. For instance, if a person from the USA is transferring an amount to his friend in India, then the bank acts as a third party who first validates that transaction and then transfers an amount after cutting their bank charges. This process takes a long time. But while using blockchain technology, the transaction takes place faster and is cheaper because no charges will be levied for the transaction process.

15.3.2.5   Consensus

Because of the consensus algorithm, every blockchain succeed. The architecture of blockchain is cleverly built, and these algorithms are major key of its structure because it assists the network in decision-making process. When a transaction gets verified by the millions of nodes, the algorithm is essential for the system to run smoothly.

15.3.2.6   Faster Settlement

The entire banking systems are slow because after finalizing all the settlements, it takes many days to process a transaction. As it is a traditional system, it can be easily corrupted. Therefore, there is need of blockchain technology because it offers faster settlement as compared to the banking system, and by using this technology, users can save their invaluable time and can transfer money comparatively faster than the banking system. This technology enables the life of a foreign worker easier by enabling them to transfer their money to their loved ones in a short period of time.

15.3.3 Public Blockchain as Sequence Decision-Making Architecture

Researchers introduced a new notion of blockchain technology in 2009. In news, a white paper is published concerning bitcoin by Satoshi Nakamoto. Bitcoin brings revolution in the entire world, as it is a digital cryptocurrency that does not require any main supervising authority. Using diver's cryptography schemes and shared consensus algorithms such as PoW, Bitcoin evolved a trust criterion between untrusted users around the entire world. Blockchain is referred as the scattered digital ledger which holds blockchain information. By using a cryptographic signature, each block gets identified in blockchain. In this technology, each block is attached to its precedent block by using its hash for building a fixed chain due to which the first block can be easily traced up.

15.3.3.1 Bitcoin Concern

Public blockchain is censured allied to scalability and seclusion as there are no privileged participants. In this, any user can connect to the networks and easily access the data on the blockchain. It also validates the new transactions. Blockchain technology has some extensible restriction related to processing rate of transactions as well as the size of the data. This technology also suffers from latency of information transmission. As the data are easy to avail by all the peers of the network, the major issues of concern in blockchain are security and privacy.

Taking consideration of predefined consensus rules, the transaction gets processed in bitcoin. Therefore, the particular functionality is allowed to process the transactions. Currently, the active nodes in bitcoin are 10,000. As bitcoin is based on distrustful environment, it allows users to execute pecuniary transactions, for example, money transfer without any third-party involvement such as any payment service or banks. Basically, it is a public blockchain which works on the consensus rules, that is, PoW whose main goal is to provide security and trust to their participants. It uses order-execute architecture to perform the transactions. That is, for finding and verifying a specific hash number, the transactions are first provided to the minors. Only after this process, the transaction is performed. The transaction takes long time to commit as verification of transactions and finding hash are done by every node in the network. Due to this limitation, several general-purpose applications are shifting from public to permissioned blockchain.

15.3.3.2 Ethereum

In 2013, a cryptocurrency researcher as well as a programmer, Vitalik Buterin suggested an open source Ethereum which is an operating system promoting smart contract performance and a distributed computing platform based on public blockchain. Ethereum works on Memory Hardness that is an improved version of Nakamoto consensus procedure, instead of employing fast processing power machines [33]. By using the bitcoin's consensus rule, that is, PoW, the substantial mining pools and large organizations can affect the network. This limitation is diminished with the dependencies of Ethereum on fast memory information movements. For executing Ethereum nodes or smart contract code, Ethereum provides the decentralized Ethereum Virtual Machine (EVM). As it is a permission-less network, any node can connect with the Ethereum network if participants download the Ethereum client to create a new account. It utilizes its own consensus rule model called EthHash PoW [34]. By using international network of nodes which are available publicly, Ethereum is capable of performing scripts. For allocating resources and preventing spam on the network, the transaction pricing-based procedure called Gas is used. The price requisite to execute a transaction on the network system is termed as Gas. The cost of the Gas is set by the miners and if it does not encounter their price threshold, then they can decline the transaction procedure. On 30 July 2015, this system went live with over 11.9 million coins premised for the crowd sale [35]. In blockchain technology, modification of data is not allowed; therefore, it consists of un-modified data of all the successfully committed transactions. It is not necessary that the bitcoin is suited in each scenario because every sector has its own needs. For controlling all the business practice and logic precisely, the general-purpose blockchain schemes are needed; hence, the blockchain technology can be easily accepted in diverse sectors. Because of the above-mentioned reasons, different organizations, banking and financial sectors are gaining their interest in permissioned blockchain scheme. Organizations that use this model are Wall Street, IBM, and Intel Corporation.

15.3.4   Platform of Permissioned Blockchain Architecture

Many venture blockchain applications are being employed in voting systems, finance sector, protecting civil infrastructure, and health industry. Permissioned blockchain system provides huge amount of availability of resources in contrast to single point failure. In permissioned blockchain system, all transactions are stored in the system because all the nodes download each block or transaction and can only be recouped when demanded from other nodes. The use of access control layer makes permissioned blockchain system different from permission-less blockchain system [36]. It limits the participants' ingress to consensus procedure and only allow the deliberate users to join the network system [37]. Permissioned blockchain system is opposite to permission-less blockchain system, through bitcoin and Ethereum, any participants can join as typified. Instead of using PoW, Quorum is the very first blockchain platform that espoused diverse consensus algorithms. The extension of Ethereum is Quorum which works as permissioned blockchain and supports smart contract with BFT and crash consensus models. Quorum is permissioned blockchain platform which gains popularity because of Ethereum buttress [38]. It becomes an effective solution for general-purpose applications such as healthcare, business and banking sectors. It also lengthened the properties in Ethereum. All the types of blockchain technology from permissioned to permissionless blockchains system have order-execute architectures. Both types of blockchain systems are having a common concern, that is, all nodes are employed for the execution of transactions which restricts the performance of the network system and produces several issues such as Denial of Service (DoS) attacks, privacy of the participants, and concurrency.

For the implementation of permissioned blockchain systems, an open source framework is employed termed as Fabric or Hyperledger Fabric which follows the execute-order-validate paradigm [39]. Ethereum and bitcoin are the two traditional frameworks which use order-execute architecture and are also responsible for slowing down the transaction processing time. The very first version of Fabric were built by two organizations, that is, IBM and Digital Asset. The two major limitations of this framework are absence of proven use cases and limited number of experts or developers able to use this framework. For all application developments, Fabric produces a smart contract interface called Chaincode. For all the general-purpose applications, Fabric becomes a flattering ledger architecture. In multiple programming languages such as Java, NodeJS, typescript & Go, Chaincode can be developed. For existing applications, it provides a Restful interface to get linked with the blockchain network. For the quick application development, Hyperledger project produces the second layer on Fabric which termed as composer. Because of various reasons, no further support is provided for the composer.

In Fabric version 1.4, many applications have been introduced. To run the Chaincode, blockchain network needs to setup an administrator who belongs to an agency for developing an application on Fabric [40]. Various security digital certificates are designed by the users for providing a secure and reliable communication between the end user and network organizations. In the blockchain network, every node is evolved with Docker containers which are established in the geographically disseminate environment. One or more services are provided by peer nodes in a network. In Chaincode, diverse applications can be assimilated which may belong to business, IoT, healthcare, and many more. The Chaincode provides the collections with various APIs. For the implementation of smart contracts, only few primary steps are needed over the blockchain network. The first step includes the implementation of Chaincode from the Chiancode Developer Kit. The validity of the contract endorses when the smart contracts get provided to the validator nodes, and then the implementation of contracts is permitted. Due to some quality facet and properties for IoT networks, diverse platforms get motif. IoT chain is the very first platform which is utilized as a decentralized network for the IoT devices. For the development purposes, it is not publicly accessible to the users. It is only employed to provide results, security facets, and other analysis and agreements to the IoT network and to differentiate outcomes with IBM-ADEPT, IT, SLOCK, IOTA, and different corresponding projects. It also fortifies PBFT and DAG (Directed Acyclic Graph) as agreements. IOTA is the second platform which is employed to initialize and store the transactions between equipment and IoT gadgets. It is a distributed ledger design which plans to supervise the transaction on the devices. Between multiple IoT devices, it acts as a public permission-less backbone which permits interoperations among them. By returning its blockchain with Tangle, IOTA should sort out the performance concern and expandability with bitcoin. Tangle is a system of nodes in which the preceding transaction gets assured by the new one. It utilizes DAG which is the main motif for the IoT system. Tangle is the major discovery of IOTA which confirms the transactions [41]. IOTA confirms that the nodes of the system are systematic, faster, well organized, and efficient than other prototypical blockchain employed in the cryptocurrencies. The main objective of DAG is to resolve the performance concern and flexibility of the system. As multiple systems are connected to Tangle, it becomes more secure, scalable, and efficient at the time of transaction process. As new transactions get confirmed by its preceding nodes, Tangle helps in minimizing the time, efforts, and memory needed to validate a transaction. Waltonchain is another platform which has the motif for IoT. It is a decentralized network which contains both the hardware and software. On newly planned blockchain structure, electronic communication gets executed and RFID is used for transmission process in it. Software contains both Waltonchain and Walton coin protocols [42].

15.3.5 Different Consensus Model

In a decentralized system, the consensus process permits the sequencing of the transactions as well as guarantee integrity of information across the geographical area. Various blockchain uses the diverse consensus models such as PoS *(Proof of Stake)*, PoW *(Proof of Work)*, Proof of Elapsed Time (PoET), Byzantine Fault Tolerance (BFT), PBFT (Practical Byzantine Fault Tolerance), and Sieve Model. The selections of these models are done on the three major key properties that is Fault Tolerance, Safety, and Liveness. All these models are explained as follows.

15.3.5.1 PoW (Proof of Work)

PoW function is a consensus model which dissuades DoS attacks as well as other various service attacks such as spam on a network. In 1993, this protocol was proposed by the Moni Naor and Cynthia Dwork. In 1999, this protocol was formalized by Markus Jakobsson [43]. Over thousands of nodes can be scaled using this consensus model. PoW needed the aggressor for solving a cryptographic or mathematical operation, a puzzle using brute forcing and also processed a winning value which is less than the defined value forwarded by the network. In PoW, a number of nodes provide a value to add block at a time and demand for a reward. As this condition produced a fork, therefore by examining the maximum amount of work done by a node or maximum value of prove of work, this condition can be solved by the network system and thus, discarded all the entreaty made by the node with a minimum PoW. It is the best suited network which needed scalability. The size of network becomes large as permission-less blockchains employ PoW because it provides the validity and reliability to the cooperating nodes. This also has some disadvantages, as for the mining process each node has to invest huge capital in buying equipment. It is more defenseless to various attacks. Master Card or VISA Card provides 10,000 transactions per second, while PoW offers only seven transactions per second which is very less and it takes more amount of time for the confirmation when in fork. Bitcoin espoused various forms of consensus models such as Monero & NameCoin, LiteCoin, and DogeCoin. In distributed systems, Byzantine Fault Tolerance, RAFT, and Paxos algorithms are used as a solution for implementing consensus models.

15.3.5.2   PoET (Proof of Elapsed Time)

According to PoET, the consensus mechanism chooses the next leader to complete the block. Trusted execution environment is employed to ensure that the election is executed in secure domain. An authenticate node insisting a leader to provide evidence from trusted execution environment by mining a block in blockchain can be easily proved by the other node. The proof has to be capitulated that it had taken shortest amount of waiting time before it permits to begin mining of the succeeding block. The major drawback of this model is that it depends on exclusive hardware.

15.3.5.3   PoS (Proof of Stake)

For handling inherent concerns in the latter, PoS was designed as a substitute of PoW. In PoS, 1 Megabyte is a maximum size in which the information of transaction is stored into a block whenever the new transaction executed. In blockchain, nodes act as an administrative body. In each block, the verification of transaction will be done by the nodes. The PoW gets replaced by the PoS as it consumes energy in adequate quantity. Rather buying an equipment to design a value, PoS advises to buy digital cryptocurrency and uses that in blockchain to purchase the feasibility of block creation. To unlock the computational challenges, computing power is needed by the mining for applying various cryptographic calculations.

15.3.5.4   BFT (Byzantine Fault Tolerance)

In decentralized distributed environment, the users frequently liaised with each other in a permission-less system. This system guarantees that it will continue to utilize where the nodes can be spiteful or breakdown. This model is used to present the diverse symptoms to various spectators. It needs low latency and operates effectively in real-time environment. Therefore, various aircrafts appraise BFT in their designs such as Boeing 777 fight control system, Boeing 777 Information

Management System. The Hyperledger Fabric is a most popular permissioned blockchain which was developed by the Linux Foundation. It relies on pluggable consensus mechanism. In central registry services, this model is developed for the registered and well-known group of users with registered identifications. The consensus mechanisms that are underpinned by Hyperledger Fabric deal with non-deterministic Chaincode (smart contract based blockchain) execution such as SIEVE model and PBFT model.

15.3.5.5 PBFT (Practical Byzantine Fault Tolerance)

PBFT was introduced to recompense the failure of Byzantine and resolving the consensus mechanism. It provides various characteristics such as encipher of information amid clients and replicas. This algorithm model uses 3n + 1 replicas to permit failures of n nodes. It sets some overhead with regard to performance and messaging over duplicate nodes. To upgrade the performance and validity, many other BFT models' approaches were proposed such as HQ, Q/U, and Zyzzyva which addressed the cost and performance concerns.

15.3.5.6 Sieve Model

In blockchain code execution, SIEVE model is a private permissioned blockchain which was developed in order to deal with the non-deterministic behaviors. The Hyperledger model uses SIEVE consensus model to permit the network system to eliminate and detect possible non-deterministic behavior requests and accomplished consensus on the output of the recommended transaction. In decentralized distributed system, if these types of operations are available inside the code, then it will provide various outputs when implemented by diverse copies. It then compares the output on the basis of two conditions. According to the first condition, discrepancy values are sieved out, if a minor discrepancy gets detected amid a small number of these copies. The second condition is that the affront's behavior gets sieved out if the discrepancy transpires over diverse processes. Table 15.2 shows the comparison of blockchain consensus on the basis of different parameters.

15.4 Blockchain for Biomedical and Healthcare Systems

All over the world, researchers and healthcare experts are scuffled with multidimensional healthcare data. Healthcare information providers are always hesitant to share the sensitive information of the patients related to medical records. As the new technologies are developing day by day, the highest priority has given to privacy and security of the medical data by the researchers. In 2015, according to the Forbes Magazine, 112 million of data records were unseemly revealed, lost, or stolen [44]. Patients, doctors, analyzers, suppliers, and the payers are the major

Table 15.2 Comparison of blockchain consensus on the basis of different parameters

	Performance	Security	Trust	Scalability	Power consumption	Transaction finality	Participation cost	Permissioned or permission-less
PoW	Low	<= 25%	Untrusted	High	High	Probabilistic	Yes	Permission-less
PoET	Medium	Unknown	Untrusted	High	Medium	Probabilistic	No	Both
PoS	High	Depends on algorithms	Untrusted	High	Medium	Probabilistic	Yes	Both
BFT (federated)	High	<= 33%	Semi-trusted	High	Low	Immediate	No	Permission-less
BFT (variants)	High	<= 33%	Semi-trusted	Low	Medium	Immediate	No	Permissioned

stakeholders in the field of healthcare. Patients are the major source of data as they generate data by using IoT wearable gadgets [45] or clinical records. Payers can be a person or an organization such as insurance companies and banks, who directly or indirectly help the patients by paying their bills of health treatments. Suppliers play an important role as they gather all the medical data-related information of the patients such as medical centers, hospitals, or blood banks. Analyzers and researchers used that medical data to improve the functioning of healthcare sector. Earlier, in the absence of blockchain technology, the different institutions provide the interoperability of healthcare information which could be classified into three different models. The first is the push model, in which the sharing of information is only feasible between two suppliers, and the third supplier cannot have ingress to the system, that is, the sharing of information is only possible between the two departments of the same hospital. The different hospital cannot ingress to that data, even though the information is shared with that hospital also. But this model fails to protect integrity of the data. The second is the pull model in which one supplier demands for the information from another supplier without systematized audit trail. For example, in an informal way, a cardiologist demands for some data from an orthopedic surgeon. The third is the view model, in which one supplier can view the information inside the medical data record delivered by the other supplier. For example, in hospital's operating room, a surgeon can ingress an X-ray record of the patient taken at urgent care center. By considering the security aspects, blockchain technology deliver a secured market to the healthcare industry. For secure ingress of the information, a formalized and standardized contract has been built by blockchain [46]. When the model based on blockchain gets employed in EHRs, it provides identity and timestamp to every workflow and distributes the copies of that with each node participated in the network [47]. This helps in identifying the patients and the treatment given to him by the doctor as well as if any updation or modification is required in the data, then it automatically get distributed to the other nodes as well participated in the network [48]. This will help the person who is accessing that information around the world. Without any human involvement, this model guarantees the integrity of data between both the end-terminals. This technology brings revolution in the healthcare industry by providing different notable opportunities such as increased capacity, consent, decentralized storage, and immutability. The first opportunity is increased capacity. As there is no need of third-party involvement and less approval complication, therefore for managing the privacy of data, the most effective technology is blockchain. The second opportunity is consent in which consensus algorithms are used to control the operations such as distribution, storage, and access. After getting approval from all the parties, the modifications can be done on the data. The third is immutability in which once the information is stored in a block, no modification or alteration can be allowed on the data. The fourth opportunity is decentralized storage. As blockchain is a decentralized network, it transparently stores the data which can be shared with the third party based on the developer's agreement and it also stores multiple copies of the data in different places of the network.

In blockchain technology, healthcare industry emerges as the most important application. In order to record, validate, analyze, and exchange the stored healthcare data, blockchain serves as a distributed ledger technology. Healthcare application such as Health Information Exchange (HIE) or health transactions among the providers, patients, and other appropriate parties is considered to be a fundamental framework and can be achieved by adopting blockchain technology. Further, these applications can be classified based on their respective key goals in order to utilize blockchain for storing data. It is also being discussed in improved insurance claim process, accelerating clinical section, and enhanced medical record management. Advanced biomedical/healthcare data ledger section is depicted to an application beyond HIE. We also discuss some key benefits and use cases of every category adopting blockchain technique which are as follows:

- *Enhanced medical record management*
  Several studies emphasize on using blockchain for exchanging medical care data in order to make an enhancement in managing the medical record, which includes Gem health network, Fatcom, MedVault, and healthcare data gateways. For managing medical records and storing healthcare data, companies such as Accenture and Deloitte are using blockchain technology. For securing over 1 million healthcare records, Estonia-based company is all set to provide a blockchain-based framework known as Guard-time.
- *Improved insurance claim process*
  One of the main tasks is to cross check the claimed transactions in order to support the healthcare financing tasks. This includes alternative payment models, smart health profile to help re-entry of Medicaid recipient, and managing constant exits, preauthorized payments, Healthcare interoperability resources for fast automatic claims, and smart contract.
- *Accelerated clinical/biomedical research*
  Some researches including Data lake, data sharing networks, MedRec, and Health bank also reveal that with the help of blockchain technology, clinical/biomedical research areas can be accelerated. In order to increase the robustness and security of distributed privacy-conserving medical care predictive modeling across multiple institutions, adoption of blockchain in Modelchain can be done.
- *Advanced biomedical/healthcare data ledger*
  Some projects and studies proposed that blockchain can exploited as a ledger for healthcare data, and also it can be utilized to store the different types of medical-care data which include precision medicine data, genomic, care plan data, and directories of patients, patient consent data, biomarker information, pharmaceutical supply chain data, and clinical trial information.

15.4.1 Need of Blockchain in Healthcare

Blockchain is an emerging technology which delivers effective solutions in different domains such as healthcare, IIoT, and business. Healthcare is a basic need of human's day-to-day life. In the past few years, blockchain technology has attained confidence as a trusted distributed system for storing and performing transaction

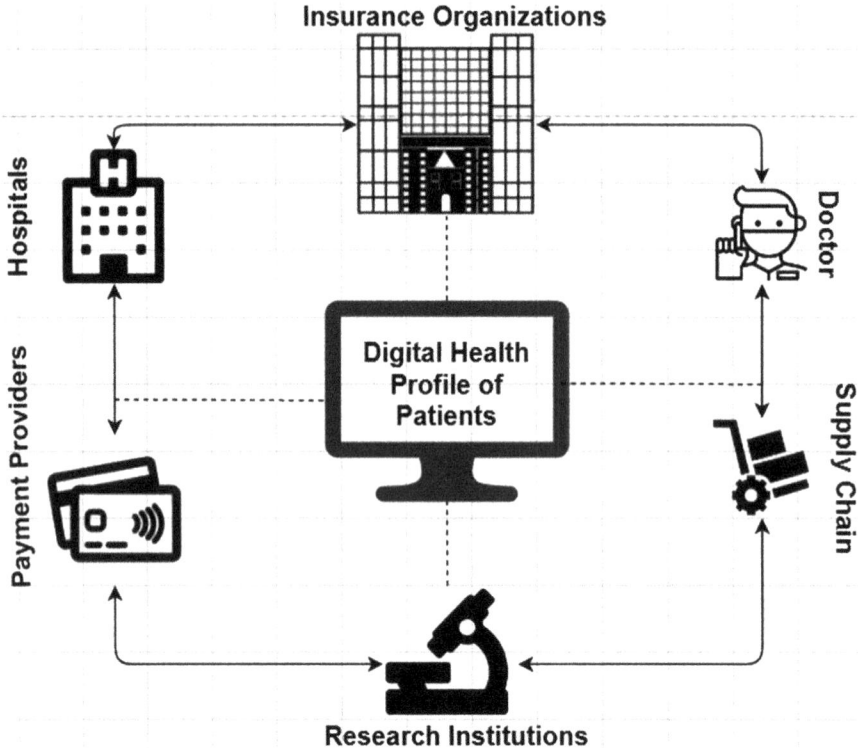

Fig. 15.2 Use of blockchain technology in healthcare

data in the form of distributed ledger [49]. In spite of focusing on the solution provided by blockchain in healthcare industry, the stakeholders are involved in questioning and discussing blockchain. This section will discuss the major issues related to existing healthcare problems and the effective solutions provided by the blockchain technology. Figure 15.2 shows the uses of blockchain technology in healthcare for sharing of data among the different stakeholders.

15.4.1.1 Securing Health Data of Patients While Exchanging Between Different Stakeholders

There are different parameters in this issue such as guarantee of data privacy, decentralized health insurance data, and ameliorate integrity of health data [50] which are explained as follows.

(i) *Guarantee of data privacy*
   The guarantee of data privacy of health record is the one of the major issues while exchanging data between collaborators such as data forwarded to

caretaker, health organizations, doctors, research and development departments, and government sectors [51].

(ii) *Decentralized health insurance data*

In most of the countries, health insurance services are provided by different private insurance organizations or social insurance system. This insurance is used to pay the charges against the healthcare treatments given to the patients by the doctors and nurses. But it does not guarantee the health service to the patients irrespective of their inhabitant country as the medical insurance data stored in decentralized network.

(iii) *Ameliorate integrity of health data*

It is difficult to maintain or ameliorate the data integrity at high level in healthcare because major operations, lab test, and doctors' prescriptions have been recommended on the basis of these records. Therefore, any errors or misconception in the reports can be led to unsuitable care or erroneous diagnosis. All these errors can be generated while sharing, exchanging, or storing record using electronic systems.

15.4.1.2 Master Patient Index

In different enterprises, this concept is used to manage accurate and consistent patient's medical data across different organizations. In global healthcare services, the major problem that arises is patient identification matching, as the integrity of medical data can be easily violated while sharing healthcare records of patients.

15.4.1.3 Limited Ingress to Medical Records

To maintain the security of the data, limited ingress to medical record is provided while sharing records with the stakeholders. So, it is difficult to investigate the different diagnosis and the reaction of prescription on patients. Therefore, this limitation builds an obstacle in the future research.

15.4.1.4 Inconsistent or Conflicting Rules and Permission in the Field of Healthcare

In every country, there are different rules and regulations related to access rights of healthcare records of the patients. This poses a challenge for the actual stakeholders to share the record at desired time as it can only be done when the data are available. This problem can be overcome by using the smart contract concept in blockchain technology.

15.4.1.5   Interoperability with Medical Record and Applications

In this category, when the participants need to store, exchange, or access the medical record and applications of a patient, it becomes a challenge against the interoperability, because before sharing of information, the trust should be established between all the stakeholders to guarantee secure access to the data. This challenge can be overcome by using blockchain technology [52].

15.4.1.6   Transactions Cost in Healthcare

There are many factors which are responsible for the transaction cost in healthcare system such as real-time processing, use of mediator between organizations, and unnecessary transmission cost. This challenge can be overcome by developing a model which delivers low-cost transaction between related stakeholders in the healthcare industry.

15.4.2   Applicability of Blockchain in Healthcare Sector

We have already discussed the existing problem in healthcare industry. According to Agbo et al. [53], the blockchain application in healthcare industry is classified into six narrow areas which are explained as follows.

15.4.2.1   Pharmaceutical Supply Chain Management

Blockchain plays a vital role in supply chain management. The pharmaceutical products are delivered in the market to the different stakeholders. Bocek et al. suggested [54] to deploy blockchain technology for delivering a secure ingress to the temperature records of the products. This will help the pharmaceutical corporations to observe the quality of their products while transportations. By using blockchain's Hyperledger Fabric policies, "a pharmaceutical turnover control system design" has been introduced by Dorri et al. [55] which is used to recognize three different nodes such as endorsing nodes, ordering nodes, and client nodes as well as role of every nodes. The ordering nodes is used in building transaction's block and update its status. The client nodes are used for the execution of transactions which is being looked after by the endorser node. The major solutions in the supply chain management and in the field of healthcare are delivered by the organization called GEM [56]. This corporation has built an operating system based on blockchain technology through which the healthcare economy data information can be accessed and shared securely with the right permissions. PHILIPS is another organization which works together with GEM to probe use cases of healthcare to know how blockchain clears the way in patient-centric strategies to the healthcare system.

15.4.2.2   Securing Healthcare Insurance Records

Zhou et al. [57] introduced a secure storage system related to healthcare insurance data using blockchain which helps insurance corporations and hospital's need of security mechanism and large storage spaces. This blockchain-based software system comprises of nodes which represent insurance corporations, records, hospitals, and servers [58]. Breteau et al. [59] have discussed the role of blockchain technology which aim to secure storage, ingress to healthcare insurance data and needs that are beneficial for the insurance corporations and insurer. HealthCoin uses blockchain technology that permits government, workers, and insurer to announce the diabetic prevention consciousness to every participants of the society [60]. Juneja et al. [61] have analyzed the use of blockchain technology to retrain, train, and allocate deep learning architecture in patient-specific Arrhythmia Classification. To share the healthcare research information, "Blockchain health," a software company, built a secured interconnection between the participants [62].

15.4.2.3   Securing Medical Records While Sharing Between Stakeholders

For every researcher, the security of essential data is becoming a challenge day by day. Whether it is a healthcare, business, or an institutional data, every information is highly vulnerable to get harmed by the attacker. As blockchain is having decentralized infrastructure, the researcher is taking it as a solution for such a problem related to data. In 2018, a new distributed blockchain structure has been introduced by Deloitte [63] for securing interoperability and supporting integration of medical data from different stakeholders. In the first stage, before using the blockchain technology in the healthcare industry, they advised to look over the four pre-conditions and can only make use of this technology after attaining these pre-conditions. In the second stage, for healthcare organizations, they advised to build a use case which can be used to authenticate and validate the transactions value or data involved in it. In the third stage, they talk about the execution of smart contract, which executes automatically after attaining these conditions. This helps in building trust between various stakeholders. In the last stage, they advised to introduce the perfect blockchain technology solutions that can be permission-less or permissioned blockchain. For transaction layer, they also explained the concept of on chain and off chain data.

In 2016, a systematic approach for exchanging health data using blockchain technology has been introduced by Peterson et al. [64]. They have discussed the issues of cross-institutional sharing and exchanging of healthcare information as this condition became a major problem due to rules and privacy concerns. First, they explained the presumption regarding involvement of various stakeholders, also discussed the structure of the healthcare blockchain and ingress of the patients in it. Then for network consensus, they proposed a hashing algorithm, that is, SHA 256 for proof of interoperability. In the year 2018, a model is introduced by Kuo et al. [65], which guarantees the privacy and security of patient information on private

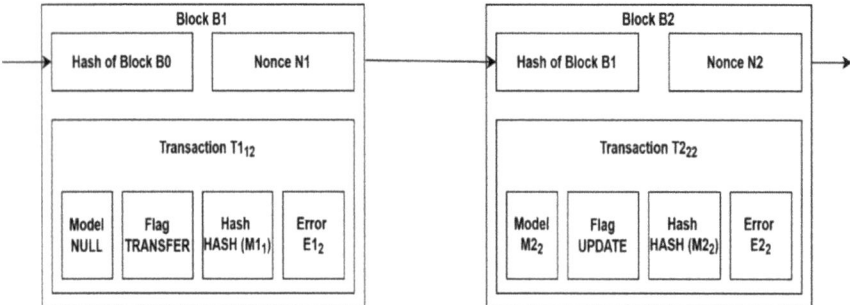

Fig. 15.3 Blockchain model containing two blocks

blockchain network using seclusion preserving machine learning algorithm. The example of this model is depicted in Fig. 15.3 using two blocks. Every block in the figure represents a transaction which comprises of hash, flag, error, and model. Then for proof of information, the researchers introduce an algorithm which takes inputs as the stakeholders, hold on and polling for a period of time. The N number of participants are taking part in transaction process, and then the output is depicted by latest online model based on machine learning.

In the last few years, many organizations have begun investigation in the block-chain technology for the different sectors such as business and healthcare. TIERION designed products and technology for the healthcare sector. In 2015, this is the first organization which successfully completed the project based on the utilization of blockchain technology in the healthcare sector. For healthcare records to online shopping, they predict this technology for the validation of range of things. They started a project named "Proof" which deploys bitcoin blockchain to demonstrate timestamp and integrity of the data.

15.4.2.4 Ethereum-Based Blockchain System to Secure Real-Time Patient Monitoring

Griggs et al. [66] introduced a secure real-time patient monitoring system based on blockchain technology. This system makes use of an Ethereum-based public blockchain which permits remote patients monitoring, that is, transmitting information to caregivers, health experts, and patients. It also provides secure storage space to store all the events of transactions. By delivering resilience to different types of manipulations, this system helps to solve the security vulnerability of real-time monitoring systems. In blockchain, the transactions can be easily traced back to its source point from where it originates. The verifications of each blocks need time, which results in delay in the process. Whereas in blockchain technology, verified blocks are unchangeable which provides privacy as well as security to patient's healthcare data.

15.5   Open Challenges and Future Research Directions

For adoption of blockchain technology in biomedical applications, some potential challenges are to be considered. In this context, the first challenge is associated with the confidentiality and transparency of data. Since, the blockchain network is a public network, it signifies that everything can be seen by everyone. Some of the main issues in blockchain is degraded confidentiality and enhanced transparency, like transparency of transferring data. Besides this, reidentification of a user by certain analysis technique and inspection using the publicly available transaction details are possible even if the end user uses hash values as addresses to create data anonymization in blockchain. So, pseudonymity is being achieved in a blockchain network. As the personal identifiable data and protected health information of a patient are the most sensitive information, this pseudonymity breaches the policy to protect it, and hence, a critical issue arises for healthcare applications. Now, another issue is associated with the scalability and transaction speed. Consider a blockchain transaction taking a longer time than usual transaction (depending on protocols), may lead to limit the scalability as the speed is constrained in these blockchain-based applications. With the help of proof-of-work protocol, we can easily figure out the transactions for bitcoin. Let us take an example, for a credit card such as Visa, there are about 150 million transactions per day. Also, on an average, there are about 3.3 transactions per second or 288,000 transactions per day for bitcoin because of the required computational workload. Because of 1 Megabyte size of block for a bitcoin, it can theoretically process only 7 transaction per second in current protocol, but 4000 transactions per second is the maximum theoretical number of transactions for a credit card such as Visa. While constructing scalable and real-time healthcare applications based on blockchain, these issues become very important. Furthermore, a threat called 51% attack is another issue which comes when we implement blockchain in an application. Blockchain network may suffer from this 51% attack, in a certain way. This attack happens when there are a greater number of malicious nodes in the network as compared to the honest one. And hence, the attacker operates the whole network. For the purpose of security in medical-care applications, this issue becomes very critical.

This section discusses about the various challenges faced by the blockchain in healthcare and their solutions which can help the industry in the future. The major challenges faced by the blockchain in healthcare sector are as follows [67]:

- Scalability is the major challenge as there are many healthcare providers who demand for the combined services between multiple hospitals. For this, IoT-based architecture is required for ensuring reliable connection between multi nodes within mobile cloud blockchain network [68]. Different providers possess different characters based on their services like doctors, clinicians, nurses, and physicians. There is a need to further increase this IoT-based system for ensuring high quality of stakeholder's experience in the future.
- Minimum network latency is an issue of concern for real time-based applications as wearable devices produced the data which is very huge in volume and leads in

congestion of traffic on cloud server. Because of the physical distance to the mobile gadgets, the traditional health services based on cloud technology faced high network latency, which is not appropriate to the time-sensitive medical application [69]. Therefore, to mitigate such an issue, mobile edge cloud could be an effective solution because with minimum network latency, it delivers medical services to the mobile user. Lightweight blockchain design is used to optimize data processing and logic unit of work for increasing efficiency.

- Privacy in data uploading is a major challenge because certain limitations exist in uploading data as sensitive information of patients are stolen without their consent. Healthcare data contain the sensitive information of the patients. There is a risk of carrying a patient data in every node. To store EHRs and PII (personally identifiable information) forever is the major challenge for the blockchain technology. Blockchain allows users to keep track of previous log history [70]. Such existing problems can be solved using involvement of reinforcement learning which is one of the suited solutions. In blockchain, decentralized, immutable, cryptographic, and independent architecture guarantees the high security to the data [71].

- Quality of service (QoS) is another challenge. It is to be guaranteed in terms of availability, flexibility, and usability. User and cloud server are to be considered for improvement in e-health system design. Using data mining and machine learning concepts, cloud-based medical records can be analyzed [72]. This helps providers to deliver instant healthcare services while keeping in view the need of security.

- It will be radical cultural move as still many doctors give consultations to the patients on paper. So, moving them from paper to electronic healthcare records is a very big task. There are many fields which are mandatory in the EHR, and doctors may leave the questions blank. Therefore, changing their working behavior is not an easy job.

- A large amount of electronic medical records of patients gets generated by the IoT wearable devices using sensor data. As architecture of blockchain is hashed and decentralized in nature, it carries finite on-chain data storage. The cost for storing information in blockchain is very high as compared to any other source. For performing different operations in blockchain such as data management, or data access, the cost is also getting higher if the size of the data is bigger. So, by keeping these factors in mind, the blockchain application get designed [73].

- Data immutability is one of the characteristics of blockchain technology which offers security to the system. But it does not provide choices such as data deletion or modification as changes are not acceptable in it. There are only two methods through which the data can be added to the blockchain. The first method is to generate a new chain and in second method, using consensus, create a new block from all nodes. Therefore, blockchain application should be developed in such a manner that there should be lowest need of information modifications to take place.

By proper implementations and designing of biomedical application system, mitigation is possible for the above discussed challenges. One of the solutions for the abovementioned issues is ModelChain. For distribution of privacy-preserving predictive models among the various healthcare institutions, ModelChain utilizes blockchain. In this case transparency is not a problem, as it only circulates the predictive framework, not the protected health information. Transactional speed of blockchain becomes negligible, as it contains some machine learning algorithms which may take a long time for execution. It also minimizes the risk of 51% attack, as it uses authorized blockchain network and hence some random malicious node will not take part in the network. A Virtual Private Network (VPN) can be used to minimize the threat of 51% attack in a blockchain network. This is possible because it deploys some component and spread the information of network on a private healthcare insurance accountability and portability Act. There are eight themes which provide different solutions to the applicability of blockchain technology in healthcare industry in the future. The first theme is blockchain as a necessity for consent management in which data exchange and confidential choices of users can be collected and stored at one place and can be accessed according to patient wishes. Experience of patient care can be improved and administrative burden can be reduced. The second theme is migration of micropayments to blockchain in which innovation can be built by utilizing easy use of universal payment interface by achieving goals to patient's outcome. Using blockchain-based payment gateway, tracking of patient's medical expanses could be simplified. The third theme is tokenization of outcomes in which tokens are used for facilitating outcomes in health sector. Outcome-based documentation method can be used for providing grants. The fourth theme is credentialed chain on providers which is one of the most critical tasks and includes maintaining health plans of patients that is to be updated on regular basis. One project related to this task involves putting demographic information on blockchain which is secure. The fifth theme is enhancement of speed by reducing electricity requirements in which speeding of logical unit of work will enhance the ease use of blockchain-based functions. The sixth theme is integrity of supply chain in which integrity of the product could be enhanced by using an approach based on pharmaceutical supply chain. The seventh theme is refinement of educational stakeholders, that is, the implementation of high use cases, because the numbers of stakeholders are educated against good and bad of blockchain. The last theme is enhancement of opportunities for data including genome in which opportunities are welcomed by data enabled people who are able to contribute for clinical research and population health-related options.

15.6   Conclusion

Blockchain plays vital role in providing privacy and security to the data. It possesses different features such as immutability, decentralized storage, and increased capacity. In this chapter, we have reviewed the proposed work of different researchers on certain parameters such as scalability, throughput, distribution of personal medical data, and confidentiality in healthcare industry from which a comparison table has been formulated. The major purpose of this chapter is to explain the need of blockchain technology in healthcare industry. For avoiding major issues related to existing healthcare system such as securing health data of patients while exchanging between different stakeholders, Master Patient Index, limited ingress to medical records, interoperability with medical record and applications, blockchain-based various solution are provided to overcome these issues which includes pharmaceutical supply chain management, securing healthcare insurance records, Ethereum-based blockchain system to secure real-time patient monitoring, and securing medical records while sharing between stakeholders. In the latter section of this chapter, we have discussed some of the open challenges and future research strategies which can help in resolving these issues faced in the healthcare industry.

References

1. S. Wang, Y. Zhang, Y. Zhang, A blockchain-based framework for data sharing with fine-grained access control in decentralized storage systems. IEEE Access **6**, 38437–38450 (2018)
2. Q. Xia, E.B. Sifah, K.O. Asamoah, J. Gao, X. Du, M. Guizani, MeDShare: Trust-less medical data sharing among cloud service providers via blockchain. IEEE Access **5**, 14757–14767 (2017)
3. T. Sharma, S. Satija, B. Bhushan, Unifying blockchain and IoT: Security requirements, challenges, applications and future trends, in *2019 International Conference on Computing, Communication, and Intelligent Systems (ICCCIS)*, (2019). https://doi.org/10.1109/icccis48478.2019.8974552
4. Z. Ying, L. Wei, Q. Li, X. Liu, J. Cui, A lightweight policy preserving EHR sharing scheme in the cloud. IEEE Access **6**, 53698–53708 (2018)
5. D.K. Soni, H. Sharma, B. Bhushan, N. Sharma, I. Kaushik, Security issues & seclusion in bitcoin system, in *2020 IEEE 9th International Conference on Communication Systems and Network Technologies (CSNT)*, (2020). https://doi.org/10.1109/csnt48778.2020.9115744
6. Blockchain in healthcare: Patient benefits and more—blockchain unleashed: IBM Blockchain Blog (2018). Retrieved from: https://www.ibm.com/blogs/blockchain/2017/10/blockchain-in-healthcare-patient-benefitsand-more/. Accessed 14 June 2020
7. A.R. Rajput, Q. Li, M.T. Ahvanooey, I. Masood, EACMS: Emergency access control management system for personal health record based on blockchain. IEEE Access **7**, 84304–84317 (2019)
8. S. Wang, D. Zhang, Y. Zhang, Blockchain-based personal health records sharing scheme with data integrity verifiable. IEEE Access **7**, 102887–102901 (2019)
9. A. Pazaitis, P.D. Filippi, V. Kostakis, Blockchain and value systems in the sharing economy: The illustrative case of Backfeed. Technol. Forecast. Soc. Chang. **125**, 105–115 (2017). https://doi.org/10.1016/j.techfore.2017.05.025
10. IBM, Blockchain for financial services means more trust for all. Accessed: 30 Oct 2018. [Online] (2018). Available: https://www.ibm.com/blockchain/industries/financial-services
11. W.J. Gordon, C. Catalini, Blockchain technology for healthcare: Facilitating the transition to patient-driven interoperability. Comput. Struct. Biotechnol. J. **16**, 224–230 (2018). https://doi.org/10.1016/j.csbj.2018.06.003
12. H. Lee, H. Kung, J.G. Udayasankaran, B. Kijsanayotin, A.B. Marcelo, L.R. Chao, C. Hsu, An architecture and management platform for blockchain-based personal health record exchange:

Development and usability study. J. Med. Internet Res. **22**(6), e16748 (2020). https://doi. org/10.2196/preprints.16748

13. E. Daraghmi, Y. Daraghmi, S. Yuan, MedChain: A design of blockchain-based system for medical records access and permissions management. IEEE Access **7**, 164595–164613 (2019)

14. S. Nakamoto, Bitcoin: A peer-to-peer electronic cash system. [Online] (2008). Available: https://bitcoin.org/bitcoin.pdf

15. M. Hölbl, M. Kompara, A. Kamisalic, L.N. Zlatolas, A systematic review of the use of blockchain in healthcare. Symmetry **10**, 470 (2018)

16. T. Varshney, N. Sharma, I. Kaushik, B. Bhushan, Authentication & encryption based security services in blockchain technology, in *2019 International Conference on Computing, Communication, and Intelligent Systems (ICCCIS)*, (2019). https://doi.org/10.1109/icccis48478.2019.8974500

17. G. Liang, S.S. Weller, F. Luo, J. Zhao, Z.Y. Dong, Distributed blockchain-based data protection framework for modern power systems against cyber attacks. IEEE Trans. Smart Grid **10**, 3162–3173 (2019)

18. P.T. Liu, Medical record system using blockchain, big data and tokenization, in *Information and Communications Security. Lecture Notes in Computer Science*, (Springer, Cham, 2016), pp. 254–261. https://doi.org/10.1007/978-3-319-50011-9_20.

19. A. Mao, Using smart and secret sharing for enhanced authorized access to medical data in blockchain (2020), https://doi.org/10.22215/etd/2020-14000

20. A. Azaria, A. Ekblaw, T. Vieira, A. Lippman, MedRec: Using blockchain for medical data access and permission management, in *2016 2nd International Conference on Open and Big Data (OBD)*, (2016). https://doi.org/10.1109/obd.2016.11

21. G.G. Dagher, J. Mohler, M. Milojkovic, P.B. Marella, Ancile: Privacy-preserving framework for access control and interoperability of electronic health records using blockchain technology. Sustain. Cities Soc. **39**, 283–297 (2018)

22. H. Li, L. Zhu, M. Shen, F. Gao, X. Tao, S. Liu, Blockchain-based data preservation system for medical data. J. Med. Syst. **42**, 1–13 (2018)

23. K. Fan, S. Wang, Y. Ren, H. Li, Y. Yang, MedBlock: Efficient and secure medical data sharing via blockchain. J. Med. Syst. **42**(8), 136 (2018). https://doi.org/10.1007/s10916-018-0993-7

24. T. Dey, S. Jaiswal, S. Sunderkrishnan, N. Katre, HealthSense: A medical use case of internet of things and blockchain, in *2017 International Conference on Intelligent Sustainable Systems (ICISS)*, (2017). https://doi.org/10.1109/iss1.2017.8389459

25. X. Yue, H. Wang, D. Jin, M. Li, W. Jiang, Healthcare data gateways: Found healthcare intelligence on blockchain with novel privacy risk control. J. Med. Syst. **40**(10), 218 (2016). https://doi.org/10.1007/s10916-016-0574-6

26. M.A. Uddin, A. Stranieri, I. Gondal, V. Balasubramanian, Continuous patient monitoring with a patient centric agent: A block architecture. IEEE Access **6**, 32700–32726 (2018)

27. L. Ismail, H. Materwala, S. Zeadally, Lightweight blockchain for healthcare. IEEE Access **7**, 149935–149951 (2019)

28. G.W. Peters, E. Panayi, Understanding modern banking ledgers through blockchain technologies: Future of transaction processing and smart contracts on the internet of money, in *Banking Beyond Banks and Money New Economic Windows*, (Springer, Cham, 2016), pp. 239–278. https://doi.org/10.1007/978-3-319-42448-4_13

29. T.T. Thwin, S. Vasupongayya, Blockchain based secret-data sharing model for personal health record system, in *2018 5th International Conference on Advanced Informatics: Concept Theory and Applications (ICAICTA)*, (2018). https://doi.org/10.1109/icaicta.2018.8541296

30. D. Metcalf, S.T. Milliard, M. Gomez, M. Schwartz, Wearables and the internet of things for health: Wearable, interconnected devices promise more efficient and comprehensive health care. IEEE Pulse **7**(5), 35–39 (2016). https://doi.org/10.1109/mpul.2016.2592260

31. S. Roy, P. Venkateswaran, Online payment system using steganography and visual cryptography, in *2014 IEEE Students' Conference on Electrical, Electronics and Computer Science*, (2014). https://doi.org/10.1109/sceecs.2014.6804449

32. T. McConaghy, R. Marques, A. Müller, D. De Jonghe, T. McConaghy, G. McMullen, R. Henderson, S. Bellemare, A. Granzotto, BigChainDB: A scalable blockchain database, BigChainDB, ascribe GmbH, Berlin, Germany, White Paper 1.0 (2016)
33. C. Cachin, M.V. Sorniotti, T. Weigold, Blockchain, cryptography, and consensus. IBM Res., Zürich, Switzerland, Tech. Rep. (2016)
34. S. Bragagnolo, H. Rocha, M. Denker, S. Ducasse, SmartInspect: Smart contract inspection technical report (2017)
35. D.O. Kondyrev, V.S. Bobrov, I.E. Efremov, V.N. Vlasov, Ethereum-based tender system. Vestnik NSU. Series: Information Technologies **15**(3), 31–39 (2017). https://doi.org/10.2520 5/1818-7900-2017-15-3-31-39
36. P. Wu, C. Cheng, C. Kaddi, J. Venugopalan, R. Hoffman, M.D. Wang, -Omic and electronic health record big data analytics for precision medicine. IEEE Trans. Biomed. Eng. **64**(2), 263–273 (2017). https://doi.org/10.1109/tbme.2016.2573285
37. J. Kwon, Tendermint: Consensus without mining (2014)
38. S. Gupta, S. Sinha, B. Bhushan, Emergence of blockchain technology: Fundamentals, working and its various implementations. SSRN Electron. J. (2020). https://doi.org/10.2139/ ssrn.3569577
39. E. Androulaki, A. Barger, V. Bortnikov, C. Cachin, K. Christidis, A.D. Caro, D. Enyeart, C. Ferris, G. Laventman, Y. Manevich, S. Muralidharan, C. Murthy, B. Nguyen, M. Sethi, G. Singh, K. Smith, A. Sorniotti, C. Stathakopoulou, M. Vukolic, S.W. Cocco, J. Yellick, Hyperledger fabric: A distributed operating system for permissioned blockchains. ArXiv, abs/1801.10228 (2018)
40. Chain of Things. (2018). Accessed: Sept 2018. [Online]. Available: https://www.blockchain-ofthings.com/
41. A. Davies, DevTeam.Space, Pros and cons of Hyperledger Fabric for blockchain networks (2018). Accessed: July 2020 [Online]. Available: https://www.devteam.space/blog/ pros-and-cons-ofhyperledger-fabric-for-blockchain-networks/
42. Waltonchain White Paper (2018) [Online]. Available: https://www.waltonchain.org/doc/ waltonchain-whitepaper_en_20180208.pdf
43. W. Wang, D.T. Hoang, P. Hu, Z. Xiong, D. Niyato, P. Wang, Y. Wen, D.I. Kim, A survey on consensus mechanisms and mining strategy management in blockchain networks. IEEE Access **7**, 22328–22370 (2019)
44. D. Munro, *Data Breaches in Healthcare Totalled Over 112 Million Records in 2015*, vol 31 (Forbes, New York, 2015)
45. S. Banerjee, T. Hemphill, P. Longstreet, Wearable devices and healthcare: Data sharing and privacy. Inf. Soc. **34**(1), 49–57 (2017). https://doi.org/10.1080/01972243.2017.1391912
46. S. Tanwar, K. Parekh, R. Evans, Blockchain-based electronic healthcare record system for healthcare 4.0 applications. J. Inform. Secur. Appl. **50**, 102407 (2020). https://doi. org/10.1016/j.jisa.2019.102407
47. N. Sharma, I. Kaushik, B. Bhushan, S. Gautam, A. Khamparia, Applicability of WSN and biometric models in the field of healthcare, in *Deep Learning Strategies for Security Enhancement in Wireless Sensor Networks. Advances in Information Security, Privacy, and Ethics*, (Information Science Reference, Hershey, 2020), pp. 304–329. https://doi. org/10.4018/978-1-7998-5068-7.ch016
48. J.J. Hathaliya, S. Tanwar, S. Tyagi, N. Kumar, Securing electronics healthcare records in healthcare 4.0: A biometric-based approach. Comput. Electr. Eng. **76**, 398–410 (2019). https:// doi.org/10.1016/j.compeleceng.2019.04.017
49. D.C. Nguyen, P.N. Pathirana, M. Ding, A. Seneviratne, Blockchain for secure EHRs sharing of mobile cloud based E-health systems. IEEE Access **7**, 66792–66806 (2019)
50. R. Guo, H. Shi, Q. Zhao, D. Zheng, Secure attribute-based signature scheme with multiple authorities for blockchain in electronic health records systems. IEEE Access **6**, 11676–11686 (2018)

51. Y. Wang, A. Zhang, P. Zhang, H. Wang, Cloud-assisted EHR sharing with security and privacy preservation via consortium blockchain. IEEE Access **7**, 136704–136719 (2019)
52. P. Zhang, J. White, D.C. Schmidt, G. Lenz, S.T. Rosenbloom, FHIRChain: Applying blockchain to securely and scalably share clinical data. Comput. Struct. Biotechnol. J. **16**, 267–278 (2018). https://doi.org/10.1016/j.csbj.2018.07.004
53. C. Agbo, Q. Mahmoud, J. Eklund, Blockchain technology in healthcare: A systematic review. Healthcare **7**(2), 56 (2019). https://doi.org/10.3390/healthcare7020056
54. T. Bocek, B.B. Rodrigues, T. Strasser, B. Stiller, Blockchains everywhere – A use-case of blockchains in the pharma supply-chain, in *2017 IFIP/IEEE Symposium on Integrated Network and Service Management (IM)*, (IEEE, Piscataway, 2017), pp. 772–777
55. A. Dorri, S.S. Kanhere, R. Jurdak, P. Gauravaram, Blockchain for IoT security and privacy: The case study of a smart home, in *2017 IEEE International Conference on Pervasive Computing and Communications Workshops (PerCom Workshops)*, (IEEE, Piscataway, 2017), pp. 618–623
56. GEMOS, The blockchain operating system (2018). Accessed: July 2020 [Online]. Available: https://enterprise.gem.co/
57. L. Zhou, L. Wang, Y. Sun, MIStore: A blockchain-based medical insurance storage system. J. Med. Syst. **42**(8), 149 (2018). https://doi.org/10.1007/s10916-018-0996-4
58. C. Manchanda, N. Sharma, R. Rathi, B. Bhushan, M. Grover, Neoteric security and privacy sanctuary technologies in smart cities, in *2020 IEEE 9th International Conference on Communication Systems and Network Technologies (CSNT)*, (2020). https://doi.org/10.1109/csnt48778.2020.9115780
59. J. Breteau, The future of blockchain in health insurance (2019). Accessed: July 2020 [Online]. Available: https://www.the-digitalinsurer.com/future-blockchain-health-insurance/
60. B. Brannan, Healthcoin—Blockchain-enabled platform for diabetes prevention (2018). Accessed: Aug 2018 [Online]. Available: https://blockchainhealthcarereview.com/healthcoin-blockchain-enabledplatform-for-diabetes-prevention/
61. A. Juneja, M. Marefat, Leveraging blockchain for retraining deep learning architecture in patient-specific arrhythmia classification, in *2018 IEEE EMBS International Conference on Biomedical & Health Informatics (BHI)*, (IEEE, Piscataway, 2018). https://doi.org/10.1109/bhi.2018.8333451
62. R. Singer, Blockchain for health research (2018). Accessed: Sept 2018 [Online]. Available: https://www.blockchainhealth.co/
63. https://www2.deloitte.com/us/en/pages/consulting/topics/blockchain.html
64. K.J. Peterson, R. Deeduvanu, P. Kanjamala, K. Mayo, A blockchain-based approach to health information exchange networks, in *Proceedings of the NIST Workshop Blockchain Healthcare*, (2016)
65. T. Kuo, L. Ohno-Machado, ModelChain: Decentralized privacy-preserving healthcare predictive modelling framework on private blockchain networks. ArXiv, abs/1802.01746 (2018)
66. K.N. Griggs, O. Ossipova, C.P. Kohlios, A.N. Baccarini, E.A. Howson, T. Hayajneh, Healthcare blockchain system using smart contracts for secure automated remote patient monitoring. J. Med. Syst. **42**(7) (2018). https://doi.org/10.1007/s10916-018-0982-x
67. M.M. Onik, S. Aich, J. Yang, C. Kim, H. Kim, Blockchain in healthcare: Challenges and solutions, in *Big Data Analytics for Intelligent Healthcare Management*, (Academic Press, London/San Diego, 2019), pp. 197–226. https://doi.org/10.1016/b978-0-12-818146-1.00008-8
68. A. Rustagi, C. Manchanda, N. Sharma, IoE: A boon & threat to the Mankind, in *2020 IEEE 9th International Conference on Communication Systems and Network Technologies (CSNT)*, (2020). https://doi.org/10.1109/csnt48778.2020.9115748
69. M.A. Khan, K. Salah, IoT security: Review, blockchain solutions, and open challenges. Futur. Gener. Comput. Syst. **82**, 395–411 (2018). https://doi.org/10.1016/j.future.2017.11.022
70. R. Casado-Vara, J. Prieto, F.D. Prieta, J.M. Corchado, How blockchain improves the supply chain: Case study alimentary supply chain. Proc. Comput. Sci. **134**, 393–398 (2018). https://doi.org/10.1016/j.procs.2018.07.193

71. B. Bhushan, N. Sharma, Transaction privacy preservations for blockchain technology, in *Advances in Intelligent Systems and Computing. International Conference on Innovative Computing and Communications*, (Springer, Singapore, 2020), pp. 377–393. https://doi.org/10.1007/978-981-15-5148-2_34

72. M. Chakarverti, N. Sharma, R.R. Divivedi, Prediction analysis techniques of data mining: A review. SSRN Electron. J. (2019). https://doi.org/10.2139/ssrn.3350303

73. C.P. Transaction, *Blockchain: Opportunities for Health Care*, Tech. Rep. 1 (Deloitte Touche Tohmatsu Ltd., London, 2018)

Index

© The Author(s), under exclusive license to Springer Nature Switzerland AG 2021 371
C. Chakraborty et al. (eds.), *Efficient Data Handling for Massive Internet of
Medical Things*, Internet of Things, https://doi.org/10.1007/978-3-030-66633-0

Lightning Source UK Ltd.
Milton Keynes UK
UKHW051655080922
408536UK00002B/12